Encyclopedia of Parkinson's Disease: Models and Modules

Volume V

Encyclopedia of Parkinson's Disease: Models and Modules
Volume V

Edited by **Kate White**

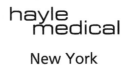

New York

Published by Hayle Medical,
30 West, 37th Street, Suite 612,
New York, NY 10018, USA
www.haylemedical.com

Encyclopedia of Parkinson's Disease: Models and Modules
Volume V
Edited by Kate White

International Standard Book Number: 978-1-63241-193-8 (Hardback)

Contents

Preface

This book aims to highlight the current researches and provides a platform to further the scope of innovations in this area. This book is a product of the combined efforts of many researchers and scientists, after going through thorough studies and analysis from different parts of the world. The objective of this book is to provide the readers with the latest information of the field.

This book on Parkinson's disease (PD) elaborates the state-of-the-art research in the field. PD is caused mainly due to the death of dopaminergic neurons in the substantia nigra. Recent PD medications treat symptoms; though none decrease the rate of dopaminergic neuron degeneration. The primary problem in development of neuroprotective therapies is a restricted comprehension of the crucial molecular mechanisms that incite neurodegeneration. The discovery of PD genes has led to the hypothesis that dysfunction of the ubiquitin-proteasome pathway and misfolding of proteins are both critical to pathogenesis of the disease. Oxidative stress and mitochondrial dysfunction, earlier labeled as responsible in the neurodegeneration of this disease may also act in part by causing the collection of misfolded proteins, along with the production of other harmful events in dopaminergic neurons. PD models based on the manipulation of PD genes should prove crucial in explaining significant characteristics of the disease, like selective vulnerability of substantia nigra dopaminergic neurons to the degenerative process. This book includes some important topics such as update on PD, oxidative stress-damage, PD & immune system and membrane binding & its implications.

I would like to express my sincere thanks to the authors for their dedicated efforts in the completion of this book. I acknowledge the efforts of the publisher for providing constant support. Lastly, I would like to thank my family for their support in all academic endeavors.

Editor

Update in Parkinson's Disease

Fátima Carrillo and Pablo Mir

Unidad de Trastornos del Movimiento. Servicio de Neurología. Instituto de Biomedicina de Sevilla (IBiS). Hospital Universitario Virgen del Rocío/CSIC/Universidad de Sevilla, Spain

1. Introduction

Parkinson's disease (PD) was first described in 1817 by James Parkinson, who described in his monograph entitled *"An Essay on the Shaking Palsy"* the description of the clinical features of this disease (Parkinson, 1817). The cardinal clinical manifestations of PD are resting tremor, rigidity, bradykinesia, and gait dysfunction. It is now appreciated that PD is also associated with many nonmotor features, including autonomic dysfunction, pain and sensory disturbances, mood disorders, sleep impairment, and dementia (Olanow et al, 2009). PD is the second most common neurodegenerative disorder, with an average age at onset of about 60 years and the mean duration of the disease from diagnosis to death is 15 years, with a mortality ratio of 2 to 1 (Katzenschlager et al, 2008). The incidence of the disease rises steeply with age, from 17 - 4 in 100 000 person years between 50 and 59 years of age to 93 - 1 in 100 000 person years between 70 and 79 years, with a lifetime risk of developing the disease of 1 - 5% (De Rijk et al, 1995). With the aging of the population and the substantial increase in the number of at-risk individuals older than 60 years, it is anticipated that the prevalence of PD will increase dramatically in the coming decades (De Lau and Breteler, 2006).

The etiology remains obscure but important genetic and pathological clues have recently been found. This monograph is designed to make a comprehensive review of all aspects of both clinical as pathophysiological and therapeutic concerning PD, as well as an update on the innovative aspects of the disease primarily focused on identifying new genetic factors and new outlook therapeutics.

2. Neuropathology

Pathologically, PD is characterized by degeneration of dopaminergic neurons in the substantia nigra pars compacta (SNc). However, cell loss in the locus coeruleus, dorsal nuclei of the vagus, raphe nuclei, nucleus basalis of Meynert, and some other catecholaminergic brain stem structures including the ventrotegmental area also exists (Damier et al, 1999). This nerve-cell loss is accompanied by three distinctive intraneuronal inclusions: the Lewy body, the pale body, and the Lewy neurite. A constant proportion of nigral neurons (3–4%) contain Lewy bodies, irrespective of disease duration. This finding is consistent with the notion that Lewy bodies are continuously forming and disappearing in the diseased substantia nigra (Greffard et al, 2010). The brain-stem shape is a spherical structure measuring 8–30µm with a hyaline core surrounded by a peripheral pale-staining halo, and is composed ultrastructurally of 7–20-nm wide filaments with dense granular material and vesicular structures. Pale bodies are large rounded eosinophilic structures that often displace neuromelanin and are the predecessor of the Lewy body.

Aggregated α-synuclein is the main component of Lewy bodies in dopaminergic neurons of all PD patients, including those in whom PD occurred sporadically. Aggregated α-synuclein in the cytosol of cells does not only occur in the Substantia nigra but already earlier, pre-symptomatically in the motor part of the Nucleus vagus, in the olfactory bulb and in the Locus coeruleus. In later stages cortical areas of the brain are also frequently involved (Braak and Tredici, 2010). In fact, these bodies are present in small numbers in almost all cases of PD (Halliday et al, 2008). Neocortical Lewy bodies are not necessarily the pathological correlate of dementia in PD (Colosimo et al, 2003; Parkkinen et al, 2005). The amount of associated cortical β-amyloid seems to be the key factor for the cognitive decline in PD (Holton et al, 2008; Halliday et al, 2008). The hypothesis that the aggregation of α-synuclein and the build up of Lewy bodies results in toxicity has been challenged.

Currently, most evidence indicates that oligomers but not the fibrils of α-synuclein that are deposited in the Lewy bodies, are the toxic species. This would also imply that the rapid conversion of α-synuclein from an oligomeric to an aggregated state, deposited in Lewy bodies, may help to detoxify the oligomeric form of α-synuclein (Goldberg and Lansbury, 2000). Fetal mesencephalic neurons implanted in patients with PD to restore dopaminergic transmission may develop Lewy bodies. The existence of different striatal level factors present in the striatal microenvironment of the host probably triggers the propagation of alpha- α-synuclein pathology. Inflammation, oxidative stress, excitotoxicity, and loss of neurotrophic support of the grafted neurons could all be important factors (Li et al, 2008, 2010). A prion hypothesis implicating permissive templating has also been proposed (Hardy 2005).

The few patients with PD of genetic origin (α-synuclein, *LRRK-2*, and *GBA* mutations) who have had autopsy have all shown changes indistinguishable from those found in patients with PD (Lees et al, 2008). Some families with *LRRK-2* mutations also have tangle pathology and non-specific neuronal loss (Gilks et al, 2005). In contrast, parkin mutations lead to nigral loss, restricted brain-stem neuronal loss, and absence of associated Lewy bodies or neurofibrillary degeneration. Heterozygous parkin carriers, however, have been associated with both Lewy body and neurofibrillary tangle pathology (Van de Warrenburg et al, 2001; Pramstaller et al, 2005).

3. Genetic of Parkinson's disease

The PD is mostly idiopathic. However, at present, genetics has taken a very important role in clinical diagnosis. The first genetic contribution to PD was made by William Richard Gowers, in 1902, with the observation of familial aggregation in some patients with PD, but it was not until 1997 that discovered the first gene mutation associated with it (*SNCA*/α-synuclein).

Today there are two kinds of Mendelian PD: autosomal dominant and autosomal recessive PD. Generally, the recessive autosomal forms are associated with PD onset age of juvenile (age of onset <40 years) and an unknown condition. Parkin (*PRKN*) is the most frequently mutated gene in early-onset PD. Dominant autosomal PD is later onset, usually appears between 50-60 years of age, and pathologically with Lewy bodies. *LRRK2* is the most frequently mutated gene in dominant PD (Lees et al, 2009).

Mutations in the glucocerebrosidase gene (*GBA*) are associated with Gaucher's disease, the most common lysosomal storage disorder. Parkinsonism is an established feature of Gaucher's disease and an increased frequency of mutations in *GBA* has been reported in several different ethnic series with sporadic PD. Heterozygous mutations in the *GBA* gene significantly increased (five times) the risk of PD (Sidransky et al, 2009). In addition, patients with heterozygous mutations in the *GBA* gene also have pathology similar to idiopathic PD, with the presence of Lewy bodies and α-synuclein aggregate. *GBA* mutations represent a significant risk factor for the development of PD and suggest that to date, this is the most common genetic factor identified for the disease (Neumann et al, 2009).

3.1 Autosomal dominant forms of Parkinson's disease

To date, there are two genes associated with dominant autosomal dominant PD: *SNCA*/α-synuclein (PARK1) and leucine rich repeat kinase 2 (*LRRK2*, PARK8).

3.1.1 *SNCA*/α-synuclein (PARK1)

SNCA located on chromosome 4q21 (PARK1) was the first gene associated with PD. First, mutations in this gene were identified in families of Greek and Italian origin in 1997 (Polymeropoulos et al, 1997). This discovery was very important, because the identification of mutations in this gene was the first evidence that PD could be due to a genetic cause. After the discovery of the first pathogenic mutation, p.Ala53Thr (Polymeropoulos et al, 1997), two mutations were identified in the *SNCA* gene: mutation in a German family p.Ala30Pro (Kruger et al, 1998) and p.Glu46Lys mutation in a Spanish family (Zarranz et al, 2004). Years later, in 2003, was discovered the first affecting the genomic triplication of *SNCA* locus in a large family with PD (known as the 'Iowa kindred') (Singleton et al, 2003). After identification of the *SNCA* triplication, duplication *SNCA* genomic locus have also been identified in familial and sporadic forms of PD (Chartier-Harlin et al, 2004).

The *SNCA* gene encodes a protein called α-synuclein. This protein consists of 140 amino acids and is highly expressed in the central nervous system. α-Synuclein is the major fibrillar component of the Lewy body (Spillantini et al, 1997). Although its function is still unknown, appears to be involved in synaptic plasticity, neuronal differentiation, and axonal transport and synaptic vesicles (Biskup et al, 2008).

Symptoms caused by mutations in the *SNCA* gene are variable, but usually comes with age at onset around 50 years and phenotypic characteristics common to Lewy body dementia, with deposits of α-synuclein fibril and / or protein Tau, where Lewy bodies are more distributed throughout the brain of what we usually see in the PD. Some patients have dementia, visual hallucinations, parkinsonism and fluctuating cognition and attention (for example, patients with the mutation p.Glu46Lys and *SNCA* locus triplication). In contrast, the families described with duplication of the *SNCA* locus appear to have a slower progression of the disease, age of onset is usually late and not have dementia (Hardy et al, 2009). These latter observations led to suggest that the evolution of the disease may be associated with a dose-related effect of the *SNCA* locus (Singleton et al, 2003).

3.1.2 *LRRK2*/Dardarin (PARK 8)

Another locus for a dominant form of PD was first mapped in a Japanese family on chromosome 12 and named PARK8 (Funayama et al, 2002). Missense mutations in the gene for *LRRK2* were found to be disease causing in 2004 (Paisan-Ruiz et al, 2004; Zimprich et al,

2004). The most common mutation is the p.Gly2019Ser, which also constitutes the most common mutation of both mendelian and sporadic PD (Healy et al, 2008). Although there are over 50 different mutations described in the gene for confirmation dardarin pathogenicity in some of these mutations are difficult (Paisán-Ruiz 2009).

LRRK2 contains 51 coding exons and encodes a protein of 2,257 amino acids called dardarin. Endogenous LRRK2 is ubiquitiously expressed within neurons and associates with membranes and lipid rafts. The protein is found in presynaptic terminals where it associates with vesicles and endosomes (Biskup et al, 2008). Its function remains unknown, although functional studies have found that certain mutants alter LRRK2 kinase activity and this activity is crucial for the toxic effect of the protein. It has also been seen that certain LRRK2 gene mutations cause neuronal death (Biskup et al, 2008). It is also believed that dardarin could be involved in vesicular traffic system (Shin et al, 2008).

Mutations in the LRRK2 gene vary greatly depending on the patient's geographical origin. There is some ethnic influence in the changes associated with the gene LRRK2. p.Arg1628Pro and p.Gly2385Arg as mutations, which, being absent in the Caucasian population, significantly increase the risk of PD in Asian populations. Both mutations are present in the normal population with a frequency of 2.65% (p.Arg1628Pro) and 1.8% (p.Gly2385Arg), but its prevalence is significantly higher in patients with PD. In addition, the mutation p.Gly2019Ser, common in the Caucasian population, is rarely identified in the Asian population (<0.1%), however, two mutations adjacent to amino p.Gly2019, p.Ile2012Thr and p.Ile2020Thr, occur more frequently in Asians than in Caucasians (Paisán-Ruiz 2009).

The clinical presentation closely resembles sporadicPD, but patients tend to have a slightly more benign course and are less likely to develop dementia and a favorable response to treatment with levodopa. Unilateral tremor is usually the first symptom of the disease, progressing slowly and benign. Patients with mutations in the LRRK2 gene are prone to develop dystonia (Healy et al, 2008). The age of onset is very variable (from 28 to 90 years old), but with an average age approaching 60 years. A person who inherits the Gly2019Ser mutation has only 28% risk of developing parkinsonism when younger than 60 years of age, but the risk rises to 74% at 79 years of age (Paisán-Ruiz 2009). p.Gly2019Ser mutation carriers have been described with no parkinsonian symptoms, suggesting the existence of incomplete penetrance associated with this mutation, and homozygous carriers without additional clinical effect caused by gene dosage (Paisán-Ruiz 2009).

3.2 Autosomal recessive forms of Parkinson's disease

Loss-of-function mutations in four genes (PRKN, DJ-1, PINK1, and ATP13A2) cause early onset recessive parkinsonism (age of onset <40 years). Parkin mutations are the second most common genetic cause of L-dopa-responsive parkinsonism, whereas mutations in the other three genes are rare.

3.2.1 *PRKN*/parkin (PARK2)

The PARK2 locus was cloned by extensive linkage analysis conducted in 13 consanguineous families from Japan in 1997. Today, mutations (> 100 different mutations) in the PRKN gene are the most common genetic cause of early-onset parkinsonism (onset age <40 years). The clinical picture associated with mutations in this gene is also similar to idiopathic PD, with a slow disease progression and response generally appropiate to treatment with levodopa.

Patients often develop dyskinesias at low doses of levodopa and generally develop dystonia. Lewy bodies are usually not a common pathology (Khan et al, 2003).

Parkin protein localizes, although not predominantly, to the synapse and associates with membranes. In general parkin is a cytoplasmic protein and functions in the cellular ubiquitination/ protein degradation pathway as an ubiquitin ligase (Kubo et al, 2001).

3.2.2 *PINK1*/PTEN-induced putative kinase 1(PARK6)

Initially, the PARK6 locus was cloned in a large Sicilian family in 2001. Three years later, pathogenic mutations in a gene called *PINK1* were identified in several Italian families (Valente et al, 2004). Symptoms caused by this gene are very similar to that described in patients with mutations in the *PRKN* gene. However, the age of onset may be more variable, reaching present even at 68 years of age, but typically has a juvenile onset (Kumazawa et al, 2008).

PINK1 encodes a primarily mitochondrial protein kinase. Mutations in the PINK1-gene are much less common than parkin mutations, and probably account for only 1 to 4 % of early-onset cases (Valente et al, 2004; Kumazawa et al, 2008; Rogaeva et al, 2004).

3.2.3 *DJ-1* (PARK7)

Mutations in the *DJ-1* gene (PARK7) are another rare cause of recessive autosomal parkinsonism (Bonifati et al, 2003; Hedrich et al, 2004). The clinical picture with early-onset and slow progression is similar to other recessive autosomal forms of PD. The normal function of DJ-1 and its role in dopamine cell degeneration is unknown, but there is evidence linking DJ-1 to oxidative stress response and mitochondrial function (Hardy et al, 2009).

3.2.4 ATP13A2-5P-type ATPase (PARK9)

The locus PARK9, *ATP13A2* was first identified in families of Chilean and Jordanian origin who had a syndrome known as Kufor-Rakeb. This disease is rare and presents with a rigid and akinetic parkinsonism and juvenile onset. Spasticity, Babinski signs, supranuclear gaze palsy and cognitive impairment are some of the clinical symptoms that often occur in this disease (Paisán-Ruiz et al, 2010). The gene encodes a protein lysosomal of 1,180 amino acids that are abundantly expressed in the brain and might act in the proteolytic degradation carried out in the lysosomes (Ramirez et al, 2006).

3.2.5 Other autosomal recessive forms of parkinsonism

Recently, mutations in the gene *PLA2G6* (phospholipaseA2 calcium-independent)(PARK 14) were also found present in individuals who had an akinetic and progressive parkinsonism. Cognitive impairment is a clinical symptom that often accompanies these patients. *PLA2G6* encodes a phospholipase enzyme of 752 amino acids. In general, the phospholipases induce changes in the composition of the membrane, activate the inflammatory cascade and alter cell signaling pathways of unknown function (Paisán-Ruiz et al, 2010).

Several familial cases with a complex parkinsonism and dystonia have been identified with mutations in the gene FBX07 (PARK15). The clinical features resembling parkinsonism caused by mutations in the *PRKN* gene. In fact, FBXO7 gene encodes a protein of 522 amino acids, which seems to be also involved in the system of ubiquitin-proteasome protein degradation (Di Fonzo et al, 2009; Paisán-Ruiz et al, 2010).

Recently, it has been shown that patients with mutations in the gene spatacsin (*SPG11*) (Non PARK locus) develop a juvenile parkinsonism similar to that caused by genes *ATP13A2*, *PLA2G6* and *FBX07*. These patients show a thinning of the corpus callosum, very characteristic signs of spastic paraplegia. The presenting symptoms of the disease are often both spasticity and parkinsonism (Paisán-Ruiz et al, 2010).

4. Clinical features

PD commonly presents with impairment of dexterity or, less commonly, with a slight dragging of one foot. The onset is gradual and the earliest symptoms might be unnoticed or misinterpreted for a long time. Fatigue and stiffness are common but non-specific complaints. Other initial symptoms are lugubrious stiff face, a hangdog appearance, a flexion of one arm with lack of swing, a monotonous quality to the speech, and an extreme slowing down. The early physical signs are often erroneously and a lag of 2 – 3 years from the first symptoms to diagnosis is not unusual. A change in a patient's writing can be present for several years before diagnosis, with a tendency to slope usually in an upward direction and for the writing to get progressively smaller and more cramped after a line or two (Lee et al, 2009).

Complaints within the first 2 years of the disease of falls (especially backwards), fainting, urinary incontinence, prominent speech, disturbed swallowing, amnesia, or delirium should raise the possibility of an alternative diagnosis.

In the late stages of PD, the face of patients is masked and expressionless, the speech is monotonous, festinant, and slightly slurred, and posture is flexed simian with a severe pill rolling tremor of the hands. Freezing of gait for several seconds can happen when attempting to enter the consulting room and, when starting to move again, the patient tends to move all in one piece with a rapid propulsive shuffle. These motor blocks lead to falls. All dextrous movements are done slowly and awkwardly, and assistance might be needed for dressing, feeding, bathing, getting out of chairs, and turning in bed. Constipation, chewing and swallowing difficulties, drooling of saliva, and urge incontinence of urine are common complaints.

Although PD has long been considered primarily a motor disorder Nonmotor symptoms (NMS) in PD are common and were recognized by James Parkinson himself. Thus, in his Essay on the Shaking Palsy in 1817, he referred to sleep disturbance, constipation, urinary incontinence and delirium (Parkinson, 1817). Numerous studies have now indicated that NMS is an integral symptom complex of PD, affecting memory, bladder and bowel, and sleep among others (Table 1) (Chaudhuri et al, 2006). It is commonly thought that NMS occur only in late or advanced PD but NMS can indeed present at any stage of the disease including early and pre-motor phase of PD. Several NMS of PD such as olfactory problems, constipation, depression and erectile dysfunction may predate the motor signs, symptoms and diagnosis of PD by a number of years (Chaudhuri et al, 2006; Tolosa et al, 2007).

Patients with PD are prone to have sleep disturbances that result in excessive daytime somnolence (EDS) and require proper identification and treatment (Comella, 2007). Sleep dysfunction in PD is usually manifest by difficulty in initiating sleep, fragmented sleep, REM behavior disorder (RBD), reversal of the sleep cycle, and EDS (Porter et al, 2008). It is possible that RBD might be early features of PD that antecede the onset of the classic motor features of the disease. In fact, in one study, RBD was found to have preceded the onset of PD symptoms in 52% of patients (Postuma et al, 2006). RBD in patients with PD is frequently seen in association with visual hallucinations (Meral et al, 2007). The presence of RBD in patients with PD is also frequently associated with neuropsychiatric problems and cognitive impairment. Even the presence of RBD in a patient with PD without dementia predicts the subsequent development of cognitive impairment (Vendette et al, 2007).

Although, troublesome dysautonomia is recognized in advanced PD, cardiac (123)I-metaiodobenzylguanidine (MIBG) imaging demonstrates early cardiac sympathetic denervation in PD (low cardiac uptake) and not multiple system atrophy (MSA) where the heart is usually visualized (Goldstein et al, 2000). Cardiac sympathetic denervation has also been found in genetic forms of PD with alpha synuclein mutation (Singleton et al, 2004).

Neuropsychiatric problems such as dementia, delirium, anxiety, and depression occur at one time or another in most patients, and can potentially be more disabling than motor dysfunction.

Risk of dementia exists, particularly in those patients who present with prominent gait and speech disorders, depression, and a poor response to L-dopa. The greatest risk factor for dementia, however, is the age of the patient and not the duration of the disease (Levy, 2007). Visuospatial difficulties, disturbances of attention and vigilance, delirium, and executive dysfunction are more common in PD than in Alzheimer's disease (Noe et al, 2004). Visual hallucinations are commonly associated with PD dementia.

Depression is pervasive in PD and affects approximately 40% of patients at least once during the course of their disease (Starkstein et al, 1992). Studies have suggested that symptoms of depression may precede the development of PD.

5. Pharmacologic treatment

5.1 Neuroprotection

Several putative neuroprotective agents have been tested in placebo-controlled clinical trials. Some clinical trials had negative outcomes despite promising theoretical or preclinical evidence. These include the antioxidant vitamin E (Parkinson Study Group, 1993), the glutamate release inhibitor riluzole (Jankovic and Hunter, 2002) , coenzyme Q10 (Shults et al, 2002), glial cell line-derived neurotrophic factor (GDNF) (Nutt et al, 2003), the antiapoptotic agents TCH346 (Olanow et al, 2006), CEP-1437 (Parkinson Study Group, 2007), and the neuroimmunophilins (Gold and Nutt, 2002) which are thought to act via a possible trophic mechanism. Conversely, some putative neuroprotective agents have demonstrated significant benefits compared with controls, but still could not be unequivocally deemed to be neuroprotective because of the possibility of confounding symptomatic or pharmacologic effects. Although it is not possible to claim with certainty that any of these drugs are neuroprotective, many are routinely used by physicians based on the hope that they might slow disease progression. These agents are considered below.

5.1.1 Selegiline

Selegiline is a selective, irreversible inhibitor of monoamine oxidase-B (MAO-B). Selegiline was the first drug to be tested as a putative neuroprotective therapy in patients with PD based on its capacity to protect dopamine neurons by inhibiting the MAO-B oxidation of MPTP and blocking the formation of free radicals derived from the oxidative metabolism of dopamine (Olanow 1996). The initial advantages shown by selegiline have not been maintained. Furthermore, evidence is insufficient to make a conclusion on the neuroprotective, as opposed to the symptomatic effect of selegiline in PD (Parkinson Study Group, 1996).

Neuropsychiatric symptoms
Depression, apathy, anxiety
Anhedonia
Attention deficit
Hallucinations, illusion, delusions
Dementia
Obsessional and repetitive behaviour (usually drug induced)
Confusion
Delirium (could be drug induced)
Panic attacks
Sleep disorders
Restless legs and periodic limb movements
REM behaviour disorder and REM loss of atonia
Non-REM sleep related movement disorders
Excessive daytime somnolence
Vivid dreaming
Insomnia
Sleep disordered breathing
Autonomic symptoms
Bladder disturbances
Urgency
Nocturia
Frequency
Sweating
Orthostatic hypotension
Coat hanger pain
Sexual dysfunction
Hypersexuality (likely to be drug induced)
Erectile impotence
Dry eyes (xerostomia)
Gastrointestinal symptoms
Dribbling of saliva
Ageusia
Dysphagia/ choking
Reflux, vomiting
Nausea
Constipation
Unsatisfactory voiding of bowel
Fecal incontinence
Sensory symptoms
Pain
Paraesthesia
Olfactory disturbance
Other symptoms
Fatigue

Diplopia
Blurred vision
Seborrhoea
Weight loss
Weight gain (possibly drug induced)

Table 1. Nonmotor features of PD

5.1.2 Rasagiline

Rasagiline is another selective, irreversible MAO-B inhibitor. There are data from studies in vitro and in animal models have shown neuroprotective capacity by rasagiline (Sagi et al, 2007; Zhu et al, 2008).

To test for a possible neuroprotective effect in patients with PD, rasagilina had been shown to have a symptomatic effect in the TEMPO study (The Rasagiline Mesylate in Early Monotherapy for PD Outpatients) (Parkinson Study Group, 2002). ADAGIO (the Effect of Rasagiline Mesylate in Early PD patients) study was designed to verify these results. It demonstrated that early treatment with rasagiline 1 mg daily provided a benefit that was not obtained with the delayed introduction of the drug. These results are consistent with rasagiline having a possible neuroprotective effect (Olanow et al, 2009).

5.1.3 Dopamine agonist

Dopamine agonists have been studied for putative neuroprotective effects in PD, based on their capacity to protect dopamine neurons from a variety of toxins (Schapira, 2002). Indeed, the dopamine agonist pramipexole has been reported to protect dopamine neurons in MPTP-lesioned primates (Iravani et al, 2006).

Clinical trials have attempted to test the capacity of dopamine agonists to provide disease-modifying effects in PD. However, Class I randomized, controlled trials with bromocriptine (Olanow et al, 1995), pramipexol (Parkinson Study Group, 2000; Parkinson Study Group, 2002), and ropinirole (Rakshi et al, 2002; Whone et al, 2003) produced no convincing evidence of neuroprotection in early PD.

5.1.4 Levodopa

The only available placebo-controlled study of levodopa in relation to neuroprotection is inconclusive about any Neuroprotective, as opposed to symptomatic effect (Fahn et al, 2004). Mortality studies suggest improved survival with levodopa therapy (Rajput 2001).

5.2 Motor symptoms treatment of PD
5.2.1 Levodopa

Levodopa is the most effective drug for the symptomatic treatment of PD and the gold standard against which new therapies must be measured. Benefits are usually seen in all stages of the disease and can be particularly noteworthy in patients with early PD, in whom the drug can control virtually all of the classic motor features. Although prediction of the therapeutic response in an individual is not possible, motor symptoms initially improve by 20 – 70%. Speech, swallowing, and postural instability can improve initially, but axial symptoms are generally less responsive and seem to escape more readily from long-term control (Fahn et al, 2004).

Levodopa exerts its symptomatic benefits through conversion to dopamine, and is routinely administered in combination with a decarboxylase inhibitor (carbidopa, benserazide) to prevent its peripheral conversion to dopamine and the resultant nausea, vomiting and orthostatic hypotension. A combination of carbidopa/levodopa and the COMT inhibitor entacapone is available. There are also sustained-release formulations of levodopa although sustained-release formulations of levodopa are not as well absorbed as regular formulations, and doses 20% to 30% higher may be necessary to achieve the same clinical effect. A gel preparation of levodopa (Duodopa) has been used for intraintestinal infusion of the agent and is used in more advanced stages of disease.

Levodopa is absorbed in the small bowel by active transport through the large neutral amino acid (LNAA) pathway, and can be impaired by alterations in gastrointestinal motility and by dietary LNAAs, such as phenylalanine, leucine, and valine, which compete with levodopa for absorption through the LNAA (Nutt et al, 1984).

Acute side effects associated with levodopa include nausea, vomiting, and hypotension, but levodopa is generally well tolerated when it is gradually increased. Levodopa is generally started at a low dose to minimize these risks. Most people can be maintained over the first 5 years of the disease on 300 – 600 mg/day levodopa. Levodopa maintain a similar level of control in de novo PD after 5 years (Koller et al, 1999), and also in more advanced PD with a duration of about 10 years and without motor fluctuations(Goetz et al, 1988).

Chronic levodopa therapy is associated with motor complications, such as dyskinesias and motor fluctuations, in the majority of patients. Motor fluctuations include delayed onset of levodopa's therapeutic effect or its wearing off between doses. Dyskinesias are involuntary choreiform movements that can involve any part of the body and sometimes impose disabling or painful postures. A meta-analysis found 40% likelihood of motor fluctuations and dyskinesias after 4–6 years of levodopa therapy (Ahlskog and Muenter, 2001). Risk factors are younger age, longer disease duration, and levodopa (Denny AP and Behari M, 1999; Fahn et al, 2004). In individual studies, the percentage of fluctuations and dyskinesia may range from 10% to 60% of patients at 5 years on disease duration, and up to 80–90% in later years (Olanow et al, 2001). Patients with PD can also experience fluctuations in such nonmotor symptoms as mood, cognition, autonomic disturbances, pain, and sensory function (Witjas et al, 2002). Levodopa may also be associated with neuropsychiatric side effects, including cognitive impairment, confusion and psychosis. Importantly, many PD features are not satisfactorily controlled by, or do not respond to, levodopa. These include freezing episodes, postural instability with falling, autonomic dysfunction, mood disorders, pain and sensory disturbances, and dementia. Levodopa treatment can also be associated with a dopamine dysregulation syndrome in which patients compulsively take extra doses of levodopa in an addictive fashion. Although levodopa has been associated with impulse control disorders (ICDs) such as hypersexuality and pathologic gambling, these behaviors have primarily been reported to be associated with dopamine agonists (Ceravolo et al, 2010). In addition, chronic levodopa treatment has been associated with punding, which is a series of repetitive and purposeless behaviors, such as collecting or assembling and disassembling objects for no apparent reason (Evans et al, 2004).

There has long been a theoretical concern that levodopa might accelerate neuronal degeneration in PD because of the potential of the drug to generate free radicals through its oxidative metabolism (Olanow et al, 2004). However, most studies in animal models and humans do not show an accelerated loss of dopaminergic neurons to long-term levodopa therapy in usual clinical doses (Olanow et al, 2004). The Earlier vs Later Levodopa Therapy in PD (ELLDOPA) study was the first double-blind, placebo-controlled trial to assess the safety and efficacy of different doses of levodopa and address the potential toxicity of levodopa in patients with PD (Fahn et al, 2004). The clinical results of this study certainly do not provide any evidence to suggest that levodopa is toxic or accelerates the development of disability in patients with PD and do not demonstrate any adverse effect of levodopa on PD progression.

5.2.2 Dopamine agonist

Dopamine agonists are a class of drugs with diverse physical and chemical properties. They share the capacity to directly stimulate dopamine receptors, presumably because they incorporate a dopamine-like moiety within their molecular configuration. Dopamine agonists have drawn particular interest as a treatment for PD because of their potential to provide antiparkinsonian effects with a reduction in the motor complications associated with levodopa. Today, dopamine agonists are also used as early symptomatic therapy to reduce the risk of developing the motor complications associated with levodopa therapy.

It is generally accepted that the shared D2-like receptor agonistic activity produces the symptomatic antiparkinsonian effect. This D2 effect also explains peripheral (gastrointestinal nausea and vomiting), cardiovascular (orthostatic hypotension) and neuropsychiatric (somnolence, psychosis, and hallucinations) side effects.

The first group of dopamine agonists used in the treatment of PD were ergot derivatives (bromocriptine, cabergoline, lisuride, pergolide, dihidroergocriptine). Numerous studies have demonstrated the effectiveness of these agents in PD as adjuncts to levodopa and shown that as monotherapy they are associated with a reduced risk of inducing dyskinesia compared with levodopa (Montastruc et al, 1994; Bracco et al, 2004; Oertel et al, 2006). However, their use has markedly declined due to the risk of valvular fibrosis and the introduction of nonergot dopamine agonists (apomorphine, pramipexole, ropinirole, rotigotine, piribedil). Although rare, cardiac dysfunction with valvular thickening and fibrosis has been reported with pergolide and cabergoline, presumably because they activate the 5HT2b receptor (Morgan and Sethi 2006; Zanettini et al, 2007; Roth BL 2007). In the nineties, nonergot dopamine agonists have largely supplanted the ergot agonists as the dopamine agonists of choice for the treatment of PD. Apomorphine is a short-acting dopamine agonist that is available in injectable form as a rescue drug for the management of "off" periods, and in some countries as an subcutaneous infusion therapy for the management of patients with advanced motor complications.

Levodopa is more efficacious than any orally active dopamine agonist monotherapy. The proportion of patients able to remain on agonist monotherapy falls progressively over time to <20% after 5 years of treatment. For this reason, after a few years of treatment, most patients who start on an agonist will receive levodopa as a replacement or adjunct treatment to keep control of motor parkinsonian signs. Over the last decade, a commonly tested strategy has been to start with an agonist and to add levodopa later if worsening of symptoms cannot be controlled with the agonist alone (Rinne et al, 1998; Parkinson Study Group 2000; Rascol et al, 2000).

From the limited data available (bromocriptine versus ropinirole, bromocriptine versus pergolide), the clinical relevance of the reported difference between agonists, if any, remains questionable (Mizuno Y et al, 1995; Korczyn et al, 1999).

Class I randomized, controlled trials demonstrate how early use of an agonist can reduce the incidence of motor complications versus levodopa (cabergoline (Bracco et al, 2004), pramipexole (Parkinson Study Group, 2000), and ropinirole (Rascol et al, 2000; Whone et al 2003). Similar conclusions were reported with bromocriptine (Montastruc et al, 1994), and pergolide (Oertel et al, 2006) in several class II studies. There is no evidence to suggest that an agonist is more effective than another in preventing or delaying the time to onset of motor complications. Dopamine agonists serve to delay the onset of motor complications by delaying the time until levodopa is required, but do not prevent motor complications once levodopa is introduced. Indeed, two studies have now shown that the time to onset of motor complications from when levodopa is introduced is the same whether levodopa is used as initial therapy or as an adjunct to the dopamine agonist (Rascol et al, 2000; Constantinescu et al, 2007).

Regarding the treatment of non-motor symptoms in PD pramipexole has shown to have an antidepressant effect in several randomized, double-blind controlled studies (Corrigan et al, 2000; Lemke et al, 2006; Bxarone et al, 2010). A recent study with transdermal rotigotine 24 hours monotherapy vs placebo has shown an improvement in nocturnal sleep disturbance (assessed by the "Modified Parkinson's Disease Sleep Scale) and early-morning motor dysfunction (Trenkwalder et al, 2011).

There are long-acting preparation of pramipexole and ropinirole with 24-hour prolonged release. Also rotigotine by transdermal administration has been shown to have constant levels of drug with a single patch daily. This allows for less fluctuation in plasma drug levels and permits drug levels to be maintained during the waking day and to drop off during the night. This may lead to better compliance and more consistent symptom response throughout the day and perhaps better nighttime symptom control. In adjunct studies, ropinirole (Pahwa et al, 2007) and pramipexol (Hauser et al, 2010) 24 hours provided improvement in UPDRS motor and quality-of-life scores comparable with the immediate release form of the drug and was well tolerated.

Dopamine agonists and all other active dopamine-mimetic medications share a common safety profile. Accordingly, side effects such as nausea, vomiting, orthostatic hypotension, confusion and psychosis, may occur with administration of any of these agents. Hallucinations and somnolence are more frequent with some agonists than with levodopa and are particularly common in elderly people or patients with cognitive impairment (Etminan et al, 2001). The ergot-derived dopamine agonists can be associated with a Raynaud's-like phenomenon, erythromelalgia, and pulmonary or retroperitoneal fibrosis (Andersohn and Garbe, 2009). These events are relatively uncommon and are not seen with the nonergot dopamine agonists. Valvular fibrosis may occur in as many as 30% of patients receiving ergot-based dopamine agonists and can lead to valvular dysfunction with the need for surgical repair in extreme cases. This has resulted in withdrawal of pergolide from the market, and a marked reduction in the use of the other ergot agonists (Zanettini et al, 2007; Roth 2007). When these agents are used, it is essential that patients be periodically monitored with echocardiography to detect valvular alterations.

Sedation with EDS and possible unwanted sleep episodes has been associated with the use of dopamine agonists. Dopaminergic medications and dopamine agonists in particular, are known to have dose-related sedative side effects (Frucht et al, 1999; Ferreira et al, 2000; Paus et al, 2003).

Other problems related to the use of dopamine agonists include weight gain (possibly related to overeating) (Nireberg and Waters, 2006), edema (especially in the lower extremities) (Kleiner-Fisman G and Fisman, 2007) and a variety of ICDs, such as pathologic gambling, hypersexuality, and compulsive eating and shopping (Weintraub et al, 2006). Risk factors for ICDs include current use of dopamine agonists, particularly in high doses, young age of PD onset, and a premorbid or family history of ICDs or depression (Voon et al, 2006). ICDs were first identified in association with pramipexole, but have now been described with ropinirole and pergolide. Interestingly, they occur much less frequently with levodopa, although punding is primarily associated with chronic levodopa treatment. The precise mechanism whereby dopamine agonists might induce these ICDs is not known. It remains to be determined if dopamine agonists are directly responsible for inducing an ICD through a particular pattern of receptor stimulation, or if there is an underlying personality disorder that becomes clinically manifest with restoration of striatal dopaminergic tone.

5.2.3 Catechol-O-methyltransferase (COMT) inhibitors

Catechol-O-methyltransferase (COMT) inhibitors reduce the metabolism of levodopa, extending its plasma half-life and prolonging the action of each levodopa dose. Administration of levodopa with a COMT inhibitor increases its elimination half-life (from about 90 minutes to about 3 hours).

Two COMT inhibitors have been approved as adjuncts to levodopa for the treatment of PD; tolcapone and entacapone. Tolcapone inhibits COMT at peripheral level and to a lesser extent at the central level whereas entacapone acts only in the periphery.

COMT inhibitors are effective when administered in conjunction with levodopa and increase interdose, trough, and mean levodopa concentrations. Administration of levodopa plus a COMT inhibitor results in smoother plasma levodopa levels and more continuous brain availability compared with levodopa alone (Muller et al, 2006). Thus, administering levodopa with a COMT inhibitor has the potential to deliver levodopa to the brain in a more predictable and stable fashion, thus decreasing the fluctuations in levodopa concentrations seen when standard levodopa is administered intermittently.

Double-blind, placebo-controlled trials have demonstrated that both tolcapone and entacapone increase "on" time, decrease "off" time, and improve motor scores for patients with PD who experience motor fluctuations. Moreover, this benefit was associated with a reduction in the mean daily dose of levodopa (Kurth et al, 1997; Parkinson Study Group, 1997). Benefits have been shown to persist for 3 years or longer (Larsen et al, 2003). In general, superior clinical benefits have been achieved with tolcapone, reflecting the increased level of COMT inhibition.

Benefits with COMT inhibitors have also been observed in stable patients PD who have not yet begun to experience motor fluctuations (Waters et al, 1997; Olanow et al, 2004).

There has also been interest in the potential of COMT inhibitors to reduce the risk for motor complications associated with standard doses of levodopa (Olanow and Stocchi, 2004). This is based on the concept that intermittent doses of short-acting levodopa leads to pulsatile stimulation of dopamine receptors and motor complications. COMT inhibitors extend the elimination half-life of levodopa and thus, if administered frequently enough, might provide continuous levodopa to the brain. Although studies in monkeys showed that administration of levodopa plus the COMT inhibitor entacapone reduced dyskinesias compared with treatment with levodopa alone (Smith et al, 2005), these results have not been observed in patients. Specifically, in a recent clinical trial, Stalevo Reduction in Dyskinesia Evaluation (STRIDE-PD), which compared the time to onset and frequency of dyskinesia in levodopa-naïve PD patients who were randomized to initiate levodopa therapy with carbidopa/levodopa compared with carbidopa/levodopa/entacapone (Stalevo), was demonstrated that patients randomized to Stalevo had an increased frequency and a shorter time to dyskinesia than did those on standard levodopa (Stocchi et al, 2010).

COMT inhibitors increase levodopa bioavailability, and hence they increase the incidence of dopaminergic adverse reactions, including nausea, and cardiovascular and neuropsychiatric complications. Diarrhoea and urine discoloration are the most frequently reported non-dopaminergic adverse reactions. Tolcapone can elevate liver transaminases, and fatal cases of liver injury are reported (Assal et al, 1998). Currently, the drug has been reintroduced to the market in many countries, but has been imposed strict safety restrictions.

5.2.4 MAO-B inhibitors

Selegiline and rasagiline inhibit the action MAO-B. MAO-B prevents the breakdown of dopamine, leading to greater dopamine availability. Mechanisms besides MAO-B inhibition may also contribute to the clinical effects (Olanow, 1996). Unlike selegiline, rasagiline is not metabolized to amphetamine, and has no sympathomimetic activity.

Selegiline was initially approved as an adjunct to levodopa in patients with motor fluctuations. However, selegiline is primarily used in early disease, based on its putative neuroprotective effects (see section on Neuroprotection) and its capacity to provide mild symptomatic benefits (Parkinson Study Group 1993). When combined with levodopa, it can enhance dopaminergic side effects and lead to increased dyskinesia and neuropsychiatric problems, particularly in the elderly.

Rasagiline has been approved for use in patients with both early and advanced PD. Rasagiline is an irreversible inhibitor of MAO-B. It is more potent and more selective than selegiline, and does not generate amphetamine or methamphetamine metabolites. TEMPO study, a class I study with rasagiline, showed improvement of both the total UPDRS and the motor subscale of the UPDRS in patients treated with rasagiline versus placebo (Parkinson Study Group 2002). Recently published data on long-term efficacy of rasagiline in patients who participated in the TEMPO study, showing maintenance of rasagiline as monotherapy in about half of patients after two years of follow-up (Lew et al, 2010). In ADAGIO study early vs delayed start rasagiline 1 or 2 mg/day were compared. The results of this study suggest that early treatment with rasagiline 1 mg/ day provides benefits that cannot be attained with later initiation of the drug, and argues for starting symptomatic treatment at an earlier time point than has conventionally been used (Olanow et al, 2009). The PRESTO (Parkinson Study Group, 2005) and LARGO (Rascol et al, 2005) study have demonstrated the benefit of rasagiline in patients with motor fluctuationes.

Safinamide is a new MAO-B inhibitor that is currently being studied as a treatment for early and advanced PD. In addition to its MAO-B inhibitor properties, it also inhibits dopamine uptake, and blocks sodium channels and glutamate release. A randomized, placebo-controlled trial of safinamide in early to midstage PD demonstrated modest antiparkinsonian effects, with benefits specifically noted in patients who were already receiving a dopamine agonist (Stocchi et al, 2004).

MAO inhibitors are generally well tolerated. Amphetamine metabolites of selegiline may induce insomnia. At the daily doses currently recommended, the risk of tyramine-induced hypertension (the cheese effect) is low. Also this reaction has not been reported with selective inhibitors of MAO-B (Heinonen EH and Myllylä, 1998). Concerns that the selegiline/levodopa combination increased mortality rates (Ben-Shlomo et al, 1998) have been allayed (Olanow et al, 1998). MAO inhibitors may also interfere with serotonin metabolism and induce a serotoninergic syndrome, although this reaction is rarely presented (Ritter and Alexander, 1997).

5.2.5 Other antiparkinsonian drugs

5.2.5.1 Anticholinergics

The precise mechanism of action of anticholinergic drugs in PD is not known although are believed to act by correcting the disequilibrium between striatal dopamine and acetyl choline activity. Some anticholinergics, e.g. benzotropine, can also block dopamine uptake in central dopaminergic neurons. The anticholinergics used to treat PD specifically block muscarinic receptors.

The use of anticholinergics has dramatically declined in the era of levodopa and dopamine agonists, but these agents are still occasionally used. Anticholinergic drugs are typically used in younger patients with PD in whom resting tremor is the dominant clinical feature and where cognitive function is preserved. Anticholinergic drugs are of little value in the treatment of other parkinsonian features such as rigidity, akinesia, gait dysfunction, or impaired postural reflexes (Cantello et al, 1986). Currently trihexyphenidyl is the most widely used of the anticholinergic drugs.

The most commonly reported side effects are blurred vision, urinary retention, nausea, constipation (rarely leading to paralytic ileus), and dry mouth. The incidence of reduced sweating, particularly in those patients on neuroleptics, can lead to fatal heat stroke. Anticholinergics are contraindicated in patients with narrow-angle glaucoma, tachycardia, hypertrophy of the prostate, gastrointestinal obstruction, and megacolon. Impaired mental function (mainly immediate memory and memory acquisition) is a well-documented central side effect that resolves after drug withdrawal. Therefore, if dementia is present, the use of anticholinergics is contraindicated (Van Herwaardenet al, 1993).

5.2.5.2 Amantadine

Amantadine's mechanism of action remains unclear. A blockade of N-methyl-D-aspartate (NMDA) glutamate receptors and an anticholinergic effect are proposed, whereas other evidence suggests an amphetamine-like action to release presynaptic dopamine stores (Kornhuber et al, 1994).

Amantadine has been shown to improve akinesia, rigidity, and tremor in placebo-controlled trials when used as monotherapy or in combination with levodopa. Early studies suggested that benefit with amantadine is transient, but some patients enjoy more sustained benefits (Butzer et al, 1975; Timberlake and Vance, 1978).

Amantadine is the only currently available agent that is capable of blocking dyskinesia without interfering with the parkinsonian response and has proven to be of considerable benefit for some patients. The utilization of amantadine, however, may be limited by its propensity to cause cognitive impairment, particularly in patients with advanced PD (Verhagen Metman et al, 1998; Metman et al, 1999).

Side effects include confusion, hallucinations, insomnia, and nightmares. These are more common in older patients, but can be seen in patients of any age. Peripheral side effects include livedo reticularis and ankle edema, although these are rarely severe enough to limit treatment. Dry mouth and blurred vision can occur and are presumed related to its peripheral anticholinergic effects.

5.3 Nonmotor symptoms treatment of Parkinson's disease (Table 2)

NMS in PD include neuropsychiatric symptoms, sleep disturbances, autonomic dysfunction, and pain or sensory problems. Such symptoms are a frequent accompaniment to the motor disability with continuing disease progression (Chaudhuri et al, 2006). Although several nondopaminergic systems within the brainstem and cortex are involved in PD, specific clinicopathological correlation for such features remains uncertain, and despite the increasing recognition of these problems, specific pharmacological therapies that target the relevant nondopaminergic neurotransmitter system are limited.

The management of dementia in PD is a pressing problem because cognitive impairment is a common and important source of disability. As dementia in PD is associated with a cholinergic deficit, trials of the cholinesterase inhibitors donepezil and rivastigmine have been carried out in patients with dementia. In these studies, both rivastigmine (Emre et al, 2004) and donepezil (Ravina et al, 2005) showed a modest but significant improvement compared with controls without worsening of parkinsonism.

The cause of psychotic symptoms in PD is probably multifactorial, involving interplay between pathological processes and dopaminergic medications. The management of hallucinations and delirium in the patient with PD must begin with a pretreatment setting eliminating those drugs that can cause hallucinations or delusions and adjusting the dose of levodopa. When the adjustments fail to eliminate or sufficiently alleviate hallucinations and/or cannot be accomplished without inducing a meaningful deterioration in PD features, neuroleptic therapy should be considered. Haloperidol, perphenazine, or chlorpromazine are effective antipsychotics, but are not recommended for patients with PD because of their capacity to block striatal dopamine D2 receptors and exacerbate parkinsonian features. The "atypical" neuroleptics are the preferred agents to use (especially clozapine (Parkinson Study Group, 1999) and quetiapine (Fernandez et al, 2003)), and can often effectively treat hallucinations and psychosis induced by dopaminergic medications. They are called "atypical" because among other factors they preferentially block limbic and cortical dopamine receptors, but are relatively devoid of D1 and D2 receptor-blocking properties (Friedman and Factor, 2000).

Anxiety and depression are extremely common in PD and frequently coexist. Both might respond to dopaminergic therapies, and anxiety in particular can be experienced when the motor effects of levodopa have worn off (ie, during an "off period). However, successful management of these mood disorders often requires treatments in addition to dopaminergic agents, which suggests that non-dopaminergic neurotransmitters are involved. The current management of depression and anxiety in PD involves the use of conventional treatments that enhance serotonergic neurotransmission, such as selective serotonin reuptake inhibitors (SSRIs) or tricyclic antidepressants. Although in clinical practice many patients with PD do experience a significant improvement in mood symptoms with these agents (whatever the exact mechanism of action), the true effectiveness in PD has not been established owing to the limited numbers of available randomised controlled trials (Weintraub et al, 2005; Chung et al, 2003). Some antidepressants, which are undergoing investigation for depression and anxiety in PD, are also selective noradrenergic reuptake inhibitors (eg, duloxetine, venlafaxine, and desipramine).

Patients with PD can experience various behavioural problems as a consequence of dopaminergic medications, including impulse control disorders, such as pathological gambling, shopping, eating, and hypersexuality,(Voon et al, 2011) and abnormal excessive motor behaviours ranging from purposeless fiddling to complex stereotypic activities, known as "punding" (Evans et al, 2004). These problems have been particularly associated with dopamine agonists, but also with levodopa. The precise mechanism whereby dopamine agonists might induce these ICDs is not known. Treatment of each patient should be individualized based on the magnitude of the ICD problem and the need for dopaminergic drugs to control PD features. The symptoms might resolve on reducing or discontinuing the dopamine agonists, although they can persist in some patients (Mamikonyan et al, 2008). Other approaches could include trials of various psychoactive agents and psychosocial interventions and referring patients for appropriate counseling services.

Sleep dysfunction in PD is usually manifest by difficulty in initiating sleep, fragmented sleep, reversal of the sleep cycle, and EDS. Sleep disturbances in PD are multifactorial and may be related to aging, parkinsonian motor dysfunction, dyskinesia, pain, nocturia, nightmares, dopaminergic and nondopaminergic medications, cognitive impairment, and a variety of specific sleep disorders, including restless legs syndrome (RLS), periodic limb movements of sleep (PLMS), RBD, and sleep apnea. Collectively, they contribute to the increase in daytime sleepiness that is so frequently found in patients with PD (Tandberg et al, 1999; Comella, 2007). Dopaminergic medications and particularly dopamine agonists can have a complex effect on sleep. Sometimes these medications cause insomnia or sleepiness. In other situations they may improve nocturnal immobility, and in this way improve the quality of sleep (Montastruc et al, 2001; Brodsky et al, 2003). Thus, dopaminergic medications can either improve or worsen sleep in patients with PD. RBD in patients with PD may be effectively treated with low-dose clonazepam (0.25 to 1.0 mg nightly). The wake-promoting drug modafinil, which possibly affects histamine release in the hypothalamus, is currently used as an option to treat excessive daytime sleepiness in patients with PD (Morgenthaler et al, 2007). Is currently being assessed two other drugs (the BF 2.649 a selective histamine H3 inverse agonist and the caffeine, a non-selective adenosine antagonist) in the treatment of EDS in PD patients.

Drugs currently used to treat orthostatic hypotension in PD include midodrine, a sympathomimetic, and fludrocortisone, a mineralocorticoid. Supine hypertension is a potential side-effect of both of these approaches. The acetylcholinesterase inhibitor pyridostigmine bromide has been suggested to reduce orthostatic hypotension with less effect on supine hypertension, although evidence is limited (Low and Singer, 2008). L-threo-3, 4- dihydroxyphenylserine is a synthetic amino acid precursor of noradrenaline that is available for freezing of gait in PD and orthostatic hypotension in autonomic failure (Mathias et al, 2001). However, few randomised controlled trials few randomised controlled trials (RCTs) of treatment for orthostatic hypotension have been undertaken specifically in PD, but rather have involved mixed populations of patients including multiple system atrophy, in which the pathophysiology of orthostatic hypotension is different. Thus, the true efficacy of treatments for orthostatic hypotension in PD remains unclear.

Urinary symptoms can be troublesome in advanced PD. Current treatments are drugs for overactive bladder symptoms, such as the muscarinic antagonists oxybutynin and tolterodine. However, such drugs are typically poorly tolerated in patients with advanced PD due to central and peripheral anticholinergic side-effects. Another muscarinic antagonist, trospium chloride, has potentially fewer central side-effects due to poor penetration of the blood – brain barrier, and is effective for treating overactive bladder symptoms (Staskin, 2006).

Postural instability is a late complication of PD which can lead to a mounting fear of falls with increasing immobilisation and dependency. Most falls in patients with PD occur in a forward or sideways direction and are due to turning difficulties, gait and postural asymmetries, problems with sensorimotor integration, difficulties with multitasking, failure of compensatory stepping, and orthostatic myoclonus (Bloem et al, 2004). Skilled physical therapy with cueing to improve gait, cognitive therapy to improve transfers, exercises to improve balance, and training to build up muscle power and increase joint mobility, is efficacious (Keus et al, 2007). Regular physical and mental exercise should be encouraged at all stages of the disease. Benzodiazepines should be avoided wherever possible because they increase the risk of falling.

Insomnia
Adjust dopaminergic drugs, sleep hygiene techniques or clonazepam
Depression
Serotonin and noradrenergic reuptake inhibitors or tricyclic antidepressants
Rapid eye movement behaviour disorders
Adjust Parkinson's disease drugs or clonazepam
Fatigue
Amantidine or selegiline
Day time sleepiness
Modafinil
Psychosis and hallucinations
Adjust Parkinson's disease drugs or antipsychotic (clozapine, quetiapine)
Constipation
Osmotic laxatives (macrogol)
Urinary urgency
Check drugs, anticholinergic bladder stabilisers, and desmopressin for nocturia
Impotence
Sildenafil, tadalafil, and vardenafil
Pain
Adjust Parkinson's disease drugs and muscle relaxants
Restless legs
Dopamine agonists
Orthostatic hypotension
Adjust Parkinson's disease drugs; increase water and salt intake; fludrocortisone, ephedrine, or midodrine
Drooling
0-5% atropine eye drops sublingually, scopoderm patch, or botulinum toxin injections into salivary glands
Excessive sweating
Adjust Parkinson's disease drugs, propantheline, propranolol, or topical aluminium creams

---

Table 2. Treatment of Non motor symptoms of PD

6. Surgical procedure for the treatment of Parkinson's disease

The capacity of surgical therapies to provide benefit for patients with PD who can no longer be satisfactorily controlled with medical therapies due to motor complications has been a major advance in the modern treatment of PD (Hallett and Litvan, 2000). Surgical therapies have historically used ablative procedures (e.g., chemical, radiofrequency, or thermal lesions) to make a destructive lesion in overactive or abnormally firing brain targets. However, ablative procedures are associated with the risk of inducing damage to neighboring structures with consequent neurologic dysfunction. The introduction in 1987 of high-frequency deep brain stimulation (DBS) procedures in PD has resolved many of these issues. High frequency stimulation of specific brain targets induces functional benefits that simulate the effects of a destructive lesion, but without the need for making a destructive brain lesion. DBS is performed by implanting an electrode with four contacts into a target site within the brain and connecting it to a pulse generator placed subcutaneously over the chest or abdomen wall. Stimulator settings can be adjusted periodically with respect to electrode configuration, voltage, frequency, and pulse width (Bergman et al, 1990; Olanow et al, 2000).

The mechanism of action of high-frequency DBS is still not clear, even more than 21 years after its introduction. The mechanism is believed to be independent of the target, because DBS mimics the effects of ablation in all targets used to date, but its effects depend on stimulation rather than on the creation of a lesion.

Patients who are thought to benefit from DBS are those affected by clinically diagnosed idiopathic PD, in whom the cardinal symptoms of the disease— bradykinesia, rigidity, and tremor— are likely to be significantly improved (Krack et al, 2003; Deuschl et al, 2006). Those who show improvement with the optimum adjustment of anti-PD drugs or suprathreshold levodopa dose (300 mg per dose) are highly likely to show a similar improvement after optimum placement of the electrodes (Charles et al, 2002). Higher baseline scores on section III (motor) of the unified PD rating scale (UPDRS) and higher baseline levodopa responsiveness are independent predictors of greater change in motor score after surgery. Midline symptoms, dysautonomic symptoms, and gait disturbance unresponsive to levodopa (ie, freezing) are only slightly improved, if at all (Xie et al, 2001).

The different surgical targets exist in the treatment of PDare as follows: - Ventral intermediate (VIM) nucleus of the thalamus: stimulation procedures in this target provide potent antitremor (Narabayashi, 1989) and antidyskinesia (Narabayashi et al, 1984) effect in PD. However, the thalamus is rarely selected as a target site today because similar benefits can be obtained with other targets that are associated with more widespread antiparkinsonian effects. Subthalamic nucleus (STN) or internal segment of the globus pallidus (GPi)—physiologic and metabolic studies indicate that neurons in both the STN and GPi are overactive in PD (Crossman et al, 1985; Mitchell et al, 1989), and that lesions of these structures provide antiparkinsonian benefits in animal models of PD (Bergman et al, 1990; Brotchie et al, 1991; Guridi et al, 1994;). Both ablation and high frequency stimulation of these targets have been shown to provide antiparkinsonian benefits as well as a profound reduction in dyskinesia (especially GPi) in patients with PD. Although the STN is currently the preferred surgical target in most centers, there is no conclusive data indicating that comparable results cannot be obtained with stimulation of the GPi (Follet et al, 2010). Patients undergoing subthalamic stimulation required a lower dose of dopaminergic agents than did those undergoing pallidal stimulation.- Pedunculopontine nucleus (PPN) — the PPN is a diffuse nucleus that extends throughout the upper brainstem. Stimulation and lesions in the PPN influence locomotion, and for this reason it has been referred to as the mesencephalic locomotor center (Pahapill and Lozano, 2000). Preliminary studies suggest that stimulation of the PPN may provide locomotor benefits for patients with PD (Stefani et al, 2007). DBS of the PPN is being actively investigated.

Side effects of DBS can be related to the surgical procedure, the device, or to the stimulation. There is a risk of hemorrhage and damage to neighboring brain structures, although risks are less than are seen with ablative procedures, particularly when performed bilaterally (Hallett and Litvan, 2000). Complications associated with the device can be related to infection or mechanical problems (e.g., lead fracture, movement of the electrode, skin erosion), and may require lead removal or reimplantation. Side effects related to stimulation are generally transient and may be controlled by adjusting the stimulation variables. The battery must be periodically replaced.

7. Recommendations for the management of Parkinson's disease

The optimal time frame for onset of therapy has not been clearly defined. Once parkinsonian signs start to have an impact on the patient's life, initiation of treatment is recommended. For each patient, the choice between the numerous effective drugs available is based in several factors. These factors include considerations related to the drug (efficacy for symptomatic control of parkinsonism/prevention of motor complications, safety, practicality, costs, etc.), and the patient (symptoms, age, needs, expectations, experience, co-morbidity, socioeconomic level, etc.).

Currently, there is no uniform proposal on initiating symptomatic medication for PD. In the past, levodopa was traditionally used to initiate therapy for PD because it was the most effective symptomatic agent, and levodopa is still commonly used as initial therapy by some physicians. Today, many movement disorder neurologists have elected to initiate symptomatic therapy with a dopamine agonist in appropriate patients, and to supplement with levodopa when satisfactory control cannot be attained with dopamine agonist monotherapy. This treatment philosophy is based on the body of laboratory and clinical information indicating that dopamine agonists are associated with a reduced risk of inducing motor complications compared with levodopa. Dopamine agonist use as as initial therapy because they delay the time until levodopa is required and permit use of lower doses of levodopa. To begin with levodopa is the preferred treatment for patients with PD with cognitive impairment, the elderly who have a reduced propensity to develop motor complications, and patients suspected of having an atypical parkinsonism who are undergoing a trial of dopaminergic therapy.

MAO-B inhibitors such as selegiline and rasagiline provide another therapeutic option in early disease. MAO-B inhibitors have been shown to provide modest antiparkinsonian effects when used as monotherapy and also delay the need for levodopa. The symptomatic effect is more modest than that of levodopa and (probably) dopamine agonists, but they are easy to administer (one dose, once daily, no titration). Furthermore the TEMPO and the ADAGIO studies suggest that early treatment with rasagiline provides benefits that cannot be attained with later introduction of the same medication (Parkinson Study Group, 2002;

Olanow et al, 2009). Although this does not establish neuroprotection and long-term studies are required to determine the effect of the drug on cumulative disability in the long run, it does indicate that earlier treatment with rasagiline may provide a better outcome, at least at the 18-month time point. For these reasons, many physicians now choose to initiate therapy in patients with early PD with an MAO-B inhibitor.

There may be advantages to initiating therapy in patients with early PD with both an MAO-B inhibitor and a dopamine agonist (not at the same time) to enhance clinical benefits and further delay the need for levodopa. However, there have been no studies as yet examining the effects of combining an MAO-B inhibitor with a dopamine agonist on the need for levodopa and the risk of inducing dyskinesia. However, subset analyses in studies testing rasagiline in advanced patients (Parkinson Study Group, 2005; Rascol et al, 2005) and preliminary studies with a new MAO-B inhibitor safinamide, (Stocchi et al, 2004) suggest that adding an MAO-B inhibitor to a dopamine agonist improves UPDRS scores.

Amantadine or anticholinergics are not routinely prescribed in patients with early PD, although some movement disorder specialists might use anticholinergics if tremor is the predominant feature in young patient with PD.

There are a variety of ways to enhance motor response in patients who experience suboptimal motor control with dopamine agonist or levodopa monotherapy. The simplest approach is to gradually raise the dose of the dopaminergic agent. However, high doses of dopamine agonists can be associated with neuropsychiatric side effects, sedation and ICDs. If patients cannot be satisfactorily controlled on an agonist, then levodopa should be added. If the patient is receiving levodopa monotherapy, increased doses might be effective. Higher doses are associated with an increased risk of motor complications, but may be justified if required to provide a satisfactory clinical response. The addition of a dopamine agonist may enhance benefit without increasing the risk of motor complications. COMT and/or MAO-B inhibitors may also be useful in managing patients with a suboptimal clinical response. The use of a subcutaneous apomorphine penject as a rescue device for unpredictable refractory off periods can also be helpful in some instances, and its fast action helps to restore confidence in patients becoming insecure about leaving home (Ostergaard et al, 1995).

Despite adjustments of the timing and dose frequency of levodopa, motor fluctuations and dyskinesias can mark the long-term therapeutic benefit. Amantadine is an effective anti-dyskinetic agent in some patients. Subcutaneous waking day apomorphine pump is a highly effective treatment for refractory motor fluctuations. Orally administered anti-parkinsonian medication should be adjusted obtain thebest results for dyskinesia reduction and off periods. Enteric administration of a soluble formulation of levodopa (Duodopa) through gastro-jejunostomy is another highly effective medical option for patients who failed to, or are reluctant to, try the apomorphine pump. Infusion therapies is based on the principle that continuous infusion of a dopaminergic agent provides more constant and physiologic activation of striatal dopamine receptors than is accomplished with intermittent administration of the same drug, and thereby reduces the risk of motor complications. Continuous infusion of either levodopa or apomorphine has been tested in patients with advanced PD and consistently been reported to reduce the frequency of motor complications (Manson et al, 2002; Antonini et al, 2007). Sustained improvement in motor performance with a great reduction in drug-induced involuntary movements can also be achieved by functional neurosurgery with bilateral deep brain stimulation of the STN or GPi.

8. Experimental approaches

Cell-based therapies have been studied based on the notion that transplantation of dopaminergic cells could replace dopamine neurons, which degenerate in PD, and restore dopaminergic function in a more physiologic manner than can be achieved with oral therapies (Lindvall and Bjo"rklund, 2004). Fetal nigral transplantation has been the best studied of these approaches to date. Numerous laboratory studies have demonstrated that embryonic dopaminergic neurons implanted into the denervated striatum can survive, extend axons, provide organotypic innervations of the striatum, produce dopamine, and provide behavioral benefits in the 6-OHDA rodent and MPTP-monkey (Olanow et al, 1996). These studies have served as the basis for initiating clinical trials in patients with PD. To date, there is no universal agreement on the optimal transplant protocol. Open-label clinical trials using a variety of different transplant regimens produced variable clinical results. Various types of cells have been used (adrenal gland, mesencephalic fetal grafts, and more recently, epithelial retinal cells). Stem cells are also being investigated, which might be better tolerated immunologically, but raise their own (oncological) problems. Despite the elegance of this approach, it is still experimental and is not currently available to patients (Morizane et al, 2008). Intrastriatal carotid body (CB) transplants have been assayed in animal models of PD to test whether they increase the striatal dopamine levels and/or exert a neuroprotective action on the nigrostriatal pathway. Currently it being studied the in vitro formation of new CB tissue derived from adult CB stem cells, given the limitations of previous studies have been presented with autotransplantation of CB in patients with PD (López-Barneo et al, 2009).

Gene delivery approaches are also being actively investigated as a possible treatment for PD. In this technology, viruses are used as vectors to introduce the DNA of a desired protein into the genome of cells within a specific brain target. Furthermore, promoters can ensure that the virus vector infects specific brain cells (e.g., TH promoter targets dopamine cells). This sequence can thus potentially result in continuous production of the desired therapeutic protein in the desired target region of the brain (Dass et al, 2006). Most human studies have used the adeno-associated virus serotype 2 (AAV-2) as the vector, as AAV-2 does not induce an immune response and permits long-term expression of the transgene. No clinically significant or unanticipated adverse events have been encountered in any of the gene therapy studies performed to date (Svendsen, 2007). Different gene therapy approaches are currently being tested in PD, e.g trophic factors such as glial-derived nerve factor (Lang et al, 2006) or neurturin (Marks et al, 2010).

9. Conclusions

The current knowledge of the disease continues to evolve and be challenged by scientific discovery. Further research on the function of the proteins identified by the susceptibility genes, the interplay of the disease process with normal ageing, and the nature of environmental triggers that unmask the disease process will be needed if we are to develop reliable biomarkers and a cure for this disabling movement disorder. Although it is producing significant progress in new therapeutic options important unmet medical needs remain, and even more effective therapeutic interventions are required for the successful management of the patient with PD. Many such agents are now in development. However, future strategies need to focus on more selective targeting of subtypes of neurotransmitter receptors to reduce side effects and optimise benefit. Finally, the development of neuroprotective agents in PD has to date focused on preventing dopamine cell loss. However, to be optimally effective, such therapies will also need to target nondopamine cells involved in the multisystem disease process.

10. References

[1] Ahlskog JE and Muenter MD(2001). Frequency of levodopa related dyskinesias and motor fluctuations as estimated from the cumulative literature. *Movement Disorders* 16, 3 (May 2001): 448–458, 0885-3185.

[2] Andersohn F, Garbe E (2009). Cardiac and noncardiac fibrotic reactions caused by ergot- and nonergot-derived dopamine agonists. *Mov Disord* 24, 1(Jan 2009):129-33, 1531-8257.

[3] Antonini A, Isaias IU, Canesi M, Zibetti M, Mancini F, Manfredi L, Dal Fante M, Lopiano L and Pezzoli G. (2007). Duodenal levodopa infusion for advanced Parkinson's disease: 12- month treatment outcome. *Mov Disord* 22, 8 (Jun 2008):1145-1149, 0885-3185.

[4] Assal F, Spahr L, Hadengue A, Rubbia-Brandt L and Burkhard PR (1998). Tolcapone and fulminant hepatitis. *Lancet* 352, 9132 (Sep 1998):958, 0140-6736.

[5] Ben-Shlomo Y, Churchyard A, Head J, Hurwitz B, Overstall P, Ockelford J and Lees AJ (1998). Investigation by Parkinson's Disease Research Group of United Kingdom into excess mortality seen with combined levodopa and selegiline treatment in patients with early, mild Parkinson's disease: further results of randomized trial and confidential inquiry. *British Medical Journal* 316, 7139 (Apr 1998): 1191–1196.

[6] Bergman H, Wichmann T and DeLong MR (1990). Reversal of experimental parkinsonism by lesions of the subthalamic nucleus. *Science* 249, 4975 (Sep 1990): 1436 - 38, 0036-8075.

[7] Biskup S, Gerlach M, Kupsch A, Reichmann H, Riederer P, Vieregge P, Wüllner U and Gasser T. (2008). Genes associated with Parkinson syndrome. *J Neuro*, 255, 5 (Sep 2008), 8-17, 0340-5354.

[8] Bloem BR, Hausdoroff JM, Visser JE and Giladi N (2004). Falls and freezing of gait in Parkinson 's disease: a review of two interconnected, episodic phenomena. *Mov Disord* 19, 8 (Aug 2004): 871-84, 0885-3185.

[9] Bonifati V, Rizzu P, van Baren MJ, Schaap O, Breedveld GJ, Krieger E, Dekker MC, Squitieri F, Ibanez P, Joosse M, van Dongen JW, Vanacore N, van Swieten JC, Brice A, Meco G, van Duijn CM, Oostra BA and Heutink P (2003). Mutations in the DJ-1 gene associated with autosomal recessive early-onset parkinsonism. *Science* 299, 5604 (Jan 2003) :256–259, 1095-9203.

[10] Braak H and Del Tredici K. (2010). Pathophysiology of sporadic Parkinson's disease. *Fortschr Neurol Psychiatr*, 78, Suppl 1 (Mar 2010), S2-4, 1439-3522.

[11] Bracco F, Battaglia A, Chouza C, , Dupont E, Gershanik O, Marti Masso JF and Montastruc JL (2004); PKDS009 Study Group. The long-acting dopamine receptor agonist cabergoline in early Parkinson's disease: final results of a 5-year, double-blind, levodopa-controlled study. *CNS Drugs* 18, 11 (Aug 2004):733–746, 1172-7047.

[12] Brotchie JM, Mitchell IJ, Sambrook MA and Crossman AR (1991). Alleviation of parkinsonism by antagonist of excitatory amino acid transmission in the medial

segment of the globus pallidus in rat and primate. *Mov Disord* 6, 2 (Jan 1991): 133–138, 0885-3185.

[13] Brodsky MA, Godbold J, Roth T and Olanow CW (2003). Sleepiness in Parkinson's disease: a controlled study. *Mov Disord* 18, 6 (June 2003):668–672, 0885-3185.

[14] Butzer JF, Silver DE and Sahs AL (1975). Amantadine in Parkinson's disease. A double-blind, placebo-controlled, crossover study with long-term follow-up. Neurology 25, 7 (Jul 1975): 603-6, 0028-3878.

[15] Bxarone P, Poewe W, Albrecht S, Debieuvre C, Massey D, Rascol O, Tolosa E, Weintraub D (2010). Pramipexole for the treatment of depressive symptoms in patients with Parkinson's disease: a randomised, double-blind, placebo-controlled trial. *Lancet Neurol* 9, 6 (Jun 2010): 573-80, 1474-4465.

[16] Cantello R, Riccio A, Gilli M, Delsedime M, Scarzella L, Aguggia M and Bergamasco B. (1986). Bornaprine vs placebo in Parkinson disease: double-blind controlled cross-over trial in 30 patients. *Ital J Neurol Sci* 7, 1 (Feb 1986): 139-43, 0392-0461.

[17] Ceravolo R, Frosini D, Rossi C and Bonuccelli U (2010). Spectrum of addictions in Parkinson's disease: from dopamine dysregulation syndrome to impulse control disorders. *J Neurol* 257(Suppl 2)(Nov 2010):S276-83, 1432-1459.

[18] Charles PD, Van Blercom N, Krack P, Lee SL, Xie J, Besson G, Benabid AL, Pollak P (2002). Predictors of effective bilateral subthalamic nucleus stimulation for PD. *Neurology* 59, 6 (Sep 2002): 932-34, 0028-3878.

[19] Chartier-Harlin MC, Kachergus J, Roumier C, Mouroux V, Douay X, Lincoln S, Levecque C, Larvor L, Andrieux J, Hulihan M, Waucquier N, Defebvre L, Amouyel P, Farrer M and Destée A. (2004). Alpha-synuclein locus duplication as a cause of familial Parkinson's disease. *Lancet* 364, 9440 (Sep 2004),1167-9, 1474-547X.

[20] Chaudhuri KR, Healy DG and Schapira AH (2006). National Institute for Clinical Excellence. Non-motor symptoms of Parkinson' s disease: diagnosis and management. *Lancet Neurol* 5, 3 (Mar 2006): 235 – 45, 1474-4422.

[21] Chung TH, Deane KH, Ghazi-Noori S, Rickards H and Clarke CE (2003). Systematic review of antidepressant therapies in Parkinson' s disease. *Parkinsonism Relat Disord* 10, 2 (Dec 2003): 59 – 65, 1353-8020.

[22] Colosimo C, Hughes AJ, Kilford L and Lees AJ. (2003). Lewy body cortical involvement may not always predict dementia in Parkinson' s disease. *J Neurol Neurosurg Psychiatry* 74, 7 (Jul 2003), 852 – 56, 0022-3050.

[23] Comella CL (2007). Sleep disorders in Parkinson' s disease: an overview. *Mov Disord* 22 (suppl 17)(Sep 2007): S367 – 73, 0885-3185.

[24] Constantinescu R, Romer M, McDermott MP, Kamp C and Kieburtz K; CALM-PD Investigators of the Parkinson Study Group (2007). Impact of pramipexole on the onset of levodopa-related dyskinesias. *Mov Disord* 22, 9 (Jul 2007):1317– 1319, 1531-8257.

[25] Corrigan MH, Denahan AQ, Wright CE, Ragual RJ and Evans DL (2000). Comparison of pramipexole, fluoxetine, and placebo in patients with major depression. *Depress Anxiety* 11, 2 (May 2000): 58-65, 1091-4269.

[26] Crossman AR, Mitchell IJ and Sambrook MA (1985). Regional brain uptake of 2-deoxyglucose in *N*-methyl-4-phenyl-1,2,3,6- tetrahydropyridine (MPTP)-induced

parkinsonism in the macaque monkey. *Neuropharmacology* 24, 6 (Jun 1985):587–591, 0028-3908.

[27] Dass B, Olanow CW and Kordower J (2006). Gene transfer of trophic factors and stem cell grafting as treatments for Parkinson's disease. *Neurology* 66, 10 suppl 4 (May 2006):S89– S103, 1526-632X.

[28] De Lau LM and Breteler MM. (2006). Epidemiology of Parkinson's disease. *Lancet Neurol* , 5, 6(june 2006), 525–535, 1474-4422.

[29] Damier P, Hirsch EC, Agid Y and Graybiel AM. (1999). The substantia nigra of the human brain. II. Patterns of loss of dopamine-containing neurons in Parkinson 's disease. *Brain* 122, 8 (Aug 1999), 1437-48, 0006-8950.

[30] Denny AP and Behari M (1999). Motor fluctuations in Parkinson's disease. *Journal of the Neurological Sciences* 165, 1(May 1999): 18–23, 0022-510X.

[31] De Rijk MC, Breteler MM, Graveland GA, Grobbee DE, van der Meché FG and Hofman A. (1995). Prevalence of Parkinson's disease in the elderly: the Rotterdam Study. *Neurology*, 45, 12 (Dec 1995), 2143–46, 0028-3878.Di Fonzo A, Dekker MC, Montagna P, Baruzzi A, Yonova EH, Correia Guedes L, Szczerbinska A, Zhao T, Dubbel-Hulsman LO, Wouters CH, de Graaff E, Oyen WJ, Simons EJ, Breedveld GJ, Oostra BA, Horstink MW and Bonifati V (2009). FBXO7 mutations cause autosomal recessive, early-onset parkinsonian-pyramidal syndrome. *Neurology* 72, 3 (Jan 2009):240-5, 1526-632X.

[32] Deuschl G, Schade-Brittinger C, Krack P, Volkmann J, Schäfer H, Bötzel K, Daniels C, Deutschländer A, Dillmann U, Eisner W, Gruber D, Hamel W, Herzog J, Hilker R, Klebe S, Kloss M, Koy J, Krause M, Kupsch A, Lorenz D, Lorenzl S, Mehdorn HM, Moringlane JR, Oertel W, Pinsker MO, Reichmann H, Reuss A, Schneider GH, Schnitzler A, Steude U, Sturm V, Timmermann L, Tronnier V, Trottenberg T, Wojtecki L, Wolf E, Poewe W and Voges J; German Parkinson Study Group, Neurostimulation Section (2006). A randomized trial of deep-brain stimulation for Parkinson's disease [published erratum in *N Engl J Med* 355, 9 (Aug 2006): 896–908, 1533-4406.

[33] Emre M, Aarsland D, Albanese A, Byrne EJ, Deuschl G, De Deyn PP, Durif F, Kulisevsky J, van Laar T, Lees A, Poewe W, Robillard A, Rosa MM, Wolters E, Quarg P, Tekin S and Lane R (2004). Rivastigmine for dementia associated with Parkinson's disease. *N Engl J Med* 351, 24 (Dec 2004):2509-18, 1533-4406.

[34] Etminan M, Samii A, Takkouche B and Rochon P (2001). Increased risk of somnolence with the new dopamine agonists in patients with Parkinson's disease. A metaanalysis of randomised controlled trials. *Drug Safety* 24, 11 (Oct 2001): 863–868, 0114-5916.

[35] Evans AH, Katzenschlager R, Paviour D, O'Sullivan JD, Appel S, Lawrence AD and Lees AJ (2004). Punding in Parkinson's disease: its relation to the dopamine dysregulation syndrome. *Mov Disord* 19, 4 (Apr 2004):397-405, 0885-3185.

[36] Fahn S, Oakes D, Shoulson I, Kieburtz K, Rudolph A, Lang A, Olanow CW, Tanner C and Marek K; Parkinson Study Group (2004). Levodopa and the progression of Parkinson's disease. *N Engl J Med* 351, 24 (Dec 2004): 2498-508, 1533-4406.

[37] Fernandez HH, Trieschmann ME, Burke MA, Jacques C and Friedman JH (2003). Long-term outcome of quetiapine use for psychosis among Parkinsonian patients. *Mov Disord* 18; 5 (May 2003):510-4, 0885-3185.

[38] Ferreira JJ, Galitzky M, Montastruc JL and Rascol O (2000). Sleep attacks and Parkinson's disease treatment. *Lancet* 355, 9212 (Apr 2000):1333-4, 0140-6736.

[39] Follett KA, Weaver FM, Stern M, Hur K, Harris CL, Luo P, Marks WJ Jr, Rothlind J, Sagher O, Moy C, Pahwa R, Burchiel K, Hogarth P, Lai EC, Duda JE, Holloway K, Samii A, Horn S, Bronstein JM, Stoner G, Starr PA, Simpson R, Baltuch G, De Salles A, Huang GD and Reda DJ; CSP 468 Study Group (2010). Pallidal versus subthalamic deep-brain stimulation for Parkinson's disease. *N Engl J Med* 362, 22 (Jun 2010):2077-91, 1533-4406.

[40] Friedman JH and Factor SA (2000). Atypical antipsychotics in the treatment of drug-induced psychosis in Parkinson's disease. *Mov Disord* 15, 2 (Mar 2000):201–211, 0885-3185.

[41] Frucht S, Rogers JD, Greene PE, Gordon MF and Fahn S (1999). Falling asleep at the wheel: motor vehicle mishaps in persons taking pramipexole and ropinirole. *Neurology* 52, 9 (Jun 1999): 1908-10, 0028-3878.

[42] Funayama M, Hasegawa K, Kowa H, Saito M, Tsuji S and Obata F (2002). A new locus for Parkinson's disease (PARK8) maps to chromosome 12p11.2–q13.1. *Ann Neurol* 51, 3 (Mar 2002), 296–301, 0364-5134.

[43] Gilks WP, Abou-Sleiman PM, Gandhi S, Jain S, Singleton A, Lees AJ, Shaw K, Bhatia KP, Bonifati V, Quinn NP, Lynch J, Healy DG, Holton JL, Revesz T and Wood NW. (2005). A common LRRK2 mutation in idiopathic Parkinson's disease. *Lancet* 365, 9457(Jan 2005), 415-16, 1474-547X.

[44] Goetz CG, Tanner CM, Shannon KM, Shannon KM and Carroll VS (1988). Controlled release carbidopa/levodopa (CR4-Sinemet) in Parkinson's disease patients with and without motor fluctuations. *Neurology* 38, 5(May): 1143–1146, 0028-3878.

[45] Gold BG, Nutt JG (2002). Neuroimmunophilin ligands in the treatment of Parkinson's disease. *Curr Opin Pharmacol* 2, 1 (Feb 2002):82– 86, 1471-4892.

[46] Goldberg MS and Lansbury PT. (2000). Is there a cause-and-effect relationship between alpha-synuclein fibrillization and Parkinson's disease?. *Nat Cell Biol* 2, 7 (Jul 2000), E115–E119, 1465-7392.

[47] Goldstein DS, Holmes C, Li ST, Bruce S, Metman LV and Cannon RO 3rd (2000). Cardiac sympathetic denervation in Parkinson disease. *Ann Intern Med* 133, 5 (Sep 2000):338–347, 0003-4819.

[48] Greffard S, Verny M, Bonnet AM, Seilhean D, Hauw JJ and Duyckaerts C. (2010). A stable proportion of Lewy body bearing neurons in the substantia nigra suggests a model in which the Lewy body causes neuronal death. *Neurobiol Aging* 31, 1(Jan 2010), 99-103, 1558-1497.

[49] Guridi J, Herrero MT, Luquin R, Guillen J and Obeso JA (1994). Subthalamotomy improves MPTP-induced parkinsonism in monkeys. *Stereotact Funct Neurosurg* 62, 1-4 (Jan 1994): 98–102, 1011-6125.

[50] Hallett M and Litvan I; Members of the Task Force on Surgery for Parkinson's Disease of the American Academy of Neurology Therapeutic and Technology Assessment Committee (2000). Scientific position paper of the Movement Disorder Society

evaluation of surgery for Parkinson's disease. *Mov Disord* 15, 3 (May 2000):436–438, 0885-3185.

[51] Halliday G, Hely M, Reid W and Morris J. (2008). The progression of pathology in longitudinally followed patients with Parkinson' s disease. *Acta Neuropathol*, 115, 4 (Apr 2008), 409-15, 0001-6322.

[52] Hardy J. (2005). Expression of normal sequence pathogenic proteins for neurodegenerative disease contributes to disease risk: permissive templating as a general mechanism underlying neurodegeneration. *Biochem Soc Trans* 33; 4 (Aug 2005), 578-81, 0300-5127.

[53] Hardy J, Lewis P, Revesz T, Lees A and Paisán-Ruiz. (2009). Genetics of Parkinson's syndromes: a critical review. *Curr Opin Genet Dev* 19, 3 (Jun 2009), 254-65, 1879-0380.

[54] Hauser RA, Schapira AH, Rascol O, Barone P, Mizuno Y, Salin L, Haaksma M, Juhel N and Poewe W (2010). Randomized, double-blind, multicenter evaluation of pramipexole extended release once daily in early Parkinson's disease. *Mov Disord* 25, 15 (Nov 2010):2542-9, 1531-8257.

[55] Healy DG, Falchi M, O'Sullivan SS, Bonifati V, Durr A, Bressman S, Brice A, Aasly J, Zabetian CP, Goldwurm S, Ferreira JJ, Tolosa E, Kay DM, Klein C, Williams DR, Marras C, Lang AE, Wszolek ZK, Berciano J, Schapira AH, Lynch T, Bhatia KP, Gasser T, Lees AJ and Wood NW (2008). Phenotype, genotype, and worldwide genetic penetrance of LRRK2-associated Parkinson's disease: a case-control study. *Lancet Neurol* 7, 7 (Jul 2008), 583–590, 1474-4422.

[56] Hedrich K, Djarmati A, Schafer N, Hering R, Wellenbrock C, Weiss PH, Hilker R, Vieregge P, Ozelius LJ, Heutink P, Bonifati V, Schwinger E, Lang AE, Noth J, Bressman SB, Pramstaller PP, Riess O and Klein C (2004). DJ-1 (PARK7) mutations are less frequent than Parkin (PARK2) mutations in early-onset Parkinson disease. *Neurology* 62, 3 (Feb 2004):389–394, 1526-632X.

[57] Heinonen EH and Myllylä V (1998). Safety of selegiline (deprenyl) in the treatment of Parkinson's disease. *Drug Saf* 19, 1 (Jul 1998): 11-22, 0114-5916.

[58] Iravani MM, Haddon CO, Cooper JM, Jenner P and Schapira AH (2006). Pramipexole protects against MPTP toxicity in nonhuman primates. *J Neurochem* 96, 5 (Mar 2006):1315–1321, 0022-3042.

[59] Jankovic J, Hunter C (2002). A double-blind, placebo-controlled and longitudinal study of riluzole in early Parkinson's disease. *Parkinsonism Relat Disord* 8, 4 (Marz 2002): 271-6, 1353-8020.

[60] Katzenschlager R and Lees AJ (2002). Treatment of Parkinson's disease: levodopa as the first choice. *Journal of Neurology* 249(Suppl. 2)(Sep 2002): II19-II24, 0340-5354.

[61] Katzenschlager R, Head J, Schraq A, Ben-Shlomo Y, Evans A and Lees AJ. Fourteen-year final report of the randomized PDRG-UK trial comparing three initial treatments in PD. *Neurology* , 71, 7 (Aug 2008), 474–80, 1526-632X.Lashley T, Holton JL, Gray E, Kirkham K, O'Sullivan SS, Hilbig A, Wood NW, Lees AJ and Revesz T. (2008). Cortical alpha-synuclein load is associated with amyloid-beta plaque burden in a subset of Parkinson' s disease patients. *Acta Neuropathol*, 115, 4 (Apr 2008), 417-25, 0001-6322.

[62] Keus SH, Bloem BR, Hendriks EJ, Bredero-Cohen AB and Munneke M; Practice Recommendations Development Group (2007). Evidence-based analysis of physical therapy in Parkinson' s disease with recommendations for practice and research. *Mov Disord* 22, 4 (Mar 2007): 451-60, 0885-3185.

[63] Khan NL, Graham E, Critchley P, Schrag AE, Wood NW, Lees AJ, Bhatia KP and Quinn N (2003). Parkin disease: a phenotypic study of a large case series. *Brain* 126, 6 (June 2003), :1279-92, 0006-8950.

[64] Kitada T, Asakawa S, Hattori N, Matsumine H, Yamamura Y, Minoshima S, Yokochi M, Mizuno Y and Shimizu N (1998). Mutations in the parkin gene cause autosomal recessive juvenile parkinsonism. *Nature* 392, 6676 (Apr 1998):605-8, 0028-0836.

[65] Kleiner-Fisman G and Fisman DN (2007). Risk factors for the development of pedal edema in patients using pramipexole. *Arch Neurol* 64, 6 (Jun 2007): 820-4, 0003-9942.

[66] Koller WC, Hutton JT, Tolosa E and Capilldeo R (1999). Immediate-release and controlled-release carbidopa/levodopa in PD: a 5-year randomized multicenter study. Carbidopa/Levodopa Study Group. *Neurology* 53, 5(Sep 1999): 1012–1019, 0028-3878.

[67] Korczyn AD, Brunt ER, Larsen JP, Nagy Z, Poewe WH and Ruggieri S (1999). A 3-year randomized trial of ropinirole and bromocriptine in early Parkinson's disease. The 053 Study Group. *Neurology* 53, 2 (Jul 1999): 364-70, 0028-3878.

[68] Kornhuber J, Weller M, Schoppmeyer K and Riederer P (1994). Amantadine and memantine are NMDA receptor antagonists with neuroprotective properties. *J Neural Transm* 43: 91–104, 0303-6995.

[69] Krack P, Batir A, Van Blercom N, Chabardes S, Fraix V, Ardouin C, Koudsie A, Limousin PD, Benazzouz A, LeBas JF, Benabid AL and Pollak P. (2003). Five-year follow-up of bilateral stimulation of the subthalamic nucleus in advanced Parkinson' s disease. *N Engl J Med* 349, 20 (Nov 2003): 1925-34, 1533-4406.

[70] Kruger R, Kuhn W, Muller T, Woitalla D, Graeber M, Kosel S, Przuntek H, Epplen JT, Schols L and Riess O. (1998). Ala30Pro mutation in the gene encoding alpha-synuclein in Parkinson's disease. *Nat Genet* 18, 2 (Feb 1998), 106–108, 1061-4036.

[71] Kubo SI, Kitami T, Noda S, Shimura H, Uchiyama Y, Asakawa S, Minoshima S, Shimizu N, Mizuno Y and Hattori N (2001). Parkin is associated with cellular vesicles. *J Neurochem* 78, 1 (Jul 2001):42–54, 0022-3042.

[72] Kumazawa R, Tomiyama H, Li Y, Imamichi Y, Funayama M, Yoshino H, Yokochi F, Fukusako T, Takehisa Y, Kashihara K, Kondo T, Elibol B, Bostantjopoulou S, Toda T, Takahashi H, Yoshii F, Mizuno Y and Hattori N (2008) Mutation analysis of the PINK1 gene in 391 patients with Parkinson disease. *Arch Neurol* 65, 6 (Jun 2008):802–808, 1538-3687.

[73] Kurth MC, Adler CH, Hilaire MS, Singer C, Waters C, LeWitt P, Chernik DA, Dorflinger EE and Yoo K (1997). Tolcapone improves motor function and reduces levodopa requirement in patients with Parkinson's disease experiencing motor fluctuations: a multicenter, double-blind, randomized, placebo-controlled trial. *Neurology* 48, 1 (Jan 1997):81– 87, 0028-3878.

[74] Lang AE, Gill S, Patel NK, Lozano A, Nutt JG, Penn R, Brooks DJ, Hotton G, Moro E, Heywood P, Brodsky MA, Burchiel K, Kelly P, Dalvi A, Scott B, Stacy M, Turner D,

Wooten VG, Elias WJ, Laws ER, Dhawan V, Stoessl AJ, Matcham J, Coffey RJ and Traub M (2006). Randomized controlled trial of intraputamenal glial cell line-derived neurotrophic factor infusion in Parkinson disease. *Ann Neurol* 59, 3 (Mar 2006):459–466, 0364-5134.

[75] Larsen JP, Worm-Petersen J, Siden A, Gordin A, Reinikainen K and Leinonen M (2003). The tolerability and efficacy of entacapone over 3 years in patients with Parkinson's disease. *Eur J Neurol* 10, 2 (Mar 2003):137–146,1351-5101.

[76] Lees AJ, Hardy J and Revesz T. (2009). Parkinson's disease. *Lancet* 373, 9680 (Jun 2009), 2055-2066, 1474-547X.

[77] Li JY, Englund E, Holton JL, Soulet D, Hagell P, Lees AJ, Lashley T, Quinn NP, Rehncrona S, Björklund A, Widner H, Revesz T, Lindvall O and Brundin P. (2008). Lewy bodies in grafted neurons in subjects with Parkinson' s disease suggest host-to-graft disease propagation. *Nat Med* 14, 5 (May 2008), 501-03, 1546-170X.

[78] Lemke MR, Brecht HM, Koester J and Reichmann H (2006). Effects of the dopamine agonist pramipexole on depression, anhedonia and motor functioning in Parkinson's disease. *J Neurol Sci* 248, 1-2 (Oct 2006): 266-70, 0022-510X.

[79] Levy G (2007). The relationship of Parkinson disease with aging. *Arch Neurol* 64, 9 (Sep 2007): 1242-46, 0003-9942.

[80] Lew MF, Hauser RA, Hurtig HI, Ondo WG, Wojcieszek J, Goren T and Fitzer-Attas CJ. (2010). Long-term efficacy of rasagiline in early Parkinson's disease. *Int J Neurosci* 120, 6 (Jun 2010): 404-8, 1563-5279.

[81] Li JY, Englund E, Widner H, Rehncrona S, Björklund A, Lindvall O and Brundin P. (2010). Characterization of Lewy body pathology in 12- and 16-year-old intrastriatal mesencephalic grafts surviving in a patient with Parkinson's disease. *Mov Disord* 25, 8, 1091-06, 1531-8257.

[82] Lindvall O and Bjo¨rklund A (2004). Cell therapy in Parkinson's disease. *NeuroRx* 1, 4 (Oct 2004):382–393, 1545-5343.

[83] Low PA and Singer W (2008). Management of neurogenic orthostatic hypotension: an update. *Lancet Neurol* 7, 5 (May 2008): 451-58, 1474-4422.

[84] López-Barneo J, Pardal R, Ortega-Sáenz P, Durán R, Villadiego J and Toledo-Aral JJ (2009). The neurogenic niche in the carotid body and its applicability to antiparkinsonian cell therapy. *J Neural Transm* 116, 8 (Aug 2009):975-82, 1435-1463.

[85] Mamikonyan E, Siderowf AD, Duda JE, Potenza MN, Horn S, Stern MB and Weintraub D (2008). Long-term follow-up of impulse control disorders in Parkinson' s disease. *Mov Disord* 23, 1 (Jan 2008): 75-80, 1531-8257 .

[86] Manson AJ, Turner K and Lees AJ (2002). Apomorphine monotherapy in the treatment of refractory motor complications of Parkinson's disease: long-term follow-up study of 64 patients. *Mov Disord* 17, 6:1235-41, 0885-3185.

[87] Marks WJ Jr, Bartus RT, Siffert J, Davis CS, Lozano A, Boulis N, Vitek J, Stacy M, Turner D, Verhagen L, Bakay R, Watts R, Guthrie B, Jankovic J, Simpson R, Tagliati M, Alterman R, Stern M, Baltuch G, Starr PA, Larson PS, Ostrem JL, Nutt J, Kieburtz K, Kordower JH and Olanow CW (2010). Gene delivery of AAV2-neurturin for Parkinson's disease: a double-blind, randomised, controlled trial. *Lancet Neurol* 9, 12 (Dec 2010):1164-72, 1474-4465.

[88] Mathias CJ, Senard JM, Braune S, Watson L, Aragishi A, Keeling JE and Taylor MD. (2001). L-threodihydroxyphenylserine (L-threo-DOPS; droxidopa) in the management of neurogenic orthostatic hypotension: a multinational, multi-center, dose-ranging study in multiple system atrophy and pure autonomic failure. *Clin Auton Res* 2001; 11, 4 (Aug 2001): 235-42, 0959-9851.

[89] etman LV, Del Dotto P, LePoole K, Konitsiotis S, Fang J and Chase TN (1999). Amantadine for levodopa-induced dyskinesias: a 1-year follow-up study. *Arch Neurol* 56, 1 (Nov 1999):1383–1386, 0003-9942.

[90] Meral H, Aydemir T, Ozer F, Ozturk O, Ozben S, Erol C, Cetin S, Hanoglu L, Ozkayran T and Yilsen M. (2007). Relationship between visual hallucinations and REM sleep behavior disorder in patients with Parkinson's disease. *Clin Neurol Neurosurg* 109, 10 (Dec 2007):862– 867, 0303-8467.

[91] Mitchell IJ, Clarke CE and Boyce S, Robertson RG, Peggs D, Sambrook MA and Crossman AR (1989). Neural mechanisms underlying parkinsonian symptoms based upon regional uptake of 2-deoxyglucose in monkeys exposed to 1-methyl-4-phenyl-1,2,3,6-tetrahydropyridine. *Neuroscience* 32, 1 (Jan 1989):213–226, 0306-4522.

[92] Mizuno Y, Kondo T and Narabayashi H (1995). Pergolide in the treatment of Parkinson's disease. *Neurology* 45, 3(Suppl. 31)(Mar 1995): S13–S21, 0028-3878.

[93] Montastruc JL, Rascol O, Senard JM and Rascol A (1994). A randomized controlled study comparing bromocriptine to which levodopa was later added, with levodopa alone in previously untreated patients with Parkinson's disease: a five year follow up. *J Neurol Neurosurg Psychiatry* 57, 9 (Sep 1994):1034 –1038, 0022-3050.

[94] Montastruc JL, Brefel-Courbon C, Senard JM, Bagheri H, Ferreira J, Rascol O and Lapeyre-Mestre M. (2001) . Sleep attacks and antiparkinsonian drugs: a pilot prospective pharmacoepidemiologic study. *Clin Neuropharmacol* 24, 3 (May-June 2001):181–183, 0362-5664 .

[95] Morgan JC and Sethi KD (2006). Pergolide-induced ergotism. *Neurology* 67, 1 (Jul 2006):104, 1526-632X.

[96] Morgenthaler TI, Kapur VK, Brown T, Swick TJ, Alessi C, Aurora RN, Boehlecke B, Chesson AL Jr, Friedman L, Maganti R, Owens J, Pancer J and Zak R; Standards of Practice Committee of the American Academy of Sleep Medicine. (2007). Practice parameters for the treatment of narcolepsy and other hypersomnias of central origin [published erratum in Sleep 2008; 31: TOC]. *Sleep* 30, 12 (Dec 2007): 1705-11, 0161-8105.

[97] Morizane A, Li JY and Brundin P (2008). From bench to bed: the potential of stem cells for the treatment of Parkinson' s disease. *Cell Tissue Res* 331, 1 (Jan 2008): 323-36, 1432-0878.

[98] Muller T, Erdmann C, Muhlack S, Bremen D, Przuntek H and Woitalla D (2006). Inhibition of catechol-O-methyltransferase contributes to more stable levodopa plasma levels. *Mov Disord* 21, 3 (Mar 2006):332–336, 0885-3185.

[99] Neumann J, Bras J, Deas E, O'Sullivan SS, Parkkinen L, Lachmann RH, Li A, Holton J, Guerreiro R, Paudel R, Segarane B, Singleton A, Lees A, Hardy J, Houlden H, Revesz T and Wood NW (2009). Glucocerebrosidase mutations in clinical and

pathologically proven Parkinson's disease. *Brain* 132, Pt 7 (Jul 2009):1783-94, 1460-2156.

[100] Narabayashi H, Yokochi F and Nakajima Y (1984). Levodopainduced dyskinesia and thalamotomy. *J Neurol Neurosurg Psychiatry* 47, 8 (Aug 1984):831– 839, 0022-3050.

[101] Narabayashi H (1989). Stereotaxic vim thalamotomy for treatment of tremor. *Eur Neurol* 29, (suppl 1)(Jan 1989):29 –32, 0014-3022.

[102] Nirenberg MJ and Waters C (2006). Compulsive eating and weight gain related to dopamine agonist use. *Mov Disord* 21, 4 (Apr 2006): 524-9, 0885-3185.

[103] Noe E, Marder K, Bell KL, Jacobs DM, Manly JJ and Stern Y (2004). Comparison of dementia with Lewy bodies to Alzheimer's disease and Parkinson's disease with dementia. *Mov Disord* 19, 1 (Jan 2004):60–67, 0885-3185.

[104] Nutt JG, Woodward WR, Hammerstad JP, Carter JH and Anderson JL (1984). The "on-off " phenomenon in Parkinson's disease. Relation to levodopa absorption and transport. *N Engl J Med* 310, 8 (Feb 1984):483– 488, 0028-4793.

[105] Nutt JG, Burchiel KJ, Comella CL, Jankovic J, Lang AE, Laws ER Jr, Lozano AM, Penn RD, Simpson RK Jr, Stacy M and Wooten GF; ICV GDNF Study Group. Implanted intracerebroventricular. Glial cell line-derived neurotrophic factor. (2003). Randomized, double-blind trial of glial cell line-derived neurotrophic factor (GDNF) in PD. *Neurology* 60, 1 (Jan 2003): 69-73, 1526-632X.

[106] Nyholm D, Nilsson Remahl AI, Dizdar N, Constantinescu R, Holmberg B, Jansson R, Aquilonius SM and Askmark H (2005). Duodenal levodopa infusion monotherapy vs oral polypharmacy in advanced Parkinson disease. *Neurology* 64, 2 (Jan 2005):216–223, 1526-632X.

[107] Oertel WH, Wolters E, Sampaio C, Gimenez-Roldan S, Bergamasco B, Dujardin M, Grosset DG, Arnold G, Leenders KL, Hundemer HP, Lledó A, Wood A, Frewer P and Schwarz J (2006). Pergolide versus levodopa monotherapy in early Parkinson's disease patients: the PELMOPET study. *Mov Disord* 21, 3 (Mar 2006): 343–353, 0885-3185.

[108] Olanow CW, Hauser RA, Gauger L, Malapira T, Koller W, Hubble J, Bushenbark K, Lilienfeld D and Esterlitz J (1995). The effect of deprenyl and levodopa on the progression of Parkinson's disease. *Ann Neurol* 38, 5 (Nov 1995): 771-7, 0364-5134.

[109] Olanow CW. Selegiline: current perspectives on issues related to neuroprotection and mortality (1996). *Neurology* 47, (6 suppl 3)(Dec 1996):S210 –S216, 0028-3878.

[110] Olanow CW, Kordower JH and Freeman TB (1996). Fetal nigral transplantation as a therapy for Parkinson's disease. *Trends Neurosci* 19, 3 (Mar 1996):102–109, 0166-2236.

[111] Olanow CW, Myllyla VV, Sotaniemi KA, Larsen JP, Pålhagen S, Przuntek H, Heinonen EH, Kilkku O, Lammintausta R, Mäki-Ikola O and Rinne UK (1998). Effect of selegiline on mortality in patients with Parkinson's disease: a meta-analysis. *Neurology* 51, 3 (Sep 1998): 825–830, 0028-3878.

[112] Olanow CW, Brin M and Obeso JA (2000). The role of deep brain stimulation as a surgical treatment for Parkinson's disease. *Neurology* 55, 12(suppl 6)(Feb 2000):60–66, 0028-3878.

[113] Olanow CW, Watts RL and Koller WC (2001). An algorithm (decision tree) for the management of Parkinson's disease: treatment guidelines. *Neurology* 56, 11 Suppl. 5 (Jun 2001): S1–S88, 0028-3878.

[114] Olanow CW and Stocchi F (2004). COMT inhibitors in Parkinson's disease: can they prevent and/or reverse levodopa induced motor complications? *Neurology* 62, 1 suppl 1 (Jan 2004):S72–S81, 1526-632X.

[115] Olanow CW, Agid Y, Mizuno Y, Albanese A, Bonuccelli U, Damier P, De Yebenes J, Gershanik O, Guttman M, Grandas F, Hallett M, Hornykiewicz O, Jenner P, Katzenschlager R, Langston WJ, LeWitt P, Melamed E, Mena MA, Michel PP, Mytilineou C, Obeso JA, Poewe W, Quinn N, Raisman-Vozari R, Rajput AH, Rascol O, Sampaio C and Stocchi F(2004). Levodopa in the treatment of Parkinson's disease: current controversies. *Movement Disorders* 19, 9 (Sep 2004): 997-1005, 0885-3185.

[116] Olanow CW, Kieburtz K, Stern M, Watts R, Langston JW, Guarnieri M and Hubble J; US01 Study Team (2004). Double-blind, placebo-controlled study of entacapone in levodopa-treated patients with stable Parkinson disease. *Arch Neurol* 61, 10 (Oct 2004):1563–1568, 0003-9942.

[117] Olanow CW, Schapira AHV, LeWitt PA, Kieburtz K, Sauer D, Olivieri G, Pohlmann H and Hubble J(2006). TCH346 as a neuroprotective drug in Parkinson's disease: a double-blind, randomised, controlled trial. *Lancet Neurol* 5, 12 (Dec 2006):1013–1020, 1474-4422.

[118] Olanow CW, Rascol O, Hauser R, Feigin PD, Jankovic J, Lang ALangston W, Melamed E, Poewe W, Stocchi F and Tolosa E; ADAGIO Study Investigators (2009) . A double-blind, delayed-start trial of rasagiline in Parkinson's disease. *N Engl J Med* 361, 13 (Sep 2009): 1268-78, 1533-4406.

[119] Olanow CW, Stern MB and Sethi K. (2009). The scientific and clinical basis for the treatment of Parkinson disease. *Neurology,* 26, 72(21 Suppl 4)(Dec 2009), S1-136, 0028-3878.

[120] Ostergaard L, Werdelin L, Odin P, Lindvall O, Dupont E, Christensen PB, Boisen E, Jensen NB, Ingwersen S and, Schmiegelow M (1995). *J Neurol Neurosurg Psychiatry* 58, 6 (Jun 1995):681-7, 0022-3050.

[121] Pahwa R, Stacy MA, Factor SA, Lyons KE, Stocchi F, Hersh BP, Elmer LW, Truong DD and Earl NL; EASE-PD Adjunct Study Investigators. (2007). Ropinirole 24-hour prolonged release: randomized, controlled study in advanced Parkinson disease. *Neurology* 68, 14 (Apr 2007): 1108-15, 1526-632X.

[122] Pahapill PA and Lozano AM (2000). The pedunculopontine nucleus and Parkinson's disease. *Brain* 123, 9 (Sep 2000):1767–1783, 0006-8950.

[123] Paisan-Ruiz C, Jain S, Evans EW, Gilks WP, Simon J, van der Brug M, Lopez de Munain A, Aparicio S, Gil AM, Khan N, Johnson J, Martinez JR, Nicholl D, Carrera IM, Pena AS, de Silva R, Lees A, Marti-Masso JF, Perez-Tur J, Wood NW and Singleton AB (2004) Cloning of the gene containing mutations that cause PARK8-linked Parkinson's disease. *Neuron* 44, 18 (Nov 2004), 595–600, 0896-6273.

[124] Paisán-Ruiz (2009). LRRK2 gene variation and its contribution to Parkinson disease. *Hum Mutat* 30, 8 (Aug 2009): 1153-60, 1098-1004.

[125] Paisán-Ruiz C, Guevara R, Federoff M, Hanagasi H, Sina F, Elahi E, Schneider SA, Schwingenschuh P, Bajaj N, Emre M, Singleton AB, Hardy J, Bhatia KP, Brandner S, Lees AJ, and Houlden H (2010). Early-onset L-dopa-responsive parkinsonism with pyramidal signs due to ATP13A2, PLA2G6, FBXO7 and spatacsin mutations. *Mov Disord* 25, 12 (Sep 2010): 1791-800, 1531-8257.

[126] Parkinson J. *An Essay on the Shaking Palsy*. London: Whittingham and Rowland for Sherwood, Neely and Jones; 1817.

[127] Parkkinen L, Kauppinen T, Pirttila T, Autere JM and Alafuzoff I (2005). Alpha-synuclein pathology does not predict extrapyramidal symptoms or dementia. *Ann Neurol* 57, 1 (Jan 2005), 82 - 91, 0364-5134.

[128] Parkinson Study Group (1993). Effects of tocopherol and deprenyl on the progression of disability in early Parkinson's disease. *N Engl J Med* 328, 21 (Jan 1993:176 –183, 0028-4793.

[129] Parkinson Study Group (1996). Impact of deprenyl and tocopherol treatment on Parkinson's disease in DATATOP subjects not requiring levodopa. *Ann Neurol* 39, 1 (Jan 1996): 29-36, 0364-5134.

[130] Parkinson Study Group (1997). Entacapone improved motor fluctuations in levodopa-treated Parkinson's disease patients. *Ann Neurol* 42, 5(Nov 1997):747–755, 0364-5134.

[131] Parkinson Study Group (1999). Low dose clozapine for the treatment of drug-induced psychosis in Parkinson's disease. *N Engl J Med* 340, 10 (Mar 1999):757–763, 0028-4793.

[132] Parkinson Study Group (2000). Pramipexole vs levodopa as initial treatment for Parkinson disease: a randomized controlled trial. Parkinson Study Group. JAMA 284, 15 (Oct 2000): 1931-8, 0098-7484.

[133] Parkinson Study Group (2002). Dopamine transporter brain imaging to assess the effects of pramipexole vs levodopa on Parkinson disease progression. JAMA 287, 13 (Jul 2002): 1653-61, 0098-7484.

[134] Parkinson Study Group (2002). A controlled trial of rasagiline in early Parkinson disease: the TEMPO Study. *Arch Neurol* 59, 12 (Dec 2002): 1937-43, 0003-9942.

[135] Parkinson Study Group (2005). A randomized placebo-controlled trial of rasagiline in levodopa-treated patients with Parkinson disease and motor fluctuations: the PRESTO study. *Arch Neurol* 62, 2 (Feb 2005):241–248, 0003-9942.

[136] Parkinson Study Group PRECEPT Investigators (2007). Mixed lineage kinase inhibitor CEP-1347 fails to delay disability in early Parkinson disease. *Neurology* 2007;69, 15 (Oct 2007):1480– 1490, 1526-632X.

[137] Paus S, Brecht HM, Köster J, Seeger G, Klockgether T and Wüllner U (2003). Sleep attacks, daytime sleepiness, and dopamine agonists in Parkinson's disease. *Mov Disord* 18, 6(Jun 2003):659-67, 0885-3185.

[138] Polymeropoulos MH, Lavedan C, Leroy E, Ide SE, Dehejia A, Dutra A, Pike B, Root H, Rubenstein J, Boyer R, Stenroos ES, Chandrasekharappa S, Athanassiadou A, Papapetropoulos T, Johnson WG, Lazzarini AM, Duvoisin RC, Di Iorio G and Nussbaum RL. (1997). α- Synuclein gene identified in families with Parkinson's disease. Science 276, 5321 (June 1997), 2045-2047, 0036-8075.

[139] Porter B, Macfarlane R and Walker R (2008). The frequency and nature of sleep disorders in a community-based population of patients with Parkinson's disease. *Eur J Neurol* 15, 1 (Jan 2008):50 –54, 1468-1331.

[140] Postuma RB, Lang AE, Massicotte-Marquez J and MontplaisirJ (2006). Potential early markers of Parkinson disease in idiopathic REM sleep behavior disorder. *Neurology* 66, 6 (Mar 2006):845– 851, 1526-632X.

[141] Pramstaller PP, Schlossmacher MG, Jacques TS, Scaravilli F, Eskelson C, Pepivani I, Hedrich K, Adel S, Gonzales-McNeal M, Hilker R, Kramer PL and Klein C . (2005). Lewy body Parkinson' s disease in a large pedigree with 77 Parkin mutation carriers. *Ann Neurol* 58: 3 (Sep 2005), 411-22, 0364-5134.

[142] Rajput AH (2001). Levodopa prolongs life expectancy and is non-toxic to substantia nigra. *Parkinsonism Relat Disord* 8, 2 (Oct 2001): 95-100, 1353-8020.

[143] Rakshi JS, Pavese N, Uema T, Ito K, Morrish PK, Bailey DL and Brooks DJ. (2002). A comparison of the progression of early Parkinson's disease in patients started on ropinirole or L-dopa: an 18F-dopa PET study. *J Neural Transm*; 109, 12 (Dec 2002): 1433-43, 0300-9564.

[144] amirez A, Heimbach A, Grundemann J, Stiller B, Hampshire D, Cid LP, Goebel I, Mubaidin AF, Wriekat AL, Roeper J, Al-Din A, Hillmer AM, Karsak M, Liss B, Woods CG, Behrens MI, Kubisch C (2006) Hereditary parkinsonism with dementia is caused by mutations in ATP13A2, encoding a lysosomal type 5 P-type ATPase. *Nat Genet* 38, 10 (Oct 2008):1184–1191, 1061-4036.

[145] Rascol O, Brooks DJ, Korczyn AD, De Deyn PP, Clarke CE and Lang AE (2000). A five-year study of the incidence of dyskinesia in patients with early Parkinson's disease who were treated with ropinirole or levodopa. 056 Study Group. *N Engl J Med* 342, 20 (May 2000): 1484–91, 0028-4793.

[146] Rascol O, Brooks DJ, Melamad E, Oertel W, Poewe W, Stocchi F and Tolosa E: LARGO study group. (2005). Rasagiline as an adjunct to levodopa in patients with Parkinson's disease and motor fluctuations (LARGO, Lasting effect in Adjunct therapy with Rasagiline Given Once daily, study): a randomised, double-blind, parallel-group trial. *Lancet* 2005;365, 9463 (Mar 2005):947–954, 1474-547X.

[147] Ravina B, Putt M, Siderowf A, Farrar JT, Gillespie M, Crawley A, Fernandez HH, Trieschmann MM, Reichwein S and Simuni T (2005). Donazepil for dementia in Parkinson's disease: a randomized, double blind, crossover study. J Neurol *Neurosurg Psychiatry* 76, 7 (Jul 2005):934 –939, 0022-3050.

[148] Renkwalder C, Kies B, Rudzinsca M, Fine J, Nikl J, Honczarenco K, et al. Rotigotine effects on early morning motor function and sleep in Parkinson's disease: a doble-blind, randomized, placebo-controlled study (RECOVER). Mov Disord 2010. [Epub ahead of print]

[149] Rinne UK, Bracco F, Chouza C, Dupont E, Gershanik O, Marti Masso JF, Montastruc JL and Marsden CD (1998). Early treatment of Parkinson's disease with cabergoline delays the onset of motor complications. The PKDS009 Study Group. *Drugs* 1998; 55(Suppl. 1)(Mar 1998): 23-30, 0012-6667.

[150] Ritter JL and Alexander B (1997). Retrospective study of selegiline antidepressant drug interactions and a review of the literature. *Ann Clin Psychiatry* 9, 1 (Mar 1997): 7–13, 1040-1237.

[151] Rogaeva E, Johnson J, Lang AE, Gulick C, Gwinn-Hardy K, Kawarai T, Sato C, Morgan A, Werner J, Nussbaum R, Petit A, Okun MS, McInerney A, Mandel R, Groen JL, Fernandez HH, Postuma R, Foote KD, Salehi-Rad S, Liang Y, Reimsnider S, Tandon A, Hardy J, St George- Hyslop P and Singleton AB (2004). Analysis of the PINK1 gene in a large cohort of cases with Parkinson disease. *Arch Neurol* 61, 12(Dec 2004):1898–1904, 0003-9942.

[152] Roth BL (2007). Drugs and valvular heart disease. *N Engl J Med* 356, 1 (Jan 2007):6 –9, 1533-4406.

[153] Shin N, Jeong H, Kwon J, Heo HY, Kwon JJ, Yun HJ, Kim CH, Han BS, Tong Y, Shen J, Hatano T, Hattori N, Kim KS,Chang S, Seol W (2008). LRRK2 regulates synaptic vesicle endocytosis. *Exp Cell Res* 314, 10 (Jun 2008),2055–2065, 1090-2422.

[154] Sagi Y, Mandel S, Amit T and Youdim MB (2007). Activation of tyrosine kinase receptor signaling pathway by rasagiline facilitates neurorescue and restoration of nigrostriatal dopamine neurons in post-MPTP-induced parkinsonism. *Neurobiol Dis* 25, 1 (Jan 2007): 35-44, 0969-9961.

[155] Schapira AH (2002). Dopamine agonists and neuroprotection in Parkinson's disease. *Eur J Neurol* 9(suppl 3)(Nov 2002):7–14, 1351-5101.

[156] Shults CW, Oakes D, Kieburtz K, Beal MF, Haas R, Plumb S, Juncos JL, Nutt J, Shoulson I, Carter J, Kompoliti K, Perlmutter JS, Reich S, Stern M, Watts RL, Kurlan R, Molho E, Harrison M and Lew M; Parkinson Study Group (2002). Effects of coenzyme Q10 in early Parkinson disease: evidence of slowing of the functional decline. *Arch Neurol* 59, 10 (Oct 2002): 1541-50, 0003-9942.

[157] Sidransky E, Nalls MA, Aasly JO, Aharon-Peretz J, Annesi G, Barbosa ER, Bar-Shira A, Berg D, Bras J, Brice A, Chen CM, Clark LN, Condroyer C, De Marco EV, Dürr A, Eblan MJ, Fahn S, Farrer MJ, Fung HC, Gan-Or Z, Gasser T, Gershoni-Baruch R, Giladi N, Griffith A, Gurevich T, Januario C, Kropp P, Lang AE, Lee-Chen GJ, Lesage S, Marder K, Mata IF, Mirelman A, Mitsui J, Mizuta I, Nicoletti G, Oliveira C, Ottman R, Orr-Urtreger A, Pereira LV, Quattrone A, Rogaeva E, Rolfs A, Rosenbaum H, Rozenberg R, Samii A, Samaddar T, Schulte C, Sharma M, Singleton A, Spitz M, Tan EK, Tayebi N, Toda T, Troiano AR, Tsuji S, Wittstock M, Wolfsberg TG, Wu YR, Zabetian CP, Zhao Y and Ziegler SG (2009). Multicenter analysis of glucocerebrosidase mutations in Parkinson's disease. *N Engl J Med* 361, 17 (Oct 2009):1651-61. 1533-4406.

[158] Singleton AB, Farrer M, Johnson J, Singleton A, Hague S, Kachergus J, Hulihan M, Peuralinna T, Dutra A, Nussbaum R, Lincoln S, Crawley A, Hanson M, Maraganore D, Adler C, Cookson MR, Muenter M, Baptista M, Miller D, Blancato J, Hardy J and Gwinn- Hardy K. (2003). Alpha-Synuclein locus triplication causes Parkinson's disease. *Science* 302, 5646 (Oct 2003), 841, 1095-9203.

[159] Singleton A, Gwinn-Hardy K, Sharabi Y, Li ST, Holmes C, Dendi R, Hardy J, Singleton A, Crawley A and Goldstein DS. (2004). Association between cardiac denervation and parkinsonism caused by alpha-synuclein gene triplication. *Brain* 127(Pt 4):768–772, 0006-8950.

[160] Smith LA, Jackson MJ, Al-Barghouthy G, Rose S, Kuoppamaki M, Olanow W and Jenner P (2005). Multiple small doses of levodopa plus entacapone produces continuous dopaminergic stimulation and reduces dyskinesia induction in MPTP-treated drug naïve primates. *Mov Disord* 20, 3(Mar 2005): 306-14, 0885-3185.

[161] Spillantini MG, Schmidt ML, Lee VM, Trojanowski JQ, Jakes R and Goedert M. (1997). Alpha-synuclein in Lewy bodies. *Nature*, 388, 6645 (Aug 1997), 839–840, 0028-0836.

[162] Starkstein SE, Mayberg HS, Leiguarda R, Preziosi TJ and Robinson RG (1992). A prospective longitudinal study of depression, cognitive decline, and physical impairments in patients with Parkinson's disease. *J Neurol Neurosurg Psychiatry* 55, 5 (May 1992):377-82, 0022-3050.

[163] Staskin DR (2006). Trospium chloride: distinct among other anticholinergic agents available for the treatment of overactive bladder. *Urol Clin North Am* 33, 4 (Nov 2006): 465 - 73, 0094-0143.

[164] Stefani A, Lozano AM, Peppe A, , Stanzione P, Galati S, Tropepi D, Pierantozzi M, Brusa L, Scarnati E and Mazzone P. (2007). Bilateral deep brain stimulation of the pedunculopontine and subthalamic nuclei in severe Parkinson's disease. *Brain* 130, 6 (Jun 2007):1596 –1607, 1460-2156.

[165] Stocchi F, Arnold G, Onofrj M, Kwiecinski H, Szczudlik A, Thomas A, Bonuccelli U, Van Dijk A, Cattaneo C, Sala P, Fariello RG; Safinamide Parkinson's Study Group (2004). Improvement of motor function in early Parkinson disease by safinamide. *Neurology* 63, 4 (Aug 2004):746 –748, 1526-632X.

[166] Stocchi F, Rascol O, Kieburtz K, Poewe W, Jankovic J, Tolosa E, Barone P, Lang AE and Olanow CW (2010). Initiating levodopa/carbidopa therapy with and without entacapone in early Parkinson disease: the STRIDE-PD study. *Ann Neurol* 68, 1 (Jul 2010): 18-2, 1531-8249.

[167] Svendsen C (2007). The first steps towards gene therapy for Parkinson's disease. *Lancet Neurol* 6, 9 (Sep 2007):754 –756, 1474-4422.

[168] Tandberg E, Larsen MD and Karlsen MD (1999). Excessive daytime sleepiness and sleep benefit in Parkinson's disease: a community-based study. *Mov Dis* 14, 6 (Nov 1999):922–927, 0885-3185.

[169] Timberlake WH and Vance MA (1978). Four-year treatment of patients with parkinsonism using amantadine alone or with levodopa. *Ann Neurol* 3, 2 (Feb 1978): 119-28, 0364-5134.

[170] Tolosa E, Gaig C, Santamaría J, Compta Y (2009). Diagnosis and the premotor phase of Parkinson disease. *Neurology* 72(7 Suppl)(Feb 2009):S12-20, 1526-632X.

[171] Trenkwalder C, Kies B, Rudzinsca M, Fine J, Nikl J, Honczarenco K, Dioszeghy P, Hill D, Anderson T, Myllyla V, Kassubek J, Steiger M, Zucconi M, Tolosa E, Poewe W, Surmann E, Whitesides J, Boroojerdi B and Chaudhuri KR; Recover Study Group. (2010). Rotigotine effects on early morning motor function and sleep in Parkinson's disease: a doble-blind, randomized, placebo-controlled study (RECOVER). *Mov Disord* 26, 1 (Jan 2011):90-9, 1531-8257.

[172] Valente EM, Abou-Sleiman PM, Caputo V, Muqit MM, Harvey K, Gispert S, Ali Z, Del Turco D, Bentivoglio AR, Healy DG, Albanese A, Nussbaum R, González-Maldonado R, Deller T, Salvi S, Cortelli P, Gilks WP, Latchman DS, Harvey RJ,

Dallapiccola B, Auburger G and Wood NW (2004). Hereditary early-onset Parkinson's disease caused by mutations in PINK1. *Science* 304, 5674 (May 2004):1158-60, 1095-9203.

[173] Van de Warrenburg BP, Lammens M, Lucking CB, Denèfle P, Wesseling P, Booij J, Praamstra P, Quinn N, Brice A and Horstink MW. (2001). Clinical and pathologic abnormalities in a family with parkinsonism and parkin gene mutations. *Neurology* 56, 4 (Feb 2001), 555-57, 0028-3878.

[174] Van Herwaarden G, Berger HJ and Horstink MW (1993). Short-term memory in Parkinson's disease after withdrawal of long-term anticholinergic therapy. *Clin Neuropharmacol* 16, 5 (Oct 1993): 438-43, 0362-5664.

[175] Vendette M, Gagnon JF, De´cary A, Massicotte-Marquez J, Postuma RB, Doyon J, Panisset M and Montplaisir J (2007). REM sleep behavior disorder predicts cognitive impairment in Parkinson disease without dementia. *Neurology* 69, 19 (Nov 2007):1843–1849, 1526-632X.

[176] Verhagen Metman L, Del Dotto P, van den Munckhof P, Fang J, Mouradian MM and Chase TN (1998). Amantadine as treatment for dyskinesias and motor fluctuations in Parkinson's disease. *Neurology* 50, 5 (May 1998):1323-26, 0028-3878.

[177] Voon V, Hassan K, Zurowski M, Duff-Canning S, de Souza M, Fox S, Lang AE and Miyasaki J (2006). Prospective prevalence of pathological gambling and medication association in Parkinson disease. *Neurology* 66, 11(Jun 2006):1750-52, 1526-632X.

[178] Voon V, Sohr M, Lang AE, Potenza MN, Siderowf AD, Whetteckey J, Weintraub D, Wunderlich GR and Stacy M (2011). Impulse control disorders in parkinson disease: A multicenter case-control study. *Ann Neurol* [Epub ahead of print].

[179] Waters CH, Kurth M, Bailey P, Shulman LM, LeWitt P, Dorflinger E, Deptula D and Pedder S. (1997). Tolcapone in stable Parkinson's disease: efficacy and safety of long term treatment. The Tolcapone Stable Study Group. *Neurology* 49, 3 (Sep 1997):665– 671, 0028-3878.

[180] Weintraub D, Morales KH, Moberg PJ, Bilker WB, Balderston C, Duda JE, Katz IR and Stern MB (2005). Antidepressant studies in Parkinson' s disease: a review and meta-analysis. *Mov Disord* 20, 9 (Sep 2005): 1161-69, 0885-3185.

[181] Weintraub D, Siderowf AD, Potenza MN, Goveas J, Morales KH, Duda JE, Moberg PJ and Stern MB (2006). Association of dopamine agonist use with impulse control disorders in Parkinson disease. *Arch Neurol* 63, 7(Jul 2006): 969-73, 0003-9942.

[182] Whone AL, Watts RL, Stoessl AJ, Davis M, Reske S, Nahmias C, Lang AE, Rascol O, Ribeiro MJ, Remy P, Poewe WH, Hauser RA and Brooks DJ (2003). Slower progression of Parkinson'sdisease with ropinirole versus levodopa: The REAL-PET study. *Ann Neurol* 54, 1 (Jul 2003): 93-101, 0364-5134.

[183] Witjas T, Kaphan E, Azulay JP, Blin O, Ceccaldi M, Pouget J, Poncet M and Chérif AA (2002). Nonmotor fluctuations in Parkinson's disease: frequent and disabling. *Neurology* 59, 3 (Aug 2002):408–413, 0028-3878.

[184] Xie J, Krack P, Benabid AL and Pollak P (2001). Effect of bilateral subthalamic nucleus stimulation on parkinsonian gait. *J Neurol* 248, 12 (Dec 2001): 1068-72, 0340-5354.

[185] Zanettini R, Antonini A, Gatto G, Gentile R, Tesei S and Pezzoli G (2007). Valvular heart disease and the use of dopamine agonists for Parkinson's disease. *N Engl J Med* 356, 1 (Jan 2007):39–46, 1533-4406.

[186] Zarranz JJ, Alegre J, Gomez-Esteban JC, Lezcano E, Ros R, Ampuero I, Vidal L, Hoenicka J, Rodriguez O, Atares B, Llorens V, Gomez Tortosa E, del Ser T, Munoz DG and de Yebenes JG. (2004). The new mutation, E46K, of alpha-synuclein causes Parkinson and Lewy body dementia. *Ann Neurol* 55, 2 (Feb 2004), 164–173, 0364-5134.

[187] Zimprich A, Biskup S, Leitner P, Lichtner P, Farrer M, Lincoln S, Kachergus J, Hulihan M, Uitti RJ, Calne DB, Stoessl AJ, Pfeiffer RF, Patenge N, Carbajal IC, Vieregge P, Asmus F, Muller-Myhsok B, Dickson DW, Meitinger T, Strom TM, Wszolek ZK and Gasser T (2004) Mutations in LRRK2 cause autosomal-dominant parkinsonism with pleomorphic pathology. *Neuron* 44, 4 (Nov 2004), 601–607, 0896-6273.

[188] Zhu W, Xie W, Pan T, Jankovic J, Li J, Youdim MB, Le W (2008). Comparison of neuroprotective and neurorestorative capabilities of rasagiline and selegiline against lactacystin-induced nigrostriatal dopaminergic degeneration. *J Neurochem* 2008; 105, 5 (Jun 2008): 1970-8, 1471-4159.

Parkinson's Disease and the Immune System

Roberta J. Ward[1], R.R. Crichton[1] and D.T. Dexter[2]
[1]Universite Catholique de Louvain, Louvain-la-Neuve,
[2]Centre for Neuroscience, Division of Experimental Medicine,
Hammersmith Campus, Imperial College London, London,
[1]Belgium
[2]UK

1. Introduction

The characteristic neuropathological markers of PD are the presence of Lewy bodies, containing modified α-synuclein amongst other proteins, in the surviving neurons, and the degeneration of neuromelanin-containing dopaminergic neurons in the substania nigra par compacta region of the brain. In addition, the progressive nature of PD is characterised by chronic innate inflammation with microglial activation, as well as astrogliosis and lymphocytic infiltration, which are implicated in both the initiation and progression of PD (Qin et al., 2007). Activation of microglial cells will increase the activity of NADPH-oxidase, (with the release of reactive oxygen and nitrogen species). In addition, mitochondrial dysfunction as well as cytotoxicity, (via glutamate release) will occur, which will contribute to the pro-inflammatory state. Abnormal proteasome function in PD contributes to the build up of α-synuclein aggregates within specific brain which will contribute to inflammation through the activation of microglia (reviewed in Crichton and Ward, 2006). Alterations in the innate and adaptive immune systems are reported in PD and will be reviewed in this chapter. Furthermore, considerable evidence over the past few years has indicated that there is a generalised inflammatory response in PD, that is present in both the brain and the periphery. Therapeutic intervention to retard such inflammation may reduce the progression of neurodegeneration in PD.

2. Immune system overview

The immune system is an intricate network of specialised tissues, which protects the host from infection. It can be divided into two interactive systems, innate and adaptive immunity.

2.1 Innate immune system and inflammation

Innate immunity is characterised by the immune system's ability to rapidly mobilize a response to an invading pathogen, toxin, or allergen, by distinguishing self from non-self. Toll like receptors, (TLRs), as well as nucleotide binding and oligomerization domain, (NOD-like receptors) and the cytoplasmic helicase retinoic acid inducible gene protein 1, (RIG-I-like receptors), are located on the phagocytic cell membranes, (e.g. macrophages and microglia) (**Figure 1**). These play a fundamental role in innate recognition of neuronal damage, by sensing pattern recognition receptors, (PRRs), on endogenous danger-associated molecules e.g. NOD-like receptors, (Reviewed in Ward et al., 2010). Activation of inflammatory gene transcription and post-translational processing will then occur. Innate immunity is present at birth, the effector cells being mostly myeloid cells, neutrophils, monocytes and macrophages, which on activation, release immunoactive substances such as cytokines, neurotrophic factors, chemokines, reactive oxygen and nitrogen species. In addition, a number of inhibitory pathways are induced during this pro-inflammatory stage, which ensure that the elevation in cytokine response does not overwhelm the host.

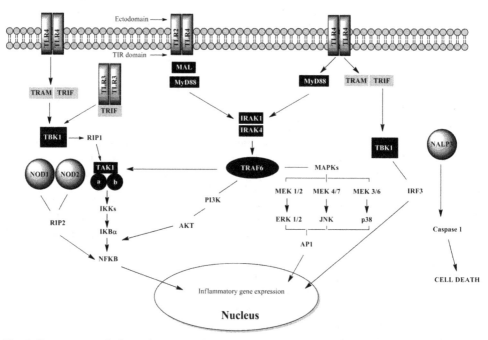

Fig. 1. Danger signals from the external environment or the cytosol are transduced through adapter protein pathways to the nucleus. TLR4 plays a major role in the activation of the immune responses.

Microglia, a subset of glial cells (the other two being oligodendrocytes and astrocytes), are regarded as the resident immuno-competent effector cells of the innate immunity in the brain. **(Figure 2).** In normal circumstances, they have two important roles; a) as surveillance cells, to regulate and supervise the removal of cell debris after neuronal death, after which the micoglia will return to their quiescent state, and b) controlling apoptosis. Microglia originate either from circulating monocytes or precursor cells that colonise the nervous system primarily during embryonic and foetal periods of development (reviewed by Chan et al., 2007). Microglia are considered to be primary mediators of neuroinflammation and, as such, have a vast repertoire of PPR as well as TLRs and phagocytic receptors. In the healthy adult brain they exist in a non-activated state, equipped with receptors for neurotransmitters, neuropeptides, hormones and immune signals. Activated microglia show a phenotypical repertoire which include the synthesis of MHC class 1 and II antigen

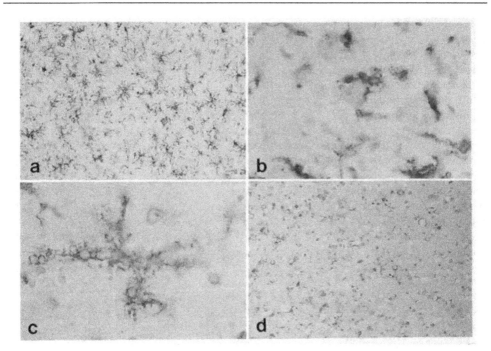

Fig. 2. Activated microglia showing highly branched processes in the ramified state.

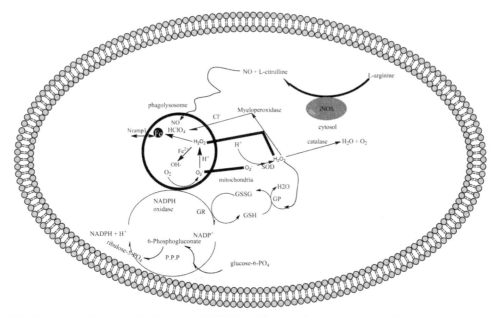

Fig. 3. Activated microglia showing NADPH oxidase activation and the subsequent generation of superoxide and nitric oxide.

presenting proteins, release cytokines such as IL-1, IL-2, IL-6. TGF-α1, CREB, the synthesis of complement components and their receptors, together with the mitogens M-CSF, GM-CSF and IL-3, **Table 1**. Cytokines are low molecular weight proteins, which modulate microglial activation by binding to their receptors, which are expressed on microglia. Pro-inflammatory cytokines e.g. IL-6, have the ability to elicit a sustained immune response while anti-inflammatory cytokines e.g. IL-10, down-regulate the immune response by binding to appropriate receptors on microglia and initiating an autocrine signalling process. Cytokine effects on the CNS function include growth promotion, inhibition and proliferation of astrocytes and oligodendrocytes, modulation of neurotransmitter release, long term potentiation which is linked to memory formation, and anxiety. Microglia also show a strong respiratory burst capacity, via NADPH oxidase, as well as the ability to release cytotoxic cytokines such as TNFα, and can produce both reactive nitrogen and oxygen species, **(Figure 3)**. In normal circumstances, the inflammatory response would be rapid, decisive and then decline. In PD it is hypothesised that microglia priming may alter brain homeostasis. Furthermore, Perry (2004) proposed that chronic exposure to pro-inflammatory signals from systemic infection during an individual's lifetime, might promote an exaggerated microglial response that could contribute to neuronal deterioration, instead of facilitating a protective homeostatic response.

Cytokines	Chemokines	Receptors	Additional factors
IL-1	IP-10	CCR2, 3, 5	MHCI, II
IL-6	MIP1a	IL10R	CD80,86
IL-10	MIP1b	IL12R	CD95, 178
IL-12	MCP1	IL18R	Complements
IL-18	IL-8	IFN R	COX-2
TNF	RANTES	F	
TGF		TGF R	Superoxide
		FCyRI-III	Hydroxyl radical
		CR1 3,4	PGE2
		Prostaglandin receptors	PGD2
			NGF, BDNF

Table 1. Changes in mRNA expression of iron genes involved in iron homeostasis in the substantia nigra and cortex of PD patients compared with controls in post mortem tissue

3. Inflammation in PD brain-innate immune response

In early studies, McGeer et al., (1998) presented evidence for neuro-inflammation in the substantia nigra, (SNc) of PD patients with high numbers of activated microglia particularly in the vicinity of the degenerating neurons. This has been substantiated in many other studies (Dauer and Przedborski 2003; Bartels and Leenders 2007; Gao and Hong 2008). Furthermore increased levels of pro-inflammatory cytokines, e.g. TNFα, IL1β, IL-2 and IL-6, as well as β2 microglobulin, epidermal growth factor, transforming growth factor, cyclooxygenase 2 and reactive oxygen and nitrogen species are evident, post mortem, in PD brains (reviewed by Qian et al., 2010), as well as the cerebrospinal fluid (Hald and Lotharius, 2005). More recently, single positron emission tomography (PET) has shown that levels of

[11C] (*R*)-PK11195, an isoquinoline carboxamide which binds selectively to the peripheral benzodiazepine receptor (PBR), (also known as the mitochondrial 18 kDa translocator protein or TSPO) a selective marker for activated microglia is significantly higher in PD patients than control subjects and correlated with dopaminergic terminal loss, as assayed by [11C] CFT BP (Ouchi et al., 2009). Whether the activation of microglia is an initial event in the development of PD or as a consequence of the degeneration of dopaminiergic neurons remains unclear. However it would seem that there is a self perpetuating cycle whereby microglia remain continuously activated and hence represent a suitable drug target. A variety of factors will contribute to this inflammatory process:

Release of ATP from damaged neurons and/or astrocytes will initiate a rapid microglial response towards the site of injury (Davalos et al., 2005), **Figure 4**. In culture it has been shown that extracellular ATP will induce rapid microglia ruffling and whole cell migration, which is mediated via G-protein-coupled P2Y receptors (Honda et al., 2001). Extracellular ATP is also released from CD4[+] helper T cells, upon stimulation of the T cell receptor. This also plays a crucial role in protracting the TCR-initiated activity of MAPK and secretion of IL-2, thus determining productive T cell activation. Recent published research indicated that ATP also inhibits the generation and function of regulatory T cells via the activation of purinergic P2X receptors (Shenk et al., 2011). Release of ATP from damaged neurons and/or astrocytes will initiate a rapid changes in astrocyte function. Activated astrocytes are present in the regions of the degenerating SNc, which will contribute to the elevated cytokine

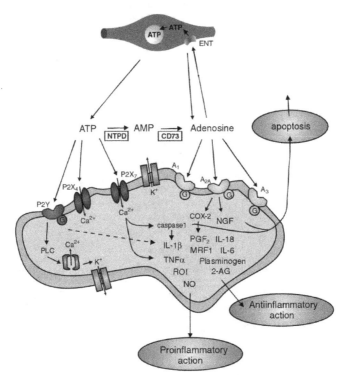

Fig. 4. Release of ATP from damaged neurons (adapted from Davalos et al., 2005).

content in this region (Forno et al., 1992). Some studies have identified a loss of astrocytes in the substatia nigra pars compacta of PD brains by comparison to controls (Damier et al., 1993). Such losses of astrocytes may imply a loss of neurotrophic support for neurons. However this has not been confirmed in other studies of PD brains (Mirza et al., 2000).

Abnormal accumulation and aggregation of α-synuclein occurs in PD. The amyloid fibril of α-synuclein will aggregate to form Lewy bodies, **Figure 5.** Such Lewy bodies will attract activated microglia (McGeer et al., 1988). Iron, which is increased in PD, will enhance intracellular aggregation of α-synuclein which leads to the formation of advanced glycation end products. In addition, there maybe an interaction between α-synuclein and Fe^{2+} to liberate hydroxy radicals, thereby contributing to the oxidative stress (Crichton & Ward, 2006).

Matrix metalloproteins, (MMPs) are proteolytic enzymes which activate microglia. Neuronal cells, in particular in dopaminergic neurons, release MMP-3 which is increased in response to various forms of cellular stress (Kim and Hwang, 2011). Thus will activate microglial cells with the production of TNFα and IL-1β as well as superoxide. The molecular mechanisms involved are unknown but may involve cleavage of surface proteins on microglial cells such as receptors, cell-cell interaction proteins, cytokines and chemokines (reviewed by Kim and Hwang 2011).

Neuromelanin, a granular dark brown pigment, is produced in catecholaminergic neurons of the SNc and locus coeruleus and is possibly the product of reactions between oxidised catechols with a variety of nucleophiles, including thiols from glutathione and proteins (Götz et al., 2004). The function of neuromelanin in the pigmented neurons is unknown but it could play a protective role via attenuation of free radical damage by binding transition metals, particularly iron. In normal individuals, the neuromelanin-iron complex is found in

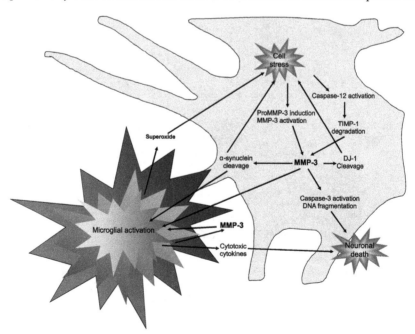

Fig. 5. Possible action of MMP-3 in neurodegeneration (adapted from Kim and Hwang, 2011)

both the SNc and locus coeruleus and increases linearly with age in the SNc. Whether the ability of the neurones to synthesis neuromelanin is impaired in PD patients is unknown, since it has been reported in some studies that the absolute concentration of nigral neuromelanin in individual neurons is less than 50% in PD with respect to age matched controls. However it is considered that when neuromelanin is released from the damaged neurons this will trigger microgliosis, microglial chemotaxis and microglial activation in PD with the subsequent release of neurotoxic mediators (reviewed in Crichton and Ward, 2006).

3.1 Stress
Stress will also have a major effect on microglial cells. Glucocorticoids are the major effector hormones of the stress system and act by binding to intracellular receptors within the cell, which are then translocated to the nucleus and act as regulators of gene expression. Generally female mammals show more robust behavioural and somatic responses to stress as well as more potent and inflammatory reactions than males (Chrousos, 2010). Stress hormones target glial cells, as well as neurons. (Jauregui-Huerta et al., 2010). Evidence that stress may contribute to the development of PD is unclear. However chronic stress will directly activate microglia as well as facilitating neuronal degeneration, which would activate microglia. Although psychological stress and glucocorticoids are reported to suppress immune function, (e.g. produce anti-inflammatory cytokines and reduce toxic radicals), possibly via glucocorticoid receptors on dopaminergic neurons, (Barcia et al., 2009), recent studies have indicated that glucocorticoids can enhance immune function in the brain (Reviewed by Jauregui-Huerta et al.,2010). This may be dependent upon the levels of glucocorticoids; i.e. high levels are pro-inflammatory while basal or low stress levels have traditional anti-inflammatory action. Such results may be important in that such stress-induced microglial activation may be involved in the progression of neurodegenerative diseases. Of the 13 epidemiological studies where the effect of stress has been studied as a possible contributory cause of PD, twelve of these studies were positive.
Serum factors, thrombin and immunoglobulins can initiate activation through protease-activated receptor 1 and Fc receptors, possibly after their passage across the BBB.

4. Polymorphisms of pro-and anti-inflammatory genes

Other contributory factors to the inflammation in PD could be functional DNA polymorphisms in some of the pro-inflammatory and anti-inflammatory cytokines which include TNF-α and IL-1β genes (Wahner et al., 2007), IL-18 607C/A polymorphism and allele 1 (C) of IL-1β (-511) (Arman et al., 2010), all of which are associated with an increased risk of PD in different populations. In contrast, the 2/2 (T/T) genotype of IL-1β (-511) may protect individuals from PD (Arman et al., 2010). Genetic variations may also be present in the HLA (human leukocyte antigen) region, where there are numerous immune related genes, which would increase the risk of PD (Hamza et al., 2010: Wahner et al., 2007). The importance of TLR4 polymorphisms in modulating the inflammatory responses has been identified.

5. Apoptosis

Neurons and glia express cellular death signalling pathways which include CD95 (Fas) /CD95L, (FasL), TNF-TNFR-1, tumor necrosis factor- tumor necrosis factor receptor 1, and TNF-related apoptosis-inducing ligand (TRAIL), with which they are able to trigger apoptosis in T cells and other infiltrating cells (Griffiths et al., 2009). Glia also express pentraxins and complement proteins. C1q, C3b and iC3b. . Hence, the rapid destruction of infiltrating T cells as well as injured neurons can be achieved by apoptosis in normal circumstances. Since apoptotic cells contain potentially neurotoxic proteins and cytokines their presence must be rapidly detected and cleared to prevent tissue damage. Such cells will express cell surface apoptotic cell-associated molecule patterns (ACAMPs) (that are comparable to PRPs), thereby identifying these cells for rapid removal from CNS to protect further damage. Failure to clear these apoptotic cells, which occurs in PD, will result in their accumulation within specific CNS tissues. Secondary necrosis of these cells will result in the release of their toxic contents thus enhancing tissue damage. Both CD47 and CD200 are expressed on microglia and are up-regulated during apoptosis, thereby inhibiting pro-inflammatory microglial cytokine expression. Apoptosis is a highly orchestrated form of cell death when a number of caspases are activated in a sequential manner. Inappropriate activation in the brain will have deleterious consequences. Apoptotic death is involved in the pathogenesis of PD.

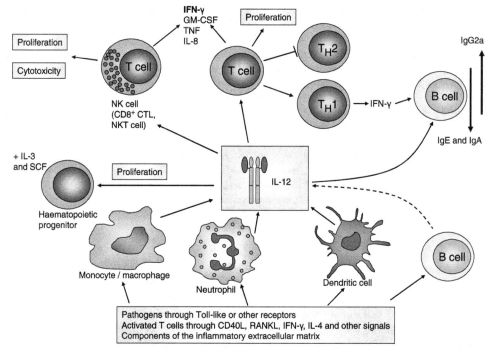

Fig. 6. Summary of the biology of Il-12 (adapted from Trinchieri, 2003)

6. Adaptive immunity and inflammation

Adaptive immunity is involved in the elimination of pathogens during the later phase of infection, (i.e. after activation of the innate immune system) and is elicited by B and T lymphocytes, which utilize immunoglobulins and T cell receptors, respectively, as antigen receptors to recognize "non self" molecules **(Figure 6)**. These receptors are generated through DNA rearrangement and respond to a wide range of potential antigens. Adaptive immunity is acquired after a longer period in later life.

Lymphocytes, B-cells and T-cells are capable of responding rapidly to these specific insults/pathogens when the insult is again encountered. This mechanism allows a small number of genes to generate a large number of different antigen receptors which are expressed on each individual lymphocyte. This information will be inherited in all of the progeny, which includes memory B cells and memory T cells to give long-lived specific immunity. B cells play an important role in the humoral immune response while T-cells are intimately involved in cell –mediated immune responses. B cells are involved in the creation of antibodies that circulate in the blood and lymph which is known as humoral immunity. There are five types of antibodies, IgA, IgD, IgE, IgG and IgM. Upon activation, B cells produce antigen specific antibodies which in conjunction with the expression of unique B cell receptor (BCR), allow the identification of specific antigens.

6.1 CD8+ T lymphocytes and cytotoxicity

Naive cytotoxic T cells are activated when their T-cell receptor (TCR) strongly interacts with a peptide-bound MHC class I molecule. This affinity will depend on the type and orientation of the antigen/MHC complex. Once activated, the cytotoxic T cell undergoes a process known as clonal expansion in which it gains functionality, and divides rapidly, to produce a donor army of "armed"-effector cells which can travel throughout the body in search of cells bearing that unique MHC Class I + peptide. CD8 refers to a transmembrane glycoprotein which is a co-receptor for the T cell receptor. CD8 will bind to class I MHC protein.

6.2 CD4+ lymphocytes

CD4+ lymphocytes, (helper T cells), are immune response mediators which play an important role in establishing and maximizing the capabilities of the adaptive immune response. These cells have no cytotoxic or phagocytic activity but orchestrate the immune response by directing other cells to perform these tasks. CD4+ T helper cells can be induced to differentiate to specific lineages according to the local cytokine milieu, towards T helper type 1 Th1, Th2, Th17 and regulatory T cell (T_{reg}) phenotypes.

Microglial activation is propagated by T-cell releasing interferon-γ. This will sensitise the microglia by upregulating the expression of various immunoregulatory molecules including CD40 on their cell surfaces. Activation of the Janus kinase/signal transducer and activator of transcription (JAK/STAT) signalling pathway plays a central role in this IFN-γ induced CD40 expression. Modulation of the JAK/STAT signalling pathway may suppress the microglial-mediated inflammation.

7. Adaptive immunity in PD

Extraneuronal nitrated α-synuclein is able to cross the BBB to the CSF where it will activate antigen presenting cells, (reviewed by Kosloski et al., 2010), i.e. naïve T cells. With appropriate co-stimulatory signals these cells will diferentiate into Teffs that will expand into different effector cell subtypes, e.g. Th1 and Th17 cells (Reviewed by Kosloski et al., 2010). Such cells will drive the disease processes towards a pro-inflammatory situation. Th1 cells express IL-2, IFN-γ and TNFα that are pro-inflammatory and will activate microglia. Th17 also elicits a pro-inflammatory effect (Kosloski et al., 2010) and will also secrete granzyme B, a cytolytic enzyme (Kebir et al., 2007). Th2 effectors release IL-4, IL-5 and IL-13 and support anti-inflammatory responses. In addition Th1, Th2 and Th17 help in the production of antibodies which specifically target modified proteins for their removal by microglia. Th1 and Th17 Teffs are synthesied in the periphery and traverse the BBB to the inflammatory foci of the nigrostriatum and identify the N-α-synuclein/major histocompatibility complex II which are presented by the antigen presenting microglia. The induction of Teffs will drive the microglia and the innate immune responses.

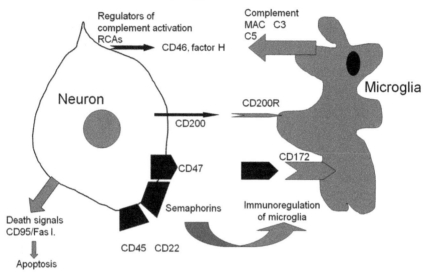

Fig. 7. Neurons express many 'self defence' proteins and receptors to prevent attack from microglia (adapted from Griffiths et al., 2010)

T cell infiltration is present in the CNS tissue of PD. Nitrated α-synuclein may activate peripheral leucocytes and mediate the adaptive immune system to potentiate mictoglial activation. Several changes in cellular and humoral immune reponses are reported to occur in the peripheral immune system of PD patients, although no clear demonstration of leucocyte involvement at the site of the neuronal damage has been reported (Brochard et al., 2009). However McGeer et al., (1998) identified cytotoxic T cells in the SNc of one PD patient while Hunot et al (1999) showed a dramatic increase of IFN-γ positive cells in brains of PD patients indicating that T cells mobilisation could be involved in the nigrostriastal injury in PD. In one further study by Brochard et al., (2009), higher densities of CD8+ and CD4+ T cell were present post mortem in PD brains. This may indicate that there are changes in the function of the blood brain barrier and that peripheral cells are entering the brain parenchyma. In a recent study, (Castellani et al., 2011) identified a subunit of CD3, part of the T receptor complex (TRC) on mature T cells, in Lewy bodies in PD. This subunit of CD3 has also been shown to be involved in dendritic outgrowth and synaptic formation thus raising the possibility that CD3 dysregulation as a pathogenic factor in PD.

8. Anti-inflammatory systems to regulate microglia activation

There are several anti-inflammatory systems that play a role in regulating microglia activation which include CD200/CD200 receptor, vitamin D receptor, peroxisome proliferator-activated receptors and soluble receptor for advanced glycation end products (Lue et al., 2020)

8.1 CD200/CD200 receptor

CD200 is a highly glycosylated protein. Its expression is primarily located to neurons and oligodentrocytes in human brain although both astrocytes and brain endothelial cells also express CD200 (Koning et al., 2007: Walker et al., 2009) With increasing age a loss of mRNA CD200 expression is reported in cells of rodents (Frank et al., 2006) which may also occur in humans. CD200R expression is found on many inflammatory cells which include macrophages, neutrophils, microglia, granulocytes, T lymphocytes, astrocytes and oligodentrocytes (Rijkers et al., 2008). The only known function for CD200 is to bind to CD200R. This ensures that the microglia remain in the resting state, **Figure 8.** The binding at the N-teminal of each of these molecules activates specific anti-inflammatory signalling pathways in CD200R expressing cells, thereby down regulating the pro-inflammatory response (Hatherley and Barclay, 2004). Loss of CD200, which is evident in PD brain regions where there is a loss of neurons, will induce an accelerated microglia response (Hoek et al., 2000) In addition, the activation of the extracellular signal-regulated kinase (ERK), c-Jun N-terminal kinase (JNK) and p38 mitogen activated protein kinase (MAPK) pathways will be inhibited by such binding (Zhang et al., 2004). Treatment of microglia and macrophages with IL-4 and IL-13 significantly increased expression of CD200R, in vitro. However expression of these cytokines was not generally detectable in brain (Walker et al., 2009). These anti-inflammatory cytokines bind to the same receptor complex and can activate the STST-6 transcription factor. Activation of STST-6 occurs in IL-4 stimulated human brain microglia which correlates with increased expression of CD200R. IL-4 exerts a powerful control over CD200 expression and hence modifies microglial activation. Therefore enhancing levels of IL-4 in the brain would be advantageous. Both statins and Vitamin D(3) will enhance IL-4 levels and thereby enhance an anti-inflammatory effect.

8.2 Vitamin D receptor (VDR)

Vitamin D3 plays a central role in immunity by a) modulating the production of several neurotrophins, (b) upregulating IL-4, and c) inhibiting the differentiation and survival of dendritic cells (Fernandes de Abreu, et al., 2009). Deficiency of vitamin D3 maybe associated with increased CNS diseases including PD (reviewed by Annweiler et al., 2009). The cellular receptor for vitamin D3, the vitamin D3 receptor (VDR), (nuclear receptor subfamily, group 1, member 1 (NR111) and calcitriol receptor is a member of the nuclear receptor family of transcription factors. Upon activation by vitamin D, the VDR forms a heterodimer with the retinoid-X-receptors which binds to hormone responsive elements on DNA, which causes an increased expression or repression of specific genes. Indirect evidence has suggested that PD have lower serum vitamin D than age matched controls (Sato et al., 2005). In a longitudinal study of 3000 participants in Finland, higher vitamin D levels were associated with a reduced risk of PD (Knekt et al., 2010).

8.3 Peroxisome proliferators activated receptors

The peroxisome proliferator-activated receptors, PPARs, belong to a superfamily of nuclear hormone receptors **(Figure 8).** Their main function is to regulate glucose and lipid metabolism and their subsequent storage. However, they also play a key role in the regulation of immune and inflammatory responses. PPARs can stimulate gene expression through binding to peroxisome-proliferator response elements, which are present in the promoter regions of target genes. The PPAR subfamily is comprised of three isoforms, PPAR-α, PARβ/δ and PPAR-γ. PPAR are activated by small lipophilic compounds and form heterodimers with the retinoid receptor-α (RXR) in the cytoplasm for full activation. Specific binding of PPAR onto DNA sequences leads to the activation of gene cascades involved in several biological processes (Reviewed by Chaturvedi and Beal, 2008). In the absence of ligands, PPAR and RXR heterodimers bind to co-repressor complexes and suppress gene transcription (Reviewed by Chaturvedi and Beal, 2008). PPARS also downgrade the production of MMPs, known activators of microglia and PPAR-γ agonists have been shown to be neuroprotective in a number of PD models.

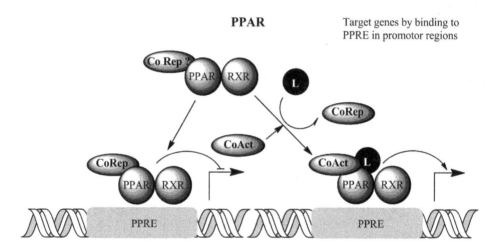

Peroxisome-proliferator-activated receptors are ligand-inducible receptors and are heterodimers with retinoid receptors (RXR).
The dimer interacts with co-activators (CoAct) or co-repressors (CoRep).

Fig. 8. Schematic representation of the PPAR signalling pathway (Adapted from Michalik et al., 2004)

9. Role of iron in inflammation in PD

There is an increased burden of iron, approximately 2 fold, compared to controls, in specific brain regions, the SNc and lateral globus pallidus of PD brains which will enhance oxidative stress (Gotz et al., 2004). H-ferritin rather than L-ferritin is present in the iron loaded SNc and lateral pallidus of PD brain (Dexter, et al., 1990) with large amounts of iron being sequestered into neuromelanin in dopaminergic neurons. Furthermore, since the SNc has a relatively high metabolic rate, with a high content of dopamine, neuromelanin, polyunsaturated fatty acids and iron, but low antioxidant protection, e.g. reduced glutathione (Sian et al., 1994) oxidative stress will be enhanced. Both reactive oxygen and nitrogen intermediates will contribute to the demise of the dopaminergic neurons, leading to the formation of lipid peroxidation products, as well as protein carbonyls and DNA damage (Alam et al., 1997). In addition, ROS, generated as a result of mitochondrial malfunction, will contribute to this toxicity. The etiology of this enhanced brain iron content may be attributable to a variety of factors which include changes in iron release mechanisms across the blood brain barrier, BBB, or perhaps more likely, a mis-regulation of iron homeostatic control in the SNc.

The control of iron homeostasis within microglia remains undefined. It is of interest that both microglia and iron deposits co-accumulate at the site of damage in PD. Whether these accumulations are a cause or effect of the disease is currently unknown. In our recent study (Ward et al., 2007) mRNA was isolated from two regions of Parkinson's brain, the SNc and the cortex, and the expression of a number of iron genes quantitated and compared with those from control post mortem material. A significant number of genes were specifically up-regulated in the substantia nigra in comparison to the cortex in the PD brains as well as controls, **Table 2.** Such up-regulation of both transferrin and transferrin receptor2 in other cell types is associated with iron deficiency, and inflammation, respectively. The high iron content of the SNc might have been expected to diminish IRP1 and IRP2 activity. However IRP-1 expression did not alter significantly whilst IRP2, which dominates post-transcriptional regulation of brain iron metabolism was up-regulated. A previous study, (Faucheux et al., 2002) reported no alteration of IRP-1 in SNc of Parkinsonian brain. The increased mRNA expression of ferroportin in SN might indicate an elevated flux of iron from certain cell types within the SNc.

Descriptor	Gene	SnM p-value	Sni	Cortex
UPREGULATED				
IRP-binding protein 1	IRP1	ns	ns	ns
IRP-binding protein 2	IRP2	0.025	ns	ns
Transferrin	Tf	0.0001	0.0030	ns
Transferrin receptor 2	TfR2	ns	0.0017	ns
Transferrin receptor 2	TfR2	ns	0.0184	ns
Ferritin H	FTH1	0.0019	ns	ns
Ferritin H pseudogene 1	FTHP1	0.0010	0.0348	ns
Ferritin L	FTL	0.0291	ns	ns
FerritinL	FTL	0.0335	ns	ns
Ferritin L	FTL	ns	0.006	ns
Caeruloplasmin	Cp	0.0276	0.0276	ns
Caeruloplasmin	Cp	ns	0.0343	ns
Caeruloplasmin	Cp	ns	0.0336	ns
Hephastin	HEPH	ns	0.009	ns
Haemochromatosis	HFE	0.0416	0.0005	ns
Haemochromatosis	HFE	ns	0.0111	ns
Haemochromatosis	HFE	ns	0.0295	ns
Haemochromatosis	HFE	ns	0.0039	ns
Ferroportin	FPN1	0.0192	ns	ns
Ferroportin	FPN1	0.0353	ns	ns
Solutecarrier family11	SLC11A2	ns	ns	0.0291
DOWNREGULATED				
Ferrochetalase		0.006	0.0223	ns
Sideroflexin 1		0.006	0.0314	ns
Friedreich ataxia		0.031	ns	ns

Table 2. Activated microglia secrete a number of factors which include cytokines, chemokines and receptors

10. Role of blood brain barrier in inflammation

The exact role played by the blood brain barrier (BBB) in excluding and permitting various molecules to cross the membrane remains an enigma. In early studies, molecular size was considered to be an important factor. However later studies have identified that passive diffusion across the blood brain barrier is very slow and that various transporters, solute carriers, as well as transcytosis, play important roles in determining whether molecules traverse the BBB. Furthermore endothelial astrocytes and neurons which are in contact with the cells of the BBB will influence intra and intercellular signalling (Neuwelt et al., 2011). The function of the BBB may be altered by inflammation in the periphery with inflammatory mediators inducing a significant paracellular leak. Immune cells are able to penetrate BBB, either at the endothelial BBB or the epithelial blood-CSF barrier. Interaction of endothelial cells with extracellular matrix will induce cross talk with adjacent cells which are pre-requisite for barrier function. For example α4β-1integrin/VCAM-1 is involved in leucocyte interaction with BBB. Inflammation and generation of ROS and RNS can acutely disrupt BBB at tight junction. Stress related pathways target nuclear transcription factors to increase P-glycoprotein expression in blood capillaries. There is altered expression of p-glycoprotein at BBB in PD.   Therefore BBB function may contribute to neuro-inflammation via deregulated entry of antigen-specific T cells, via compromised removal of toxic products of neuronal damage and death and lead to disease progression via signalling of systemic inflammation. It remains unclear whether there is BBB leakage in PD patients. Polymorphism in the P-glycoprotein drug transporter MDR1 gene association and ABCB1 gene encoding the P-glycoprotein may alter the properties of the BBB in PD patients (Reveiwed by Neuwelt et al., 2011).

11. Inflammation in the periphery

Possible biofluids which can be used in the search for pertinent PD biomarkers are the cerebrospinal fluid, plasma and urine. It would be advantageous clearly to identify markers which precede the degeneration of nigrostriatal dopaminergic neurons. For example it is known that an impaired sense of smell is prevalent prior to and during the clinical motor stages of PD. Odour discrimination performance strongly correlates with risk of future PD (Berendse and Ponsen, 2009). In addition reduced striatal dopamine transporter SPECT imaging was also identified in subjects, who later developed PD. Biomarkers which correlated with these early physical symptoms would be of paramount important for early therapeutic intervention. In a small study of 84 subjects, (Chen et al., 2008), plasma inflammatory biomarkers were assessed approximately 4 years before PD diagnosis, IL-6 was associated with a greater risk of PD. Other inflammatory markers such as C-reactive protein, fibrinogen, and TNF-α were not related with risk. In contrast, analysis of serum and cerebrospinal fluid from PD patients which have active and progressive PD, it was not surprising that increased levels of the inflammatory cytokines TNFα, IL-1β, IL-2, IL-4, IL-6 and interferon γ were observed (Bacia et al., 2009). Similarly, increased oxidative damage is involved in the progression of PD and plasma levels of F(2)-Isoprostanes, hydroxyeicosatetraenoic acid products, 7 beta and 27-hydroxycholesterol, 7 ketocholesterol, F(4)-neuroprostanes and urinary 8-hydroxy-2'-deoxyguanosine were elevated in PD patients while plasma levels of phospholipase A(2) and platelet activating factor acetylhydrolase activities were lower (Seef et al., 2010).

CSF may be the most promising biological fluid since it is in closer contact with degenerating neurons. The assay of both alpha-synuclein and DJ-1 have been shown to be good biomarkers for PD but larger clinical trials as to their potential use are needed. Although some studies have advocated the assay of a pattern of inflammatory cytokines, further investigations are required to ascertain their specificity for PD.

Plasma homocysteine was increased in PD patients (Obeid et al., 2009) while platelet levels of amyloid precursor proteins and alpha synuclein may be pertinent markers of methylation. In addition various polymorphisms have been identified in the genes of TNFα and its receptor, as well as IL-1α and IL-1β (Wahner et al., 2007). All of these studies have been on small numbers of PD patients. However other studies have not confirmed the associations of such polymorphisms with PD disease (Reviewed by Hirsch and Hunot, 2009) which may indicate that such polymorphisms are involved in susceptibility to the causative agent of PD. More importantly such polymorphisms may reflect the basal levels of the inflammatory status of an individual or reflect the ability of phagocytic cells to respond to an inflammatory stimulus.

Various changes in antibodies have been identified in the serum of PD patients although these have not been confirmed in all studies (reviewed by Hirsch and Hunot, 2009). Increased numbers of circulating CD4+ bright and CD8+ dull lymphocytes are detectable in the serum of PD patients (Hisanaga et al., 2001). Since the counts of these lymphocytes increase after viral infection, this could indicate that viral infections contribute to the pathogenesis of PD.

12. Therapeutic aspects

There have been some discussions as to whether improvements in the ability of the immune system to respond to the inflammatory turmoil maybe of importance in preventing the progression of PD. Probiotics, are dietary supplements which contain beneficial bateria, (lactobacillus and bifidobacterium), or yeast. They are administered in different quantities to allow for colon colonization. They help by stimulating health promoting flora as well as suppressing pathogenic colonisation and disease. It is claimed that probiotics will strengthen the immune system to combat allergies, stress and possibly neurodegenerative diseases (Saraf et al., 2010).

12.1 Anti-inflammatory agents

Some epidemiological studies have indicated that people who regularly use anti-inflammatory drugs have less risk of developing clinical PD (Chen et al 2003., Chen., 2005), although this has not been confirmed in other studies (Ton et al., 2006; Bornebroek et al., 2007; Hancock et al., 2007). Anti-inflammatory drugs may retard the progression of the degeneration although it remains to be elucidated whether their use would be an additional therapy in diagnosed PD patients. Inhibition of inflammation is associated with reduced neuronal impairment in various PD models (Gao et al., 2003; Wu et al., 2003) as discussed below.

Non-steroidal anti-inflammatory (NSAI) drugs act by inhibiting the enzyme cyclooxygenase COX-1 and COX-2. While aspirin will inhibit both COX-1 and COX-2, ibuprufen will inhibit COX-2 only. COX-2 is specifically involved in dopaminergic degeneration. COX-2 inhibitors have been demonstrated to specifically inhibit microglia activation. NSAI may be effective in decreasing the incidence of PD which has been associated with the COX-inhibiting effect of these compounds (Chen et al., 2005). Minocycline may be effective in delaying PD progression by suppressing the formation of IL-1β and the activation of NADPH-oxidase and iNOS which are potent activators of microglia (NINDS 2006; Couzin 2007). The presence of polymorphisms of pro-inflammatory genes such as COX-2 genes may provide a genetic predisposition to initiate microglial activation.

12.2 Antioxidants
Antioxidants may reduce the progression of the neurodegenerative process. Lipoic acid is a universal antioxidants. Lipoic acid in its reduced form dihrolipoic acid is active against ROS and will reduce oxidative stress. (De Araujo et al., 2011). However peripherally administered antioxidant will need to be targeted to specific regions of the brain where oxidative stress occurs.

12.3 Vitamins and mineral
Micronutrients such as the Vitamins A, B_6, B_{12}, C, D and E, folic acid as well as iron, zinc, copper and selenium, are involved in the synergy to support the protective properties of the immune system and most are also essential for antibody production (Maggini et al., 2007). Supplementation with these micronutrients may enhance immunity.

12.4 Steroid hormones
Steroid hormones, such as 17 beta oestradiol or progesterone protect against dopaminergic degeneration which may explain why woman are less affected by PD. In addition oestrogens may reduce inflammatory processes in the brain (Reviewed by Barcia et al., 2009) diminishing glial cell activation around dopaminergic neurons possibly mediated by differential expression of oestrogen receptors on glial cells and neurons (Reviewed by Barcia et al., 2009).

12.5 Flavonoids
Flavonoids, a group of phenolic phytochemicals are abundant in various spices, vegetables and fruit. Several medicinal properties have been ascribed to flavonoids which include anti-oxidants, anti-inflammatory and anti carcinogenic. Apigenin and its phase I metabolite, luteolin reduce CD40 and CD40L expression on dentritic cells and basophils. In our recent investigation of apigenin and luteolin in cultured microglia it was demonstrated that both of these compounds significantly reduced CD40 expression induced by IFN-γ. This was paralleled by significant decreases in the release of pro-inflammatory cytokines IL-6 and TNFα by microglia. Such changes were due to inactivation of STAT1 (Datla et al., 2001, 2007; Zbarsky et al., 2005).

12.6 Taurine and taurine prodrugs
In our recent studies we have shown that taurine has an anti-inflammatory action by stabilistaion of IkappaBα in macrophages and microglia (Ward et al., 2011). This in turn will reduce NFkappaB translocation to the nucleus and will prevent the release of pro-inflammatory cytokines. In earlier animal studies the protective effect of taurine in the 6-hydroxy dopamine model was reported (Ward et al., 2006). In the later studies, prodrugs of taurine have been developed, notably ethane-β-sultam, which reduce microglial activation in the brain of an animal model of neurodegeneration (Ward, Della Corte, Dexter unpublished data).

12.7 Iron chelators

The iron content of the SNc increases in the brains of PD patients and is associated with the progression of the inflammatory process. Hence, it's chelation may prevent the progression of the disease. Two clinically used iron chelators, namely the hexadendate, deferrioxamine and the tridendate chelator deferasirox have been investigated for their efficacy to induce neuroprotection in the 6-hydroxy dopamine (6-OHDA) animal model of PD. Acute administration of desferrioxamine, 0.4 mM or desferasirox, 1 mM, via a microdialysis probe into the striatum immediately prior to a dose of 6-OHDA, prevented the generation of hydroxyl radicals, as well as reducing bio-available iron. Intraperitoneal injection of the iron chelators, desferasirox, 20 mg/kg or desferrioxamine, 30 mg/kg or deferriprone 10mg/kg, to the 6-OHDA rat model, significantly attenuated the loss of tyrosine hydroxylase positive cells as well as elevating dopamine content in the lesioned striatum (Dexter et al., 2010). Such results would confirm that the administration of these chelators show therapeutic efficacy and should be considered to be an additional therapy for the treatment of PD. Clinical trials of deferiprone are now underway in a group of drug-naïve PD patients.

12.8 MMP-3 inhibitors

The development of selective MMP-3 inhibitors has proved difficult. It is unlikely that relatively large peptide based inhibitors of MMP-3 would cross BBB. Doxycycline, a tetracycline derivative that crosses the BBB can down regulate cell stress induced MMP-3 expression and release and can therefore attenuate apoptosis in dopaminergic neurons (Cho et al., 2009). Minocycline protection of neurones from a variety of insults may in part be due to down regulation of MMP-3. However early clinical trials in PD patients were stopped because of unwanted side effects (NINDS NET-PD Investigators 2008). Preliminary studies of ghrelin, glycitein and exendin-4 have also shown down regulation of MMP-3 expression (reviewed by Kim and Hwang, 2011).

12.9 PPAR modifications

Several non-steroidal anti-inflammatory drugs bind to PPAR-α and PPAR-γ. thereby activating their receptors. PPAR regulate the transcriptional activity of several transcription factors which include NFkappaB, the signal transducer factor-1 (STAT) and the activating transcription factor-1, ATF-1 and ATF-4. PPAR function by competing with NFkappaB for binding to the overlapping series of co-activators, i.e. cAMP-response element-binding protein (CREB), and inhibiting the NFkB mediated inflammatory response. PPAR also directly interacts with p65/p50/IkBα suppressing the DNA binding activity of NFkB. PPAR also inhibit NFkB and AP-1 signal-dependent transcriptional activation of inflammatory genes by transrepression (Reviewed by Chaturvedi and Beal, 2008). Modulation of iNOS and cyclooxygenase may also occur. PPAR may play a role in improving mitochondrial function. The neuro-protective role of PPAR agonists have been evaluated in PD patients. Agonists such as pioglitazone and rosiglitazone, may be able to protect against oxidative stress, apoptosis and inflammation in CNS (Reviewd by Chaturvedi and Beal, 2008).

13. Inflammation in animal models of PD

Activation of microglia has been identified in the SNc and /or striatum in various animal models of PD, which include the MPTP and lipopolysaccharides models (reviewed by Marinova-Mutafchieva et al., 2009). In addition, in the medial forebrain bundle axotomised model, brain activation of microglia precedes neuronal loss (Gao et al., 2003). In the 6-hydroxy dopamine models significant microglia activation was evident 48h after it's administration as well as NADPH- derived free radicals prior to dopamine cell death in the SNc. In our recent studies unilateral injection of 6-OHDA into the medial forebrain bundle, activation of microglia occurred rapidly, which selectively adhered to degenerating axons dentrites and apoptotic dopamine neurons in the SNc after 7 days.(Dexter et al 2011). After this time, there was a progressive loss of tyrosine hydroxlase positive neurons. These results indicated that microglia activation precedes dopamine neuronal cell loss. Furthermore neurons undergoing degeneration may be removed prematurely by microglia phagocytosis. (Marinova-Mutafchieva et al., 2009). In vitro it has also been shown that the toxicity of LPS to immortalised dopaminergic neurons was evident only when microglia were present in the cell culture (Gao et al., 2003). These results clearly indicate that activated microglia play an important role in the early stage of the disease pathogenesis.

This review has confirmed that in PD there is a persistent and progressive inflammation both in the periphery and brain which is caused by changes in both the innate and adaptive immune systems which fuel the degeneration. The factors involved in the initiation of this cycle remains unknown. Although therapeutic intervention may diminish such inflammatory pathways, the goal for future researchers will be to identify the cause of such perturbations. Only then will there be the opportunity to develop new drugs which will cure PD.

14. References

Alam ZI., Jenner A., Daniel SE., Lees AJ., Cairns N., Marsden CD., Jenner P., Halliwell B. J Neurochem. (1997) Oxidative DNA damage in the parkinsonian brain: an apparent selective increase in 8-hydroxyguanine levels in substantia nigra J Neurochem 69:1196-203

Annweiler C., Allali G., Allain P., Bridenbaugh S., Schott AM., Kressig RW., Beauchet O. (2009) Vitamin D and cognitive performance in adults: a systematic review. Eur J Neurol 16: 1083-1089.

Arman A., Isik N., Candan F., Becit KS., List EO. (2010) Association between sporadic Parkinson disease and interleukin-1 beta-511 gene polymorphisms in the Turkish population. Eur Cytokine Netw 21: 116-121.

Barcia C., Ros F., Carrillo MA., Aguado-Llera D., Ros CM., Gomez A., Nombela C., de Pablos V., Fernandez-Villalba E., Herrero M-T. (2009) Inflammatory responses in Parkinsonism in Birth, Life and death of dopaminergic neurons in the substatia nigra G di Giovanni et al Eds J Neural Transm 73: 245-252.

Bartels AL., Leenders KL. (2007) Neuroinflammation in the pathophysiology of Parkinson's Disease: evidence from animal models to human in vivo studies with [11C]-PK11195 PET. Mov Disord 22: 1852-1856.

Berendse HW., Ponsen MM. (2009) Diagnosing premotor Parkinson's Disease using a two-step approach combing olfactory testing and DAT SPECT imaging. Parkinsonism Relat Disord 15 Suppl 3: S26-S30.

Bornebroek M., de Lau LM., Haag MD., Koudstaal PJ., Hofman A., Stricker BH., Breteler MM. (2007) Non-steroidal anti-inflammatory drugs and the risk of Parkinson's disease. Neuroepidemiology 28: 193-196.

Brochard V., Combadiere B., Prigent A. et al., (2009) Infiltration of CD4+ lymphocytes into the brain contributes to neurodegeneration in a mouse model of Parkinson Disease J Clin Invest 119: 182-192.

Castellani RJ., Nugent SL., Morrison AL., Zhu X., Lee HG., Bajic V. et al (2011) CD3 in Lexy pathology: does the abnormal recall of neurodevelopmental processes underlie Parkinson's Disease J Neural Transm 118: 23-26

Chan WY., Kohsaka S., Rezaie P.(2007) The origin and cell lineage of microglia: new concepts. Brain Res Rev. 53:344-54

Chaturedi RK,, Beal MF. (2008) PPAR: a therapeutic target in Parkinson's Disease. J Neurochem 106: 506-518.

Chen H., Zhang BY., Hernan MA., Schwarzschild MA., Willett WC., Colditz GA., Speizer FE., Ascherio A. (2003) Non-steroidal anti-inflammatory drugs and the risk of Parkinson's disease. Arch Neurol 60: 1059-1064.

Chen H., Jacobs E., Schwarzschild MA., McCullough ML., Calle EE., Thun MJ., Ascherio A. (2005) Non-steroidal anti-inflammatory drug use and the risk for Parkinson's disease Ann Neurol 58: 963-967.

Chen H., O'Reilly EJ., Schwarzschild MA., Ascherio A. (2008) Periphereal inflammatory markers and risk of Parkinson's disease. Am J Epidemiol 167: 90-95.

Chrousos GP., (2010) Stress and sex versus immunity and inflammation Sci Signal 3 pe36.

Cho Y., Son HJ., Kim EM., Choi JH., Kim ST., Ji IJ., Choi DJ., Joh TH., Kim YS., Hwang O (2009) Doxycycline is neuroprotective against nigral dopaminergic degeneration by a dual mechanism involving MMP-3 Neurotox Res 16: 361-371.

Couzin J. (2007) Clinical research. Testing a novel strategy against Parkin's disease Science 315: 1778.

Crichton RR., Ward RJ. (2006) Metal based neurodegeneration. Publ Wiley and Sons. Pp 1-269.

Crichton RR., Dexter DT., Ward RJ. (2008) Molecular-based neurodegenerative diseases: from molecular mechanisms to therapeutic strategies Coordination Chemistry Reviews 252:1189-1199.

Crichton RR., Dexter DT., Ward RJ. (2008) Molecular-based neurodegenerative diseases: from molecular mechanisms to therapeutic strategies. Coordination Chem Reviews 252:1189-1199

Damier P., Hirsch EC., Zhang P., Agid Y., Javoy-Agid F. (1993) Glutathione peroxidase, glial cells and Parkisnon's Disease Neuroscience 52: 1-6.

Datla KP., Christidou M., Widmer WW., Rooprai HK., Dexter DT. (2001) Tissue distribution and neuroprotective effects of citrus flavonoid tangeretin in a rat model of Parkinson's disease. Neuroreport.2:3871-5

Datla KP., Zbarsky V., Rai D., Parkar S., Osakabe N., Aruoma OI., Dexter DT.(2007) Short-term supplementation with plant extracts rich in flavonoids protect nigrostriatal dopaminergic neurons in a rat model of Parkinson's disease. J Am Coll Nutr.;26:341-9

Dauer W., Przedborski S. (2003) Parkinson's disease: mechanisms and models Neuron: 889-909.

Davelos D., Grutzendler J., Yang G., Kim JV., Zuo Y., Jung S. et al. (2005) ATP mediates rapid microglial response to local brain injury in vivo. Nat Neuroscience 8: 752-758.

De Araujo DP., Lobato Rde F., Cavalcanti JR., Sampaio LR., Araujo PV., Silva MC., Neves KR., Fonteles MM., Sousa FC., Vasconcelos SM (2011) The contributions of antioxidant activity of lipoic acid in reducing neurogenerative progression of Parkinson's disease: a review.Int J Neurosci 121: 51-57.

Dexter DT., Carayon A., Vidailhet M., Ruberg M., Agid F., Agid Y., Lees AJ., Wells FR., Jenner P., Marsden CD. (1990) Decreased ferritin levels in brain in Parkinson's diseaseJ Neurochem. 55:16-20.

Dexter DT., Statton SA., Whitmore C., Freinbichler W., Weinberger P., Tipton KT., Della Corte L., Ward RJ., Crichton RR. (2011) Clinically available iron chelators induce neuroprotection in gthe 6-OHDA model of Parkinson's disease after periphereal administration. J Neural Transm 118:223-231.

Forno LS., DeLanney LE., Irwin I., Di Monte D., Langston JW. (1992) Astrocytes and Parkinson's disease. Prog Brain Res 94: 429-436.

Frank MG., Barrientos RM., Biedenkapp JC., Rudy JW., Warkins LR., Maier SF. (2006) mRNA up-regulation of MHC II and pivotal pro-inflammatory genes in normal brain aging. Neurobiol Aging 27; 717-722.

Faucheux BA., Martin ME., Beaumont C., Hunot S., Hauw JJ., Agid Y., Hirsch EC. (2002) Lack of up-regulation of ferritin is associated with sustained iron regulatory protein-1 binding activity in the substantia nigra of patients with Parkinson's disease. J Neurochem. 83:320-30.

Fernandes de Abreu DA., Eyles D., Féron F. (2009) Vitamin D, a neuro-immunomodulator: implications for neurodegenerative and autoimmune diseases. Psychoneuroendocrinology. Suppl 1:S265-77.

Gao HM., Liu B., Zhang W., Hong JS. (2003) Novel; anti-inflammatory therapy for Parkinson's disease. Trends Pharmacol Sci 24: 395-401.

Gao HM., Hong JS. (2008) Why neurodegenerative diseases are progressive: uncontrolled inflammation drives disease progression Trends Immunol 29: 357-365.

Götz ME., Double K., Gerlach M., Youdim MB., Riederer P. (2004) The relevance of iron in the pathogenesis of Parkinson's disease Ann N Y Acad Sci. 1012:193-208.

Griffiths MR., Gasque P., Neal JW. (2009) The multiple roles of the innate immune system in the regulation of apoptosis and inflammation in the brain. J Neuropathol Exp neurol 68: 217-226.

Hald A., Lotharius J. (2005) Oxidative stress and inflammation in Parkinson's disease: Is there a causal link? Exp Neurol 193: 279-290.

Hamza TH., Zabetian CP., Tenesa A., Laederach A., Montimurro J., Yearout D. et al. (2010) Common genetic variation in the HLA region is associated with late-onset sporadic Parkinson's disease Nat Gener 42: 781-785.et al., 2010

Hancock DB., Martin ER., Stajich JM., Jewett R., Stacy MA., Scott BL., Vance JM., Scott WK. (2007) Smoking, caffeine and non-steroidal anti-inflammatory drugs in families with Parkinson's disease Arch Neurol 64: 576-580.

Hirsch E., Hunot S. (2009) Neuroinflammation in Parkinson's disease: a target for neuroprotection. Lancet Meurology 8: 382-397.

Hatherley D., Barclay AN. (2004) The CD200 and CD200 receptor surface cell surface proteins interact through their N-terminal immunoglobulin-like domains. Eur J immunol 34: 1688-1694.

Hisanaga K., Asagi M., Itoyama Y., Iwasaki Y. (2001) Increase in peripheral CD4 bright+ CD adult T cells in Parkinson's disease Arch Neurol 58: 1580-1583.

Hoek RM., Ruuls SR., Murphy CA., Wright GJ., Goddard R., Zurawski SM., Blom B., Homola ME., Streit WJ., Brown MH., Barclay AN., Sedgwick JD. (2000) Downregulation of the macrophage lineage through interaction with OX2 (CD200) Science 290: 1768-1771.

Honda S., Sasaki ., Ohsawa K., Imai Y., Nakamura Y. et al. (2001) Extracellular ATP or ADP induce chemotaxis of cultured microglia through Gi/o-coupled P2Y receptors. J Neurosci 21: 1975-1982.

Hunot S., Dugas N., Faucheux B., Hartmann A., Tardieu M., Debré P., Agid Y., Dugas B., Hirsch EC. (1999) FcepsilonRII/CD23 is expressed in Parkinson's disease and induces, in vitro, production of nitric oxide and tumor necrosis factor-alpha in glial cells. J Neurosci 19: 3440-3447

Jauregui-Huerta F., Ruvalcaba-Delgadillo Y., Gonzalez-Castaneda R., Garcis-Estrada J., Gonzalez-Perez O., Luguin S. (2010) Responses of glial cells to stress and glucocorticoids. Curr Immunol Rev 6: 195-204.

Kebir H., Kreymborg K., Ifergan I., Dodelet-Devilliers A., Cayrol R. et al (2007) Human Th17 lymphocytes promote blood brain barrier disruption and central nervous system inflammation Nat Med 13: 1173-1175.

Kim E-M., Hwang O. (2011) Role of matrix metalloproteinase-3 in neurodegeneration. J Neurochem 116: 22-32.

Knekt P., Kikkinen A., Rissanen H., Marniemi J., Saaksjarvi K., Heliovaara M. (2010) Serum vitamin D and the risk of Parkinson disease. Arch Neurol 67: 808-811

Koning N., Swaab DF., Hoek RM., Huitinga I. (2009) Distribution of the immune inhibitory molecules CD200 and CD200R in the normal central nervous system and multiple sclerosis lesions suggest neuron-glia and glia-glia interactions J Neuropathol Exp Neurol 68: 159-167

Koning N., Bo L., Hoek RM., Huitinga I. (2007) Downregulation of macrophage inhibitory molecules in multiple sclerosis lesions. Ann Neurol 62: 504-514

Kosloski LM., Ha DM., Huttler JA., Stone DK., Reynolds AD., Gendelman HE., Mosley RL (2010)Adaptive immune regulation of glial homeostasis as an immunization strategy for neurodegenerative diseases J Neurochem 114: 261-276.

Lue LF., Kuo YM., Beach T., Walker DG. (2010) Microglia activation and anti-inflammatory regulation in Alzheimer's disease Mol Neurobiol 41:115-128.

McGeer PL., Itagaki S., Boyes BE.,McGeer EG. (1998) Reactive microglia are positive for HLA-DR in the substantia nigra of Parkinson's and Alzheimer's disease brains. Neurology 38: 1285-1291.

Maggini S., Wintergerst ES., Beveridge S., Hornig DH. (2007) Selected vitamins and trace elements support immune function by strengthening epithelial barriers and cellular and humoral immune responses B J Nutrition 98: Suppl 1, S29-S35.

Marinova-Mutafchieva L., Sadeghian M., Broom L., Davis JB., Medhurst AD., Dexter DT. (2009) Relationship between microglial activation and dopaminergic neuronal loss in the substantia nigra: a time course study in a 6-hydroxydopamine model of Parkinson's disease. J Neurochem 110: 966-975.

Michalik L., Desvergne B., Wahli W. (2004) Peroxisome-proliferator-activated receptors and cancers: complex stories Nature Rev Cancer 4: 61-70.

Mirza B., Hadberg H., Thomsen P., Moos T. (2000) The absence of reactive astrocytosis is indicative of a unique inflammatory process in Parkinson's Disease Neuroscience 95:425-432.

Neuwelt EA., Bauer B., Fahlke C., Fricker G., Iadecola C., Janigro D., Leybaert L. et al (2011) engaging neuroscience to advance translational research in brain barrier biology Nature Reviews neuroscience 12: 169-182.

NINDS, NET-PD (2008) Investigators A randomised double-blind futility clinical trial of creatine and minocycline in early Parkinson disease Neurology: 66: 664-671.

Obeid R., Schadt A., Dillmann U., Kostopoulos P., Fassbender K., Herrmann W. (2009) Methylation status and neurodegenerative markers in Parkinson disease. Clin Chem 55: 1852-1860

Ouchi Y., Yagi S., Yokokura M., Sakamoto M. (2009) neuroinflammation in the living brain of Parkinson's disease. Parkinsonism Related Disord 15S3 S200-S204.

Perry VH. (2004) The influence of systemic inflammation in the braim: implications for chronic neurodegenerative disease, Brain Behav Immun 18: 407-413

Praczko T., Kostka T. (2006). Infections in the elderly. Part II Prevention and treatment. Wiad Lek 59: 692-696.

Qin L., Wu X., Block ML., Liu Y., Bresse GR., Hong JS., Knapp DJ., Crews FT. (2007) Systemic LPS causes chronic neuroinflammation and progressive neurodegeneration. Glia 55: 453-462.

Rijkers ES., de Ruiter T., Baridi A., Veninga H., Hoek RM., Meyaard L. (2008) The inhibitory CD200R is differentially expressed on human and mouse T and B lymphocytes.Mol Immunol. 2008 Feb;45(4):1126-35.

Sato Y., Honda Y., Iwamoto J., Kanoko T., Satoh K. (2005) Abnormal bone and calcium metabolism in immobilized Parkinson's disease patients Mov Disord. 20:1598-603

Seef RC., Lee CY., Tan JJ., Quek AM., Chong WL., Looi WF., Huang SH., Wang H., Chan YH., Halliwell B. Oxidative damage in Parkinson disease: Measurement using accurate biomnarkers. Free Radic Biol Med 48: 560-566.

Saraf K., Shashikanth MC., Priy T., Sultana N., Chaitanya NC. (2010) Probiotics--do they have a role in medicine and dentistry J assoc Physicians India 58: 488-490

Shenk U., Frascoli M., Proietti M., Geffers R., Traggiai E., Buer J., Ricordi C., Westendorf AM., Graasi F., (2011) ATP Inhibits the Generation and Function of Regulatory T Cells Through the Activation of Purinergic P2X Receptors. Sci Signal 4: ra12.

Sian J., Dexter DT., Lees AJ., Daniel S., Agid Y., Javoy-Agid F., Jenner P., Marsden CD. (1994) Alterations in glutathione levels in Parkinson's disease and other neurodegenerative disorders affecting basal ganglia. Ann Neurol. 36:348-55

Ton TG., Heckbert SR., Longstreth WT Jr, Rossing MA., Kukull WA., Franklin GM., Swanson PD., Smith-Weller T., Checkoway H. (2006) Non-steroidal anti-inflammatory drugs and risk of Parkinson's disease Mov Disord 21: 964-969.

Trinchiere G. (2004) Interleukin-12 and the regulation of innate resistance and adaptive immunity Nature Rev Immunology 3: 133-146.

Wahner AD., Sinsheimer JS., Bronstein JM., Ritz B. (2007) Inflammatory cytokine gene polymorphisms and increased risk of Parkinson disease. Arch Neurol 64: 836-840.

Walker DG., Sing-Hernandez JE., Campell NA., Lue LF. (2009) Decreased expression of CD200 and CD200 receptor in Alzheimer's Disease: a potential mechanism leading to chronic inflammation. Exp Neurol 215:5-19.

Ward R., Cirkovic-Vellichovia T., Ledeque F., Tirizitis G., Dubars G., Datla K., Dexter D., Heushling P., Crichton R. (2006) Neuroprotection by taurine and taurine analogues. Adv Exp Med Biol. 583:299-306.

Ward RJ., Crichton RR., Taylor DL., Della Corte L., Srai SK., Dexter DT. (2010). Iron and the immune system. J Neural Trans 118: 15-28.

Ward RJ, Lallemand F., De Witte P., Crichton RR., Piette J., Della Corte L., Hemmings K., Page M., Taylor D., Dexter DT. (2011)Anti-inflammatory actions of taurine analogues in phagocytic cells Biochem Pharmacol 81: 743-751

Wu DC., Teismann P., Tieu K., Vila M., Jackson-Lewis V., Ischiropoulos H. etal (2003) NADPH oxidase mediates oxidative stress in the 1-methyl-4-phenyl-1,2,3,6-tetrahydrapyridine model of Parkinson's disease Proc Natl Acad Sci USA 100: 6145-6150.

Zbarsky V., Datla KP., Parkar S., Rai DK., Aruoma OI., Dexter DT.(2005) Neuroprotective properties of the natural phenolic antioxidants curcumin and naringenin but not quercetin and fisetin in a 6-OHDA model of Parkinson's disease. Free Radic Res.;39:1119-25

Zhang S., Cherwinski H., Sedgwick JD., Phillips JH. (2004) Molecular mechanisms of CD200 inhibition of mast cell activation. J Immuno 173(11):6786-93

3

Timing Control in Parkinson's Disease

Quincy J. Almeida
Sun Life Financial Movement Disorders Research & Rehabilitation Centre,
Wilfrid Laurier University
Canada

1. Introduction

Internal generation and modulation of timing may be an important underlying yet unrecognized mechanism of many symptoms in Parkinson's disease. It has been recently debated whether the basal ganglia or cerebellum might contribute to overall timing control during movement execution. As seen in basal ganglia disorders such as Parkinson's disease (PD) and Huntington's disease (HD), timing dysfunction is present and contributes to the ability to control everyday movements. In some cases, timing deficits may be associated with very debilitating movement impairments such as speech festination, balance control (falling) and freezing of gait.

One interesting example is how the 'shuffling gait' that is typical of PD can be improved with visual step cues spaced appropriately apart, even when dopaminergic medications are withdrawn. While this is a well known fact, it is important to consider whether the observed improvements in stride length may be the result of a spatiotemporal trade-off (Morris et al., 2001; 1994b). That is, while a larger stride length can be achieved with the use of visual step cues, a subsequent timing deficit (i.e. gait rhythmicity becoming even slower) may also result. However, unlike spatial parameters of movement like step length, timing dysfunction is resistant to the typical dopaminergic treatments used in Parkinson's disease (Blin et al., 1991). Thus, research has argued that spatiotemporal trade-off may be the result of a shift of focus to specific spatial components of movement (Georgiou et al., 1993; Zijlstra et al., 1998), while temporal control is simultaneously sacrificed. Alternatively, the inability to modulate timing during movement may be part of an underlying deficit in the ability to process interoceptive sources of feedback that guide the control of movement. If this were the case, then internal timing would be an important direction for therapeutic interventions which might have the potential to improve motor symptoms in PD.

Within this chapter we will examine timing deficits in upper limb repetitive and coordinated movements and also timing during gait in PD. Further, to evaluate how attention and processing of sensory feedback may contribute to timing control, we will take a close look at new methodologies to investigate timing control during gait in Parkinson's disease. Specifically we will evaluate the ability of individuals with PD (while "On" and "Off" their dopaminergic medication) to modulate spatial and temporal components of gait in self-paced, and temporally-cued conditions using an auditory stimulus, and further to determine whether this modulation is dependent on the dopaminergic system. The concept of evaluating timing error will also be introduced as a potential way to better understand the motor symptoms of PD. The results of these studies will be discussed with respect to how the timing deficits might be an important underlying factor that contributes to the typical motor symptoms seen in Parkinson's disease.

2. Timing during upper limb movements

Control of upper limb movements is essential for many activities of daily living, and represents an area of concern for individuals with Parkinson's disease (PD). Many of the well known motor symptoms including tremor, rigidity and bradykinesia have an associated timing control deficit that has the potential to influence the execution of upper limb movements. For example, the dysfunctional motor output that leads to co-contraction of agonist and antagonistic muscles and hence the symptom of rigidity, has the potential to influence any sort of rhythmic movement behaviour that requires timing. Functionally, timing deficits could be reflected in upper limb tasks like typing or handwriting, where it has been commonly reported that 'hastening' (i.e. increased temporal frequency of tapping) is necessary to synchronize rhythmic hand movements requiring a frequency greater than 2Hz with tremor frequency of the hands (Freund, 1989).

It is also notable that many of the standard upper limb clinical tests, rate slowness as the low end of the severity spectrum while greater timing variability (in finger tapping, opening and closing hands, and wrist pronation-supination) represents an increased severity of motor symptoms. In these sorts of tests, the more the timing variability, the greater the severity of motor symptoms is rated.

As early as 1954, Schwab, Chafetz and Walker demonstrated that individuals with PD lacked the ability to maintain two concurrent voluntary motor activities. These observations were made during a rhythmic ergogram-squeezing task with one hand while connecting points on a triangle with the other. Results of this study indicated that the PD participants could do each task very well in isolation, but were unable to maintain both tasks at the same time. They concluded that individuals with PD have difficulty internally regulating continuous rhythmic movements, although the possibility that cognitive resource limitations associated with dual tasking needs to be considered. Since then, internal timing deficits have been commonly reported during upper limb movements in PD (Freeman et al., 1993; Nakamura et al., 1978; OBoyle et al., 1996; Pastor et al., 1992; Yahalom et al., 2004; Ziv et al., 1999).

2.1 Timing during upper limb tapping movements

One of the simplest movements to evaluate clinical timing deficits is tapping. Due to its continuous rhythmical nature, timing deficits would be easily identified. It also the ideal type of clinical test for identifying unilateral deficits, since slowing of tapping frequency and increased in tapping variability are easy to recognize. O'Boyle et al. (1996) examined self-paced finger tapping in PD and found that relative to control participants, patients were unable to maintain their own self-selected frequency. Although, PD is typically associated with bradykinesia, they demonstrated that PD participants tapped faster during the self-paced tapping task when compared to healthy control participants. Additionally, they demonstrated that PD had a higher timing variability during the tapping task, which is interesting in itself, since self-paced timing might be considered the optimal state for the motor system to internally generate movement. Similarly, Pastor et al. (1992) examined rhythmic flexion-extension movements of the wrist and identified less accurate timing during movements at 2 and 2.5 Hz (but not slower required frequencies) in PD relative to healthy control participants.

In addition, they demonstrated that individuals who had moderate or severe PD were less accurate at all frequencies. The authors suggested that deficits were related to impairment in an internal timekeeper, and it could be argued that progressive neurodegeneration continues to further degrade timing control. This has been supported by other rhythmic unimanual tapping research in PD (Nakamura et al., 1978; Ziv et al., 1999).

Perhaps one of the most thorough evaluations of internal versus external timing control during upper limb tapping was published by Yahalom *et al.* (2004). Their group investigated a number of controlled frequencies that were both internally and externally generated. In this set of studies, self-paced tapping would have been considered as a baseline, and internally-generated tapping would have been considered the 'as fast as possible' frequency of tapping. External timing would have been evaluated by modifying the frequency required by an external auditory metronome. Results revealed that PD had difficulty with internally generated fast rhythmical movements (i.e. slowed tapping) but externally or self-paced was preserved. In contrast to other studies, these findings might be difficult to interpret since self-paced movements might also be argued to be internally driven movements, whereas the deficits identified during fast rhythmical tapping movements might simply be the influence of the cardinal symptom of bradykinesia. One potentially interesting method of evaluating these sorts of deficits further, would be to externally pace movement at a pace that is faster than the internally-generated fast pace. If participants are still unable to match the fast required frequencies, it might be concluded that attempting to distinguish between externally and internally driven movements would be pointless. The other potential method to evaluate timing control would be to evaluate timing error (or timing accuracy) during the tapping, relative to the timing of the metronome. This alternative might be argued to be a better indicator of control, and will be discussed in the upcoming section on timing control during gait.

The other benefit of evaluating timing control in a motor skill as simplistic as tapping, is that unimanual tapping can easily be combined with other tasks. For example, unimanual tapping can easily be combined with the contralateral limb to evaluate bimanual finger tapping, or in some cases, lip tapping in internally and externally-paced situations in PD (Konczak et al., 1997a). In these experiments, results indicated that PD performed all tasks with reduced tapping amplitude and an increased variability. And that this performance was largely influenced by hastening. Their overall conclusion was essentially a replication other researchers who argue that deficits in PD are associated with an internal cueing deficit. Oddly, since external cueing did not improve these impairments, the authors concluded that external cueing may have further negative effects of repetitive movements (Konczak et al., 1997a), although it might be important to evaluate how dopaminergic treatment response influences timing control during both internally and externally driven rhythmic movements, in order to make stronger conclusions on whether or not the basal ganglia are associated with internal versus external timing.

2.2 Timing during sequential upper limb movements

Generally research suggests that movement execution deficits observed with PD become even more pronounced when they involve coordination of multiple sequences of limb actions (Benecke et al, 1987). In a study involving a two-segmented movement, while individuals with PD displayed a marked delay between movement segments, the movement kinematics were similar to those of healthy control participants (Weiss et al.,

1997). One interpretation of these results is that individuals with PD have difficulty timing a switch between the sequential steps of a motor program, while others might argue that online integration of upcoming movement might represent a deficit in the ability to utilize sensory information in a closed-loop fashion to control movement. In a similar study Roy et al., (1993), observed a marked deficit during movement when participants with PD were required to produce different sequences of movements, as opposed to repeating the same sequence of movement repetitively. This finding would suggest that the difficulty making transitions between motor steps are accentuated in situations where different actions must be planned to complete the movement sequence (Brown & Almeida, 2011).

In contrast, Curra et al.,(1997) argue that individuals with PD may encounter a delay in the timing of movement execution when required to process a greater quantity of information per unit of time. In their sequential line drawing task, Parkinson's patients encountered more difficulty than healthy control participants in completing a full drawing sequence. However, when it was required to produce each segment with a step-wise cueing of the drawing sequence, PD patients were able to improve their performance. The results of these studies support the notion that individuals with PD may suffer from an attentional overload when selecting and preparing appropriate motor steps required for executing a movement sequence (Brown et al., 1993; Jones et al., 1994; Robertson & Flowers, 1990), while timing control itself is not impaired.

Sequencing difficulties of individuals with PD have also been documented in bimanual situations. Horstink (1990) noted that individuals with PD were unable to coordinate two separate plans of action for the upper limbs. While this perspective supports the idea of attentional overload, it may be of further interest since other studies of interlimb coordination have demonstrated that coordination deficits are not apparent when the movement tasks for each upper limb are related to a common goal. For example, Stelmach used a discrete bimanual targeting task in in-phase and anti-phase conditions of varying distances (Stelmach & Worringham, 1988). Unlike the findings of studies with different motor tasks for each limb, their results indicated that individuals with PD were able to coordinate movements as a single unit, and that deficits beyond typical bradykinesia were only present for asymmetrical movements. A detailed review of timing deficits that have been identified during bimanually coordinated movements is discussed further in the next section.

A number of studies have since confirmed that interlimb coordinated movements that involve a common goal between the limbs are less impaired in PD. This would suggest that strategies that help create a single movement goal for coordinated actions between two limbs may have important benefits in working toward improved coordination of timing between limbs. This may have even more important implications for basal ganglia disorders that are primarily or initially unilateral in nature, such as hemi-Parkinsonism, hemiballismus and even unilateral stroke of the basal ganglia. In therapeutic settings, important benefits might be achieved if interventions take into consideration coordinated movements that require both limbs to work together toward a common goal.

2.3 Timing during coordinated upper limb movements

A wide variety of deficits have been found in individuals with PD during bimanual coordination. The most common measures used to describe coordination impairment are the accuracy and variability of the relative phase relationship between the upper limbs. Coordination accuracy and variability were found to be worse in PD during both symmetrically performed (in-phase) movements while greater impairments were identified during non-symmetrical, unidirectional (anti-phase) movements (Serrien et al., 2000). PD were also found to have poorer coordination accuracy and greater variability during anti-phase (but not in-phase) during a medial-lateral sliding task (see Figure 1) and a pronation-supination task of the forearms (Almeida et al., 2002; Byblow et al., 2000).

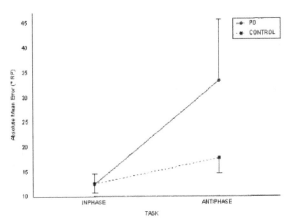

Fig. 1. Coordination accuracy as represented by absolute mean error in PD and healthy age-matched control participants *(Almeida et al., Movement Disorders, 2002)*

It is interesting to note however, that these results may be dependent on temporal parameters and requirements of the task. Some researchers would argue that timing demands might impose movement coordination to be dynamically self-organized. For example, Byblow and colleagues failed to identify coordination deficits in PD (Byblow et al., 2002), but it was proposed that this was a result of individuals with PD selecting a preferred frequencies of 1.02 Hz compared to a self-selected1.56 Hz in healthy controls during a pronation-supination task. Similarly, no differences in relative phase were seen using a frequency of 0.6 Hz with wrist flexion-extension movements (Byblow et al., 2003). Together these experiments suggest that an externally-driven demand imposed by a fast paced metronome is critical to establish coordination deficits. Coordination performance has also been investigated using the number of successful trials. Individuals with PD were shown to have more unsuccessful trials during in-phase at high frequencies and anti-phase at low frequencies than healthy age-matched controls during bimanual circular drawing (Ponsen et al., 2006).

Coordination (i.e. accuracy and stability) involves the temporal and spatial coupling of the limbs (Swinnen, 2002). However (as previously mentioned), the individual assessment of amplitude and frequency are important to consider in bimanual coordination in PD due to the possible contributions of motor symptoms including bradykinesia (slowness of movement) and hypometria (reduced size of movement) (see section 2) to voluntary movement. In addition to coordination deficits, impairments in amplitude and frequency have been documented in individuals with PD while performing bimanual tasks. Smaller amplitudes were seen during both in-phase and anti-phase at a frequency of 1 Hz (Swinnen et al., 1997). During symmetrical (in-phase) triangle drawing, smaller amplitudes were seen but only symmetrical patterns were used (Swinnen et al., 2000). Smaller amplitudes of movements were found predominantly with increasing the frequency from below to above the spontaneous transition frequency (Byblow et al., 2002). More variable amplitude was seen across all conditions for individuals with PD (Serrien et al., 2000). Amplitudes were found to be more variable in symmetrical triangle drawing (Swinnen et al., 2000). However, conflicting evidence has also found that amplitudes were not more variable during a cyclical flexion-extension task (Swinnen et al., 1997). The reason for this finding is unclear but it was suggested that the novel task used in this experiment could have resulted in variability of amplitude to be high across all participants.

Timing deficits as represented by a failure to follow a required frequency of movement has been even more commonly found in individuals with PD during bimanual coordination tasks. The frequency of movements in PD participants was found to be slower than healthy controls (see Fig. 2) only at a frequency of 1.75 Hz but not at 0.75 or 1.25 Hz (Almeida et al., 2002). Longer cycle durations were found in PD participants either when both arms moved 80 degrees or when one moved 80 while the other moved 40 degrees but not during movements of 40 degrees (Serrien et al., 2000). Longer cycle durations were also seen during both in-phase and anti-phase at 1 Hz (Swinnen et al., 1997). During symmetrical triangle drawing, longer cycle durations were seen with a goal of 1.5 seconds per cycle (Swinnen et al., 2000). As such, there may be value to evaluating error in ability to follow a required frequency. This notion will be considered during gait in more detail below.

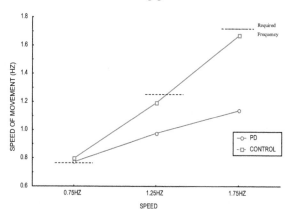

Fig. 2. Timing relative to required frequency during upper limb coordinated movements *(adapted from Almeida et al., Movement Disorders, 2002)*

In order to better appreciate timing deficits during coordinated limb actions, it may be valuable to consider what temporal demands might produce greater variability. For example, coordinated movements were found to be more variable at 1.0 Hz regardless of the complexity of required movement phase (Johnson et al., 1998). A slower and longer time to reach peak velocity as well as a longer time to reach peak negative and positive acceleration was seen in PD (Lazarus & Stelmach, 1992). A more variable frequency was seen at higher speeds and to a greater extent during anti-phase (Ponsen et al., 2006). More variability was seen in cycle durations during a cyclical flexion-extension task (Swinnen et al., 1997) and during in-phase triangle drawing (Swinnen et al., 2000). Thus, the use of auditory feedback to augment movement timing and performance has been controversial during upper limb bimanually coordinated movements in PD. Pacing was provided from a metronome for half of the 20-second trials during an bimanual coordination task, and no difference in coordination, speed or size of movements was seen with the metronome (Almeida et al., 2002). Similarly, no effects of auditory cueing were seen on temporal, spatial, pattern switching or coordination in a bimanual coordination task (Byblow et al., 2000). Furthermore, no differences were seen in temporally regulating symmetrical bimanual triangle drawing with or without a metronome (Swinnen et al., 2000). Based on this evidence, it appears that auditory cueing does not negatively influence coordination performance in PD. However, research demonstrated that external cues from a metronome improved accuracy and stability of bimanual coordination during in-phase coordination but caused individuals with PD to switch from anti-phase to in-phase during anti-phase trials (Johnson et al., 1998). They suggested that this may have increased the complexity of the task. However, this may also have been the contribution of increased attentional demand as proposed by Almeida *et al.* (2003). Thus, it remains unclear whether timing devices such as an external auditory metronome might negatively affect coordination performance in PD. It is suggested that externally pacing devices may increase attentional demands or affect coordination through sensorimotor integration deficits.

3. Gait and timing control in Parkinson's

In comparison to upper limb pointing movements where eye-hand coordination is critical to our normal experience of executing a goal-directed movement, gait may be of particular interest when considering movement deficits because the lower limbs likely require greater integration of a variety of sensory inputs that are not as visually-based. To be explicit, while vision may be important in identifying the goal of a locomotor task or to evaluate how locomotion through the environment progresses, each lower limb can be efficiently controlled by spinal circuitry without a specific dependence on the visual system to monitor the trajectory and progression of each individual step throughout gait. In fact, while the upper limb motor system develops from childhood with a heavy dependence on visual guidance for reaching, pointing and grasping movements, would revert back to a greater dependence on vision in any neurologically-impaired state. Thus, it is important to consider how timing control might be differentially influenced in lower limb (in contrast to upper limb) systems.

3.1 Typical gait deficits associated with Parkinson's

Although the control of gait may be one of the motor system's most useful and versatile capabilities, the contribution of the different sensory systems in a purposeful gait task is not often considered in PD or other basal ganglia disorders. That is, while upper limb pointing studies have been used to evaluate sensory guidance of goal-directed movement (as described above), investigations of gait in PD have spent more time attempting to quantify the unusual characteristics of PD gait rather than examining similar issues during goal-directed locomotion.

Traditionally, research into the gait deficits of PD has focused on differences between PD patients "On" and "Off" their dopaminergic medications, in self-paced walking tasks. Research has well documented the responsiveness of certain gait parameters to dopaminergic therapy in PD. The most typical finding is that both velocity and step length improve with dopaminergic treatment during conditions of self-paced locomotion in PD (O'Sullivan et al., 1998). As such, these studies have been interpreted as evidence that only spatial impairments (e.g. decreased stride length) improve with dopaminergic treatment while temporal characteristics remain unchanged (Blin et al., 1991; Morris et al., 2001), thus concluding that the basal ganglia are involved in scaling movement amplitude (Morris, et al., 1998). The assumption would be that scaling of movement amplitude may be processed through the basal ganglia/supplementary motor-premotor cortex loop, while movement rhythmicity must be controlled by other neural structures such as the brainstem, spinal cord and cerebellum. This conclusion however may be premature, since these types of experiments do not specifically evaluate how individuals with PD are able to incorporate timing cues into an on-going locomotor behaviour.

In contrast, temporal characteristics such as cadence have been demonstrated to show no specific response to medications during self-paced locomotion (Blin et al., 1991; Morris et al., 1994a; O'Sullivan et al., 1998). Since step length and gait velocity both increase in response to drug therapy, while timing (which according to physics, is the only other factor that can contribute to gait slowness) is thought to remain constant, it is not surprising that researchers have been quick to assert that the underlying mechanism responsible for gait disturbance in PD involves the scaling and regulation of stride length.

Interestingly, many of the latest studies examining individuals with PD have determined that stride length regulation may not be the only contributing factor to gait disturbance. Hausdorff and colleagues have proposed that temporal measures, and specifically their stride-to-stride variability may be critical to evaluate since they have been demonstrated to be significantly associated with an increased fate of falling in PD (Hausdorff et al., 1998; Schaafsma et al., 2003). In both of these studies, stride-to-stride variability was investigated during self-paced gait over a large sampling period (80m). Although this variability was responsive to dopaminergic medication, individuals with PD in the "On" state were still considerably more variable than healthy control participants. Increased step-to-step timing variability has also been identified more frequently in those patients who experience episodes of freezing during gait (Hausdorff et al., 2003). This may have important implications for understanding the role of the basal ganglia in the control of timing, in light of recent research that has demonstrated dysfunctional cadence in the three steps proceeding an episode of freezing (Nieuwboer et al., 2001). As suggested by Morris and colleagues, hypokinesia and freezing are aggravated by a number of different ambulatory tasks (Morris et al., 2001) and so it is important to examine other gait tasks that involve a variety of goals rather than step length modulation, in response to visual cues.

However, there are a number of research groups that have argued that gait in PD can be improved through the use of timing cues (Earhart, 2009). Thaut and colleagues (Thaut et al., 1999) have acknowledged that important differences between timing associated-rhythm and auditory stimulation through music exist, but the argument that music might lead to auditory priming of timing control is an interesting one. Researchers have pointed about the suggested benefits of dance therapies such as tango (Hackney et al., 2007) and non-partnered dance (Hackney & Earhart) in PD. Thus, the potential for timing therapy to improve motor control in PD requires further consideration.

3.2 Freezing of gait and timing mechanisms in Parkinson's

Interestingly, severe gait impairments during the on-going execution of movement may also be clinically evident as freezing and are most commonly identified in the gait of individuals with PD. Clinical evaluations have revealed that 14% of impairments associated with freezing phenomena occur during movement execution rather than more common initiation problems (Giladi et al., 1992). Each example described in the study involves a shift in the sensory feedback experience, which may have resulted in an interruption in the on-going movement pattern. Examples include difficulty changing between a climbing and normal gait when reaching the last step of a staircase; continuing gait into an elevator before the door suddenly closes; maintenance of a consistent gait pattern over a change in floor texture and, difficulty switching between forward and side-ways step patterns. Common to these cases of severe movement impairment is the requirement for coordination between the lower limbs with feedback from the visual and proprioceptive senses, which provides a rationale for an examination into gait control in individuals with PD, and it may be important to consider how timing demands might contribute to these sorts of severe gait deficits.

Recent research has identified increases in timing variability as a marker that occurs prior to a freezing of gait episode (Hausdorff et al., 2003), and this has been used to predictably identify situations in which freezing of gait might most commonly occur. For example, our own research has identified an increase in timing variability prior to an unusually narrow doorway (Almeida & Lebold, 2010), and this can be identified in only those patients with PD who experience freezing of gait. Although more research is needed on this topic, anecdotal reports from patients who experience freezing of gait, suggest that if they focus on a single goal (such as timing there steps to dance through a doorway), that freezing episodes can be overcome. And so, in order to fully appreciate the potential underlying mechanisms for gait disturbance, it is important to decipher how gait parameters are modified while attempting to achieve a locomotor goal. As we will discuss later, modulating timing relative to an external rhythm might be such a locomotor goal.

3.3 External cueing and gait in Parkinson's

The most common goal-oriented locomotor task employed to evaluate gait characteristics is the ability to follow or match gait characteristics to an external stimulus. Borrowed from the practice of physical therapy, external cueing has been argued to be a useful tool to bypass deficits associated with basal ganglia dysfunction (Rubinstein et al., 2002). The most universally known example is the improvement in step length that can be seen when visuospatial cues are provided in the form of parallel line in the path of a walk (Azulay et al., 1999; Azulay et al., 1996), compared to the typical shuffling and short-stepped gait of PD. Other sensory cues have also been studied and demonstrate improvements to the cadence (rate of stepping) and overall gait velocity, as a result of auditory cueing (Howe et al., 2003; McIntosh et al., 1997; Thaut et al., 2001), in spite of the fact that cadence control has been suggested to be intact in PD (Iansek & Morris, 1997; Morris et al., 1994b). Large clinical trials are now underway that are more thoroughly investigating the use of auditory cues as a therapeutic intervention for PD (Rochester et al., 2009). In many cases, when the instructions are specific to focusing on the timing of the task, PD performance can be improved with auditory cueing (Ringenbach et al., 2009).

4. Neural correlates of timing control in Parkinson's

Imaging research has implicated the basal ganglia, and specifically the putamen in the neural network involved in timing control during movement (Harrington, Haaland, & Knight, 1998; Rao et al., 1997). Interestingly, the nigrostriatal projections to the putamen are believed to be involved in the loop producing motor dysfunction in PD. These projections are part of a feedback loop between motor cortex, striatum, pallidum, thalamus and supplementary motor cortex (SMA) (Alexander et al.,1986), and are likely involved in the internal regulation of well-practiced, repetitive movements (Almeida et al., 2003). This parallel circuit may play a vital role in the sensorimotor integration of proprioceptive feedback from the limbs with other external stimuli. Integration of proprioceptive feedback and other sensory cues may be a critical aspect of internal guidance of movement that is rarely considered. Bearing this perspective in mind, a sample PD population with a dysfunctional timing neural network might be expected to demonstrate measurable deficits in temporal variability of gait such as cadence, step time and support time when integrating an auditory timing metronome, but not in tasks involving a self-selection of pace.

4.1 An integrated approach toward understanding timing control in gait

As previously mentioned, one of the most important ways to decipher the contribution of the basal ganglia system to movement control is to evaluate motor performance in a neurodegenerative population such as PD, when the patients are in the On and Off medication states. This allows us to make inferences about how movement control changes when the dopaminergic system has an opportunity to contribute to performance. And so, while we know that spatial parameters such as movement amplitude are strongly influenced by dopaminergic status, there would be a reasonably strong rationale to evaluate how timing control might also be influenced by dopamine. Thus, some of our own research has been focused on utilizing tasks that focus on the locomotor goal of modulating or maintaining timing in a movement task.

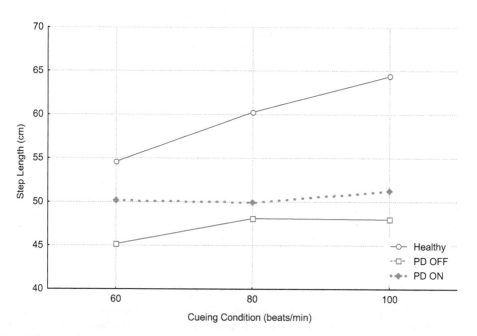

Fig. 3. Externally-paced step length for healthy participants, PD "Off " and "On". *(adapted from Almeida et al., Movement Disorders, 2007)*

Since some of our previous research has suggested that auditory timing cues may not be beneficial to upper limb repetitive and coordinated movements in PD (Almeida et al., 2002), we have been attempting to specifically evaluate the ability of individuals with PD (while "On" and "Off" their dopaminergic medication) to integrate an auditory timing cue to modulate the rhythmicity of gait. By manipulating dopaminergic status, we were able to acquire an important glimpse into whether this modulation might be dependent on dopaminergic system involvement (Almeida et al., 2007). As can be seen in Figure 3, only healthy control participants have a resulting increase in step length, when an increase in stepping frequency is prompted by an external timing device. In contrast, while PD participants show the expected step length increase (in response to dopaminergic medication), the same modulation of step length that occurs in healthy participants (when required to increase stepping frequency) does not occur.

This was the first study to demonstrate that while temporal characteristics were unaffected in the self-paced gait of PD patients (regardless of dopaminergic status and in comparison to healthy), PD patients "On" their regular dopaminergic therapy were more variable than both PD "Off" medication and healthy participants when required to integrate an external cue into the regular gait cycle. In fact, none of the timing measures (cadence, step time, double support time) yielded significant between-group differences during self-paced gait, although significant differences were apparent with the provision of external cue.

One of the most intriguing findings of this study (see figure 4a,b) was that temporal measures such as cadence, step time, and double support time identified that only the PD "Off" group now behaved similar to healthy participants, while PD "On" had greater difficulty maintaining appropriate timing in the two slowest cueing conditions (i.e. the PD "On" group performed least like the healthy age-matched participants). At 100 steps per minute, one might have expected that the behavioral response might become more automatically driven, implying less opportunity for supraspinal control. Thus, it might be expected that temporal differences between groups would be minimized. For example researchers have shown that galvanic vestibular stimulation has less of an effect at faster speeds of locomotion than during slower speeds (Jahn et al., 2000) arguing that the gain of this sensory regulation is down regulated at the higher speeds.

4.2 A novel proposal for evaluating timing control in gait

Given that timing modulation differences can be identified between the PD "On" and "Off" states, it seems important to determine whether these dopa-responsive changes are a specific issue of voluntary *control* over timing. One very common method identified for evaluating control and performance during upper limb tasks (described above) is to evaluate accuracy or error of performance. However, there have been very few applications to timing control during gait.

Thus, in order to apply measures of error to timing control during, the goal of our most recent research has been aimed at evaluating the influence of dopaminergic status on timing error (Almeida & Lebold, 2010). This can be achieved by comparing the specific goal of timing a heel strike on the ground relative to the auditory-paced signal from an external auditory metronome. Hence, a timing error could be calculated, with the prediction that if the basal ganglia truly contribute to temporal control, there should be identifiable differences in timing error that are specifically dependent on dopaminergic status.

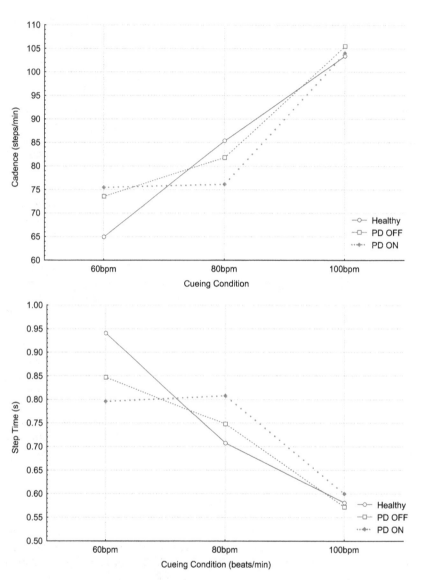

Fig. 4. a) Cadence of gait for the healthy participants, PD "Off " and "On" in the externally-cued conditions, b) Step time for the healthy participants, PD "Off " and "On" in the externally-cued conditions. *(adapted from Almeida et al., Movement Disorders, 2007)*

To test this hypothesis, eighteen PD participants were tested "On" and "Off" dopaminergic medication (consistent with our previous protocols), as well as a group of ten healthy, age-matched control participants. We required all participants to walk in 4 conditions paced by an auditory metronome (5 blocked trials per condition) over a computerized data-collecting and pressure-sensitive carpet (GAITRite®, CIR Systems, Inc., Clifton, New Jersey).

Conditions included self-paced Gait (SP), 30% slower than self-paced gait (-30% SP), 10% slower than self-paced gait (-10% SP) and 10% faster than self-paced gait (+10% SP), and timing error was calculated by comparing the onset of heel strike to the onset of the auditory cue, and averaged over the course of the trial. The error calculating software was created by CIR Systems, Inc., in collaboration with the researchers with the potential aim of creating a new clinical measure to evaluate neurological populations.

Perhaps more interestingly, the primary outcome measure, timing error identified a significant interaction ($F(4,56)=4.87$; $p<.0019$) between medication state and trial. Post hoc analysis revealed that while healthy control participants had a consistently lower timing error than PD, PD "Off" dopaminergic medication were initially less errorful (and behaved more like healthy control participants than PD "On"), but that with practice PD "On" gradually improved timing error while PD "Off" did not (Figure 6).

In addition, PD "Off" were identified to walk with overall greater step-to-step timing variability than PD "On". This difference in variability was specifically identified in the slowest paced condition. Together, the overall interpretation of these findings is that timing variability (which has been linked to falls) and timing error measures reveal an interaction with medication state, suggesting that the basal ganglia may play a role in incorporating sensory timing cues into online control of gait in individuals with PD. Evaluating timing error may be in an important clinical indicator of motor control in PD and other neurological populations.

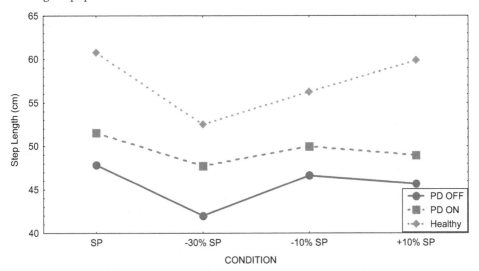

Fig. 5. Regardless of dopaminergic status, PD do not scale step length to the same extent as healthy control participants.

5. Conclusion

Deficits in timing control are evident in both unimanual and bimanual movements, across both the upper and lower limbs. Several methods of identifying timing deficits have been identified, with the important of error and variability being highlighted as important factors that reflect motor control deficits in PD. Although it is clear that amplitude is influenced by basal ganglia dysfunction, it is important to consider how timing may be sacrificed in tasks where amplitude cues are the focus of the task. Similarly, the results of our own research suggest that amplitude (and specifically step length control) appears to be sacrificed when attention must be focused on the goal of modulating timing relative to an external auditory cue. Thus, consideration of sensory-related timing issues in PD may be an important approach in exercise rehabilitation interventions for PD and other basal ganglia-disordered populations.

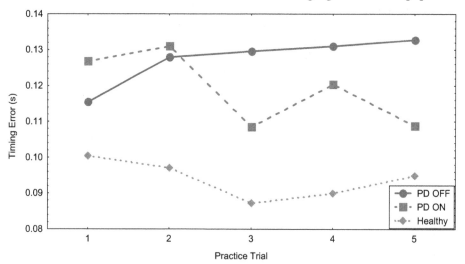

Fig. 6. A significant interaction between medication and trial revealed that with experience utilizing the metronome patients in the OFF state significantly increase their timing error, whereas PD ON improve timing error with practice.

The findings of our own studies on temporal characteristics of gait are consistent with the view that the basal ganglia may be involved in the neural network for precise modulation of timing of repetitive movement relative to external stimuli (Harrington et al., 1998; Rao et al., 1997) and are suggestive of an underlying mechanism for basal ganglia involvement in sensorimotor processing during movement.

In PD, where projections to specific basal ganglia nuclei (such as the putamen) that are implicated in the neural timing system are known to be affected, studies of repetitive finger tapping and lip movements have quantified a basic timing deficit (Freeman et al., 1993; Harrington et al., 1998; Konczak et al., 1997b; O'Boyle et al., 1996). Yet, external cues are heralded to be a potential method of overcoming basal ganglia-related movement impairments (Rubinstein et al., 2002) and a means of enhancing motor performance (Howe et al., 2003; McIntosh et al., 1997; Thaut et al., 2001). As seen in our studies, although provision of external auditory cues may improve certain characteristics of hypokinetic gait such as velocity and cadence, it may also contribute to greater step-to-step variability in PD which can lead to increased risk of falls, lack of stability and may lead to further impairments such as freezing of gait (Hausdorff et al., 1998; Hausdorff et al., 2003).

It is this within-trial variability that may provide insight into the sensorimotor mechanism underlying timing deficits in PD. Perhaps most interesting is the finding that group differences in variability (related to external cueing) are observable in measures of step time and double support time. This may be critically important to consider, in light of recent research that has identified the relationship between step time variability and falls (Schaafsma et al., 2003) and freezing (Hausdorff et al., 2003) in PD. Double support time has been considered an important indicator of abnormal balance control in healthy, older adults and those with cerebellar dysfunction, as well as those with basal ganglia disease (Hausdorff et al., 1998). Increased double support time in medicated PD patients, in light of increased temporal variability may be representative of additional proprioceptive sampling that is required to verify that external cues are being used appropriately. Bearing in mind that the greatest increase in timing variability can be identified in PD "On", this may reflect an increased dependency on proprioceptive feedback for sensorimotor integration with the external stimuli in order to improve timing, with a faulty yet functioning basal ganglia providing input into the neural network for timing. It may be that the basal ganglia are specifically involved in interpreting and integrating proprioception during repetitive and automated movements such as gait. Therefore in timing modulation tasks, where the importance of proprioceptive integration is critical, differences between participants "On" and "Off" their dopaminergic medications can be identified.

Further in support of our view, it should be pointed out that all three groups experienced the most variability in timing at the slowest cueing condition, when there is the greatest opportunity to sample and integrate proprioceptive information with the auditory cues while maintaining balance. In the PD "Off" medication group, performance across temporal measures may approach that of healthy individuals because the basal ganglia loop is not centrally involved when medications are withdrawn. Under these circumstances, a mode of control similar to that for visual cues may be employed.

Finally, timing error was introduced as a novel and potentially interesting method of identifying timing control deficits. Although future research is necessary, evaluating timing error may be an important clinical indicator of disruptions to normal timing control in PD and other neurological disorders.

6. Acknowledgment

Some of this research has been supported by the research grants from the Natural Science and Engineering Research Council of Canada, the Parkinson's Society of Canada, and the Canadian Foundation for Innovation. The author would also like to acknowledge the support of Sun Life Financial to complete research at the Movement Disorders Research & Rehabilitation Centre at Wilfrid Laurier University, Canada.

7. References

Alexander, G. E., DeLong, M. R., & Strick, P. L. (1986). Parallel organization of functionally segregated circuits linking basal ganglia and cortex. *Annu Rev Neurosci, 9*, 357-381.

Almeida, Q. J., Frank, J. S., Roy, E. A., Patla, A. E., & Jog, M. S. (2007). Dopaminergic modulation of timing control and variability in the gait of Parkinson's disease. *Mov Disord, 22*(12), 1735-1742.

Almeida, Q. J., & Lebold, C. A. (2010). Freezing of gait in Parkinson's disease: a perceptual cause for a motor impairment? *J Neurol Neurosurg Psychiatry, 81*(5), 513-518.

Almeida, Q. J., Lebold, C.A. . (2010). *Basal Ganglia Contributions to Timing Control in Parkinson's: Attentional vs. Motor Mechanisms* Paper presented at the 3rd International Congress on Gait and Mental Function, Washington, United States.

Almeida, Q. J., Wishart, L. R., & Lee, T. D. (2002). Bimanual coordination deficits with Parkinson's disease: the influence of movement speed and external cueing. *Mov Disord, 17*(1), 30-37.

Almeida, Q. J., Wishart, L. R., & Lee, T. D. (2003). Disruptive influences of a cued voluntary shift on coordinated movement in Parkinson's disease. *Neuropsychologia, 41*(4), 442-452.

Azulay, J. P., Mesure, S., Amblard, B., Blin, O., Sangla, I., & Pouget, J. (1999). Visual control of locomotion in Parkinson's disease. *Brain, 122 (Pt 1)*, 111-120.

Azulay, J. P., Van Den Brand, C., Mestre, D., Blin, O., Sangla, I., Pouget, J., & Serratrice, G. (1996). [Automatic motion analysis of gait in patients with Parkinson disease: effects of levodopa and visual stimulations]. *Rev Neurol (Paris), 152*(2), 128-134.

Blin, O., Ferrandez, A. M., Pailhous, J., & Serratrice, G. (1991). Dopa-sensitive and dopa-resistant gait parameters in Parkinson's disease. *J Neurol Sci, 103*(1), 51-54.

Brown, M. J., & Almeida, Q. J. (2011). Evaluating dopaminergic system contributions to cued pattern switching during bimanual coordination. *Eur J Neurosci, 34*(4), 632-640.

Byblow, W. D., Lewis, G. N., & Stinear, J. W. (2003). Effector-specific visual information influences kinesthesis and reaction time performance in Parkinson's disease. *J Mot Behav, 35*(2), 99-107.

Byblow, W. D., Summers, J. J., Lewis, G. N., & Thomas, J. (2002). Bimanual coordination in Parkinson's disease: Deficits in movement frequency, amplitude, and pattern switching. *Movement Disorders, 17*(1), 20-29.

Byblow, W. D., Summers, J. J., & Thomas, J. (2000). Spontaneous and intentional dynamics of bimanual coordination in Parkinson's disease. *Human Movement Science, 19*(2), 223-249.

Earhart, G. M. (2009). Dance as therapy for individuals with Parkinson disease. *Eur J Phys Rehabil Med, 45*(2), 231-238.

Freeman, J. S., Cody, F. W., & Schady, W. (1993). The influence of external timing cues upon the rhythm of voluntary movements in Parkinson's disease. *J Neurol Neurosurg Psychiatry, 56*(10), 1078-1084.

Freund, H. J. (1989). Motor dysfunctions in Parkinson's disease and premotor lesions. *Eur Neurol, 29 Suppl 1*, 33-37.

Georgiou, N., Iansek, R., Bradshaw, J. L., Phillips, J. G., Mattingley, J. B., & Bradshaw, J. A. (1993). An evaluation of the role of internal cues in the pathogenesis of Parkinsonian hypokinesia. *Brain, 116*, 1175-1587.

Giladi, N., McMahon, D., Przedborski, S., Flaster, E., Guillory, S., Kostic, V., & Fahn, S. (1992). Motor blocks in Parkinson's disease. *Neurology, 42*(2), 333-339.

Hackney, M. E., & Earhart, G. M. Effects of dance on gait and balance in Parkinson's disease: a comparison of partnered and nonpartnered dance movement. *Neurorehabil Neural Repair, 24*(4), 384-392.

Hackney, M. E., Kantorovich, S., Levin, R., & Earhart, G. M. (2007). Effects of tango on functional mobility in Parkinson's disease: a preliminary study. *J Neurol Phys Ther, 31*(4), 173-179.

Harrington, D. L., Haaland, K. Y., & Hermanowicz, N. (1998). Temporal processing in the basal ganglia. *Neuropsychology, 12*(1), 3-12.

Harrington, D. L., Haaland, K. Y., & Knight, R. T. (1998). Cortical Networks Underlying Mechanisms of Time Perception. *J. Neurosci., 18*(3), 1085-1095.

Hausdorff, J. M., Cudkowicz, M. E., Firtion, R., Wei, J. Y., & Goldberger, A. L. (1998). Gait variability and basal ganglia disorders: stride-to-stride variations of gait cycle timing in Parkinson's disease and Huntington's disease. *Mov Disord, 13*(3), 428-437.

Hausdorff, J. M., Schaafsma, J. D., Balash, Y., Bartels, A. L., Gurevich, T., & Giladi, N. (2003). Impaired regulation of stride variability in Parkinson's disease subjects with freezing of gait. *Exp Brain Res, 149*(2), 187-194.

Howe, T. E., Lovgreen, B., Cody, F. W., Ashton, V. J., & Oldham, J. A. (2003). Auditory cues can modify the gait of persons with early-stage Parkinson's disease: a method for enhancing parkinsonian walking performance? *Clin Rehabil, 17*(4), 363-367.

Iansek, R. T., & Morris, M. (1997). Rehabilitation of gait in Parkinson's disease. *J Neurol Neurosurg Psychiatry, 63*(4), 556-557.

Jahn, K., Strupp, M., Schneider, E., Dieterich, M., & Brandt, T. (2000). Differential effects of vestibular stimulation on walking and running. *Neuroreport, 11*(8), 1745-1748.

Johnson, K. A., Cunnington, R., Bradshaw, J. L., Phillips, J. G., Iansek, R., & Rogers, M. A. (1998). Bimanual co-ordination in Parkinson's disease. *Brain, 121*, 743-753.

Konczak, J., Ackermann, H., Hertrich, I., Spieker, S., & Dichgans, J. (1997a). Control of repetitive lip and finger movements in Parkinson's disease: Influence of external timing signals and simultaneous execution on motor performance. *Movement Disorders, 12*(5), 665-676.

Konczak, J., Ackermann, H., Hertrich, I., Spieker, S., & Dichgans, J. (1997b). Control of repetitive lip and finger movements in Parkinson's disease: influence of external timing signals and simultaneous execution on motor performance. *Mov Disord, 12*(5), 665-676.

Lazarus, J. A. C., & Stelmach, G. E. (1992). Interlimb Coordination in Parkinsons-Disease. *Movement Disorders, 7*(2), 159-170.

McIntosh, G. C., Brown, S. H., Rice, R. R., & Thaut, M. H. (1997). Rhythmic auditory-motor facilitation of gait patterns in patients with Parkinson's disease. *J Neurol Neurosurg Psychiatry, 62*(1), 22-26.

Morris, M., Iansek, R., Matyas, T., & Summers, J. (1998). Abnormalities in the stride length-cadence relation in parkinsonian gait. *Mov Disord, 13*(1), 61-69.

Morris, M. E., Huxham, F., McGinley, J., & Iansek, R. (2001). Gait disorders and gait rehabilitation in Parkinson's disease. *Adv Neurol*, 347-361.

Morris, M. E., Iansek, R., Matyas, T. A., & Summers, J. J. (1994a). Ability to modulate walking cadence remains intact in Parkinson's disease. *J Neurol Neurosurg Psychiatry, 57*(12), 1532-1534.

Morris, M. E., Iansek, R., Matyas, T. A., & Summers, J. J. (1994b). The pathogenesis of gait hypokinesia in Parkinson's disease. *Brain, 117 (Pt 5)*, 1169-1181.

Morris, M. E., Iansek, R., Matyas, T. A., & Summers, J. J. (1996). Stride length regulation in Parkinson's disease. Normalization strategies and underlying mechanisms. *Brain, 119 (Pt 2)*, 551-568.

Nakamura, R., Nagasaki, H., & Narabayashi, H. (1978). Disturbances of Rhythm Formation in Patients with Parkinsons-Disease .1. Characteristics of Tapping Response to Periodic Signals. *Perceptual and Motor Skills, 46*(1), 63-75.

Nieuwboer, A., Dom, R., De Weerdt, W., Desloovere, K., Fieuws, S., & Broens-Kaucsik, E. (2001). Abnormalities of the spatiotemporal characteristics of gait at the onset of freezing in Parkinson's disease. *Mov Disord, 16*(6), 1066-1075.

O'Boyle, D. J., Freeman, J. S., & Cody, F. W. (1996). The accuracy and precision of timing of self-paced, repetitive movements in subjects with Parkinson's disease. *Brain, 119 (Pt 1)*, 51-70.

O'Sullivan, J. D., Said, C. M., Dillon, L. C., Hoffman, M., & Hughes, A. J. (1998). Gait analysis in patients with Parkinson's disease and motor fluctuations: influence of levodopa and comparison with other measures of motor function. *Mov Disord, 13*(6), 900-906.

OBoyle, D. J., Freeman, J. S., & Cody, F. W. J. (1996). The accuracy and precision of timing of self-paced, repetitive movements in subjects with Parkinson's disease. *Brain, 119,* 51-70.

Pastor, M. A., Jahanshahi, M., Artieda, J., & Obeso, J. A. (1992). Performance of Repetitive Wrist Movements in Parkinsons-Disease. *Brain, 115,* 875-891.

Ponsen, M. M., Daffertshofer, A., van den Heuvel, E., Wolters, E., Beek, P. J., & Berendse, H. W. (2006). Bimanual coordination dysfunction in early, untreated Parkinson's disease. *Parkinsonism Relat Disord, 12*(4), 246-252.

Rao, S. M., Harrington, D. L., Haaland, K. Y., Bobholz, J. A., Cox, R. W., & Binder, J. R. (1997). Distributed Neural Systems Underlying the Timing of Movements. *J. Neurosci., 17*(14), 5528-5535.

Ringenbach, S. D., van Gemmert, A. W., Shill, H. A., & Stelmach, G. E. Auditory instructional cues benefit unimanual and bimanual drawing in Parkinson's disease patients. *Hum Mov Sci.*

Rochester, L., Burn, D. J., Woods, G., Godwin, J., & Nieuwboer, A. (2009). Does auditory rhythmical cueing improve gait in people with Parkinson's disease and cognitive impairment? A feasibility study. *Mov Disord, 24*(6), 839-845.

Rubinstein, T. C., Giladi, N., & Hausdorff, J. M. (2002). The power of cueing to circumvent dopamine deficits: a review of physical therapy treatment of gait disturbances in Parkinson's disease. *Mov Disord, 17*(6), 1148-1160.

Schaafsma, J. D., Giladi, N., Balash, Y., Bartels, A. L., Gurevich, T., & Hausdorff, J. M. (2003). Gait dynamics in Parkinson's disease: relationship to Parkinsonian features, falls and response to levodopa. *J Neurol Sci, 212*(1-2), 47-53.

Serrien, D. J., Steyvers, M., Debaere, F., Stelmach, G. E., & Swinnen, S. P. (2000). Bimanual coordination and limb-specific parameterization in patients with Parkinson's disease. *Neuropsychologia, 38*(13), 1714-1722.

Stelmach, G. E., & Worringham, C. J. (1988). The control of bimanual aiming movements in Parkinson's disease. *J Neurol Neurosurg Psychiatry, 51*(2), 223-231.

Swinnen, S. P. (2002). Intermanual coordination: from behavioural principles to neural-network interactions. *Nat Rev Neurosci, 3*(5), 348-359.

Swinnen, S. P., Steyvers, M., Van Den Bergh, L., & Stelmach, G. E. (2000). Motor learning and Parkinson's disease: refinement of within-limb and between-limb coordination as a result of practice. *Behav Brain Res, 111*(1-2), 45-59.

Swinnen, S. P., Van Langendonk, L., Verschueren, S., Peeters, G., Dom, R., & De Weerdt, W. (1997). Interlimb coordination deficits in patients with Parkinson's disease during the production of two-joint oscillations in the sagittal plane. *Mov Disord, 12*(6), 958-968.

Thaut, M. H., Kenyon, G. P., Schauer, M. L., & McIntosh, G. C. (1999). The connection between rhythmicity and brain function. *IEEE Eng Med Biol Mag, 18*(2), 101-108.

Thaut, M. H., McIntosh, K. W., McIntosh, G. C., & Hoemberg, V. (2001). Auditory rhythmicity enhances movement and speech motor control in patients with Parkinson's disease. *Funct Neurol, 16*(2), 163-172.

Yahalom, G., Simon, E. S., Thorne, R., Peretz, C., & Giladi, N. (2004). Hand rhythmic tapping and timing in Parkinson's disease. *Parkinsonism & Related Disorders, 10*(3), 143-148.

Zijlstra, W., Rutgers, A. W., & Van Weerden, T. W. (1998). Voluntary and involuntary adaptation of gait in Parkinson's disease. *Gait Posture, 7*(1), 53-63.

Ziv, I., Avraham, M., Dabby, R., Zoldan, J., Djaldetti, R., & Melamed, E. (1999). Early-occurrence of manual motor blocks in Parkinson's disease: a quantitative assessment. *Acta Neurologica Scandinavica, 99*(2), 106-111.

4

Free Radicals, Oxidative Stress and Oxidative Damage in Parkinson's Disease

Marisa G. Repetto, Raúl O. Domínguez,
Enrique R. Marschoff and Jorge A. Serra
School of Pharmacy and Biochemistry,
University of Buenos Aires (UBA) / PRALIB – CONICET
Argentina

1. Introduction

Parkinson's disease (PD) is an adult-onset disease of unknown etiology, with a prevalence of 0.3% in the entire population, affecting more than 1% of humans over 60 years of age. Primary degeneration occurs in pigmented dopamine-containing neurons in the *pars compacta* of the *substantia nigra*, with projections to the striatum and typical motor signs that appear with a loss of 60% of the dopaminergic neurons of the brain area. While 90-95% of PD cases have no known genetic basis, approximately 5-10% arises from inherited mutations (Farooqui & Farooqui, 2011). While the actual physiopathology of PD remains uncertain, it is currently suggested that the molecular mechanism of the vulnerability of dopaminergic neurons in the *substantia nigra* involves monoamine oxidase-mediated abnormal dopamine metabolism, hydrogen peroxide generation, and abnormal mitochondrial and proteosomal dysfunctions along with microglia cell activation which may be closely associated with neurodegenerative process. The loss of dopaminergic neurons in the *substantia nigra* may be related to resting tremor, rigidity, bradykinesia, postural instability, and gait disturbance in PD patients. Also associated with PD neuropathology are disrupted iron homeostasis, intracellular deposition of proteins in Lewy bodies, and oxidative stress and neuronal damage.

PD is considered the paradigm of α-synucleinopathies within the spectrum of neurodegenerative diseases that exhibit α-synuclein in cytosolic protein aggregates (Navarro et al., 2009).

There is evidence that oxidative stress participates in the neurodegeneration (Lustig et al., 1993; Famulari et al., 1996; Repetto et al., 1999; Fiszman et al., 2003; Domínguez et al., 2008); neutrophils express a primary alteration of nitric oxide release in PD patients, where reactive oxygen species and oxidative stress parameters are more probably related to the evolution of PD (Gatto et al., 1996; Gatto et al., 1997; Repetto & Llesuy, 2004). Peripheral markers of oxidative stress in red blood cells of neurological patients could be a reflection of the brain condition and suggests that oxygen free radicals are partially responsible for the damage observed in PD living patients (Serra et al., 2001; Repetto, 2008). Other reports suggest that mitochondrial dysfunction and impairment of the respiratory complexes are associated with the neuronal loss (Boveris & Navarro, 2008). Moreover, increased mDNA deletions were recognized in nigral neurons in PD (Bender et al., 2006).

1.1 Clinical criteria diagnosis in idiopathic Parkinson's disease

The differential diagnosis of parkinsonian syndromes is considered one of the most challenging in clinical neurology. Despite published consensus operational standards for the diagnosis of idiopathic Parkinson's disease (PD) and the various parkinsonian disorders, such as secondary Parkinson's disease, progressive supranuclear palsy, multiple system atrophy and corticobasal degeneration, the clinical separation of PD requires the application of strict diagnostic criteria.

The diagnosis of the specific secondary Parkinsonism was based on the constellation of clinical features suggestive of a secondary etiology (Gibb et al., 1988; Quinn, 1989; Dalakas et al., 2000; Schrag et al., 2002), namely: Manifestations and suspected etiologies of non PD, Vascular Parkinsonism, Drug-induced Parkinsonism, Multiple System Atrophy, Lewy body dementia, Toxin exposure (carbon-monoxide poisoning), Progressive supranuclear palsy, Hemiparkinsonism – hemiatrophy, Juvenile Parkinsonism with dystonia and hemiatrophy, Walking apraxia-ataxia frontal lobe, Action or postural tremor prominent (essential tremor) and the Stiff person syndrome.

While the clinical characteristics of the Parkinson syndrome facilitate the diagnosis, which is easy in the advanced stages in the paucisymptomatic forms or at the early stages the diagnosis becomes more difficult.

In the absence of a biological marker diagnosis in life can only be performed by clinical criteria. In recent decades the criteria used were not universally recognized, and the PD could be over diagnosed. In a study carried out between 1999 and 2000 (Serra et al., 2001) patients were recruited if they had, at least, two cardinal symptoms of PD according to clinical criteria (Hughes et al., 1992) and, additionally, Hoehn and Yahr stage 1 to 3 (Hoehn & Yahr, 1967), to assess the severity at presentation and progression. Patients also required a history of positive response to levodopa therapy.

Currently, the diagnosis of PD follows the United Kingdom Brain Bank Criteria, which demands bradykinesia and one additional symptom, *i.e.*, rigidity, resting tremor or postural instability. The latter is not a useful sign for the early diagnosis of PD, because it does not appear before Hoehn and Yahr stage 3. Other symptoms of PD which precede the onset of motor disturbances are hyposmia, REM sleep behavioral disorder, constipation and depression. The clinical diagnosis of PD can be supported by levodopa or apomorphine tests. Imaging studies such as cranial CT or MRI are helpful to distinguish PD from atypical or secondary Parkinson's disease.

In the last decade the Unified Parkinson's Disease Rating Scale (UPDRS) is the most widely used clinical rating scale for PD. Authors unanimously considered the concept of a single clinical rating scale to be an important tool for clear and consistent communication among movement disorder colleagues (Fahn et al., 1987; Movement Disorder Society Task Force, 2003).

1.2 Biochemical mechanisms associated to Parkinson's disease

The degradation processes of macromolecules, such as serotonin, norepinephrine, dopamine, and other neurotransmitters of dopaminergic neurons in *substantia nigra*, catalyzed by monoamine oxidase are critically important not only for the regulation of emotional behavior, but also for other neural functions. As a consequence, the brains of PD patients are subject to high levels of oxidative stress. The dopaminergic cell loss and disease progression are accompanied by the accumulation of high iron levels, associated with aggregation of α-synuclein (especially in the mutated form found in familial Parkinson's disease). Increasing evidence indicates that multiple biochemical and cellular factors are involved in neuronal death in PD, some of them involve protein dyshomeostasis, mitochondrial impaired function and metal-induced toxicity. These processes contribute to the oxidative stress and damage and inflammatory response in brain of PD patients (Farooqui & Farooqui, 2011). The current views on PD consider that this disease is not only characterized by *substantia nigra* dysfunction but that it also involves the frontal cortex with a cognitive decline at the early stages of Parkinsonism (McNamara et al., 2007). Oxidative damage and mitochondrial dysfunction in the human frontal cortex are considered factors that lead to impaired cognition in PD patients.

1.2.1 Protein dyshomeostasis

The neuropathological hallmarks of PD include the presence of Lewy bodies mostly composed of α-synuclein, a presynaptic protein that not only plays an important role in neuropathology of PD, but is also known to bind divalent metals as iron (Fe) and copper (Cu), which accelerates the aggregation of α-synuclein to form various toxic aggregates *in vitro*. Although the normal biological function of this protein remains to be elucidated, it is clear that regulation of its expression is essential for healthy neuronal function. Even a 1.5 fold elevation in its expression is sufficient to produce Lewy body disease (Sigletton et al., 2003). Membrane-bound α-synuclein may play a role in fibril formation. Overexpression of α-synuclein impairs mitochondrial function and increases oxidative stress. This prion protein has a neuroprotective function by acting as antiapoptotic factor that inhibits the mitochondria-mediated apoptosis by preventing the formation of the permeability pore of the inner mitochondrial membrane (Opazo et al., 2003; Kozlowski et al., 2009).

These effects are associated to mitochondrial dysfunction due to decreased activity of cytochrome c oxidase and to the increased production of reactive oxygen species, which in turn triggers mitochondria-mediated apoptotic neurodegeneration (Rossi et al., 2004; Spencer et al., 2009).

1.2.2 Mitochondrial impaired function

Neurochemically, PD is characterized by mitochondrial dysfunction and brain mitochondrial oxidative damage. There are also consistent observations of the impaired functioning of mitochondrial respiratory transport chain at the site of complex I (NADH CoQ10 reductase), from PD brain, particularly in the *substantia nigra*, with consequent aggregation and accumulation of α-synuclein (Opazo et al., 2003; Friedlich et al., 2009) and in frontal cortex in PD patients (Boveris & Navarro, 2008). The inhibition of complex I observed in PD has an etiological impact. The question then arises as to the origin of the complex I-deficiency in PD. It could result from an environmental toxin or an acquired or inherited mtDNA mutation(s) (Petrozzi et al., 2007).

The molecular mechanism involved in the inactivation of complex I is likely accounted by the sum of peroxinitrite mediated reactions, reactions with free radical intermediates of the lipid peroxidation process and amine-aldehyde adduction reactions. The inhibitory effects on complex I lead synergistically to denaturation of the protein structure and to further increases of superoxide anion (O_2^-) y peroxinitrite production at the vicinity of complex I (Navarro et al., 2009; Navarro & Boveris, 2009).

Inhibition of complex I creates an environment of oxidative stress that ultimately leads to the aggregation of α-synuclein with the consequent neuronal death. Complex I dysfunction, also called "complex I syndrome" results in complex I inactivation, reduced oxygen (O_2) uptake and ATP formation, increased O_2^- formation, oxidative stress and lipid peroxidation, events that lead to neuronal depolarization and contribute to excitotoxic neuronal injury (Opazo et al., 2003; Kozlowski et al., 2009; Navarro & Boveris, 2009). Mitochondrial dysfunction in the human frontal cortex is to be considered a factor contributing to impaired cognition in PD in comparison to age-matched healthy controls. The mitochondrial impairment observed in frontal cortex in PD patients is properly described as a reduced frontal cortex respiration, with marked decrease in complex I activity, associated with oxidative damage, the latter determined by the increased content of phospholipids and protein oxidation products (Navarro et al., 2009).

Deficient complex I function would likely increase production of superoxide anion by impairing electron flow from NADH to ubiquinone, promoting oxidative stress through subsequent superoxide dismutase and Fenton chemistry. Similar deficits in respiratory transport chain complex I have also been reported in peripheral cells (myocytes and platelets).

Mitochondrial metabolic abnormalities, DNA mutations and oxidative stress contribute to ageing, the greatest risk factor for neurodegenerative diseases. Somatic mitochondrial DNA mutations have been reported in PD brain. These findings are important because the mitochondrial DNA encodes components of the respiratory transport chain complexes, and such mutations may impair efficient electron flow from NADH to molecular oxygen (Friedlich et al., 2009). Further, mitochondrial abnormalities occur early in most of the neurodegenerative disorders, and the evidence of specific interactions of disease-related proteins with mitochondria represents ultimate proof of mitochondrial involvement in neurodegeneration.

Mitochondria are targets of metal toxicity, and in many cases a close link between metal-induced oxidative stress, and damage and mitochondrial dysfunction has been established (Navarro & Boveris, 2004, Navarro & Boveris, 2009; Navarro et al., 2009, Navarro et al., 2010).

1.2.3 Transition metals toxicity

Increasing evidence indicates that metal-induced toxicity is associated with the etiology of neurodegenerative diseases. Two main mechanisms are currently considered likely to be the mechanism for redox active metals: a Haber-Weiss reaction and a depletion of major sulfhydryls, reduced glutathione and protein –SH groups (Repetto & Boveris, 2011).

The cellular and tisular levels of transition metals are apparently determined by regulatory proteins and metallochaperons that control metal capture, transport and storage. The major consequences of metal dyshomeostasis are mitochondrial dysfunction, oxidative stress and mitochondrial genomic damage which enhanced activation of the apoptotic machinery (Kozlowski et al., 2009).

Transition metals including iron (Fe) mediated oxidative damage to cellular components through the one-electron transfer called the Fenton reaction ($Fe^{2+} + H_2O_2 \longrightarrow Fe^{3+} + OH \cdot + OH^-$), which leads to production of the unstable hydroxyl radical (OH.) that will oxidize nucleic acid, protein, carbohydrate and lipid, whichever is proximate (Halliwell & Gutteridge, 1984). Disrupted iron metabolism is implicated in PD, iron levels are increased in the PD *substantia nigra*, associated with α-synuclein pathology, substantial iron deposits are associated with neuronal loss, gliosis and Lewy body pathology. Iron sequestered in

Lewy bodies and other pathobiologic pools of iron in PD brains has the potential to promote Fenton chemistry and oxidative damage to macromolecules. Evidence of oxidative damage to macromolecules is abundant in post-mortem PD tissue, with proteins, nucleic acids, lipids and sugars, all showing evidence of oxidative modification.

The mitochondria of Fe-treated rats show lower respiratory control in association with higher resting (state 4) respiration. This mitochondrial uncoupling elicited by Fe-treatment does not affect the phosphorylation efficiency or the ATP levels, indicating a mild degree of uncoupling in Fe overload (Pardo Andreau et al., 2009).

The Fe accumulation in *substantia nigra* (with up to 255% increases) results in oxidative stress; oxidative damage, decreased reduced glutathione levels and increased dopamine neuronal toxicity (Kozlowski et al., 2009). The Fe-induced oxidative damage to mitochondria contributes to the cellular death mechanisms, arising from a diminished respiratory chain activity and ATP production. The significant reduction in transferrin levels, observed in patients with Parkinson's diseases, is a factor contributing to increase Fe concentrations (Kozlowski et al., 2009; Spencer et al., 2011).

Fe and Cu are prevalent in human tissues, including the brain, and altered levels of these essential metals have been found in brain tissues of patients with neurodegenerative diseases (Repetto & Boveris, 2011). Because approximately 20% of the total Cu is stored in the nucleus, DNA is the major target for copper-catalyzed oxidations. Accumulation of oxidative DNA base modifications, produced by dopamine and other catecholamine neurotransmitters and neurotoxins, is associated with elevated copper (Cu) levels in the presence of O_2^- and H_2O_2 and potentially results from one-electron oxidation and/or the site-attack of hydroxyl radicals via a DNA-Cu(I)OOH complex. Because accumulation of oxidative DNA has been reported as a major contributing factor to genomic instability and mitochondrial dysfunction in aging and neurodegenerative disorders as Alzheimer and PD, it probably contributes to neuronal death associated with these degenerative processes (Spencer et al., 2011).

1.2.4 Oxidative stress and oxidative damage

The concept of oxidative stress is defined as an imbalance with increased oxidants or decreased antioxidants (Sies, 1991). As an imbalance situation, it implies that in the normal physiological condition there is a balance, or a controlled situation of quasi-equilibrium between oxidants and antioxidants. Oxidants are continually produced as secondary products of respiration and oxidative metabolism and antioxidants are continually reacting with oxidant molecules. In the oxidative stress condition, oxidants increase or antioxidants decrease in a progressive and continuous form, sometimes including adaptive responses that involve the synthesis of antioxidants and antioxidant enzymes and that confer elasticity and reversibility to the biological situation of oxidative stress (Boveris et al., 2008). They defined the intracellular oxidative stress as a situation where increases of the steady-state concentrations of any intermediate produces an increase in oxidant intermediates, an increase in the chain reaction rate and a decrease in intracellular antioxidants.

The brain is particularly susceptible to oxidative stress due to its high-energy demand and the specialized redox activities of neurons. Although the brain only constitutes 2 to 3% of total body mass, it utilizes 20% of basal oxygen supplied to the body. Low level of oxidants are needed for normal cellular functions, including, but not restricted to the regulation of neuronal excitability via redox-sensitive ion channels, synaptic plasticity, gene transcription, and the activity of enzymes controlling protein phosphorylation. At higher concentrations, oxidants cause neuronal membrane damage. The biological targets of oxidants include membrane proteins, unsaturated lipids and DNA.

Oxidative stress promotes aggregation and accumulation of α-synuclein, characteristic of Parkinson's disease (Kozlowski et al., 2009; Opazo et al., 2003). The series of observed changes include glycation protein oxidation, lipid peroxidation, depletion of antioxidants and nucleic acid oxidation (Famulari et al., 1996; Gatto et al., 1996; Gatto et al., 1997; Repetto et al., 1999; Fiszman et al., 2003; Boveris et al., 2008; Repetto, 2008). It has been proposed that oxidative damage favors the aggregation of α-synuclein in sporadic PD.

According to a now classical definition, antioxidants are molecules which, when present in small concentrations compared to the biomolecules that are supposed to protect, can prevent or reduce the extent of oxidative destruction of biomolecules. They can prevent initiation or intercept the lipid peroxyl radical involved in the propagation phase. In human plasma there are transition metal binding proteins in order to prevent metal catalysis; on the other side, cell membranes and lipoproteins contain lipophilic antioxidants, which are able to react with lipid peroxyl radicals, eventually terminating the chain reaction of lipid peroxidation. The implication of free radicals in various pathological processes has been detected in an increasing number of human diseases. The assay of oxidative stress parameters has brought substantial insights into the pathogenesis of many diseases in humans, by demonstrating the involvement of free radicals and/or the decrease of antioxidants.

1.2.5 Lipid peroxidation

Lipid peroxidation is a chain reaction initiated by the hydrogen substraction or addition of an oxygen radical, resulting in the oxidative damage of polyunsaturated fatty acids (PUFA). Since polyunsaturated fatty acids are more sensitive than saturated ones, it is obvious that the activated methylene (RH) bridge represents a critical target site. Molecular oxygen rapidly adds to the carbon-centered radical (R·) formed in this process, yielding to lipid peroxyl radical (ROO·). The formation of peroxyl radicals leads to the production of organic hydroperoxides, which, in turn, can subtract hydrogen from another PUFA. This reaction is termed propagation, implying that one initiating hit can result in the conversion of numerous PUFA to lipid hydroperoxides. In sequence of their appearance, alkyl, peroxyl and alkoxyl radicals are involved. The resulting fatty acid radical is stabilized by rearrangement into a conjugated diene that retains the more stable products including hydroperoxides, alcohols, aldehydes and alkanes. Lipid hydroperoxide (ROOH) is the first, comparatively stable, product of the lipid peroxidation reaction. In conditions in which lipid peroxidation is continuously initiated it gives non-radical products (PNR), destroying two radicals at a time. In the presence of transition metal ions, ROOH can give rise to the generation of radicals capable of re-initiating lipid peroxidation by redox-cycling of these metal ions (Halliwell & Gutteridge, 1984).

Lipid peroxidation can have significant downstream effects and possibly play a major role in cell signaling pathways. For example, the mitochondrion lipid cardiolipin makes up to 18% of the total phospholipids and 90% of the fatty acyl chains are unsaturated. Oxidation of cardiolipin may be one of the critical factors initiating apoptosis by liberating cytochrome c from the mitochondrial inner membrane and facilitating permeabilization of the outer membrane. The release of cytochrome c activates a proteolytic cascade that culminates in apoptotic cell death (Navarro & Boveris, 2009).

Many of these products can be found in biological fluids, as well as addition-derivatives of these very reactive end-products. As a result of lipid peroxidation a great variety of aldehydes can be produced, including hexanal, malondialdehyde (MDA) and 5-hydroxynonenal (Repetto, 2008). Oxidation of an endogenous antioxidant reflects an oxidative stress that is evaluated by measuring the decrease in the total level of the antioxidant or the increase in the oxidative form. The only way not to be influenced by nutritional status is to measure the ratio between oxidized and reduced antioxidants present in blood. The published literature provides compelling evidence that MDA represents a side product of enzymatic PUFA-oxygenation and a secondary end product of non enzymatic (autoxidative) fatty peroxide formation and decomposition. Conceptually, these two facts indicate that MDA is an excellent index of lipid peroxidation. With biological materials, it appears prudent to consider the TBARS test more than an empirical indicator of the potential occurrence of peroxidative lipid damage and not as a measure of lipid peroxidation (Repetto, 2008).

1.2.6 Inflammation

Among neural cells, neurons are particularly vulnerable to oxidative damage, not only as a consequence of mitochondrial dysfunction (Boveris & Navarro, 2008), but also due to inactivation of glutamine synthetase, which reduces the uptake of glutamate by glial cells and increases glutamate availability at the synapse producing excitotoxicity. Oxidative damage to lipids and protein of neuronal membrane affects activities of membrane-bound enzymes, ion channels and receptors. Glial cell´s response to oxidative stress-mediated neurodegenerative process is extremely complex. Astrocytes may play a dual function, either protecting neurons from excitotoxicity through glutamate uptake system, or contributing to the extracellular glutamate via reversed glutamate transporter. They may contribute to the inflammatory response by transforming themselves into activated microglia and also release matrix metalloproteinase's, oxidants, prostaglandin E_2 and proinflammatory cytokines such as TNF-α and IL-β1 (Farooqui & Farooqui, 2011). In addition, at the site of neurodegenerative process, neural and non-neural cells express and secrete cytokines, chemokine and complement proteins, which also play important roles in induction, propagation and maintenance of inflammatory response. Cytokines are major effectors of the inflammatory response; they produce their effects by interacting with specific membrane associated receptors. Although physiological levels of cytokines are necessary for normal neuronal function and survival, the increased secretion of cytokines during neurodegenerative process may be detrimental to neurons.

Nitric oxide (NO) is a free radical and potent biological effectors regulating blood vessel dilatation and immune function and serve as a neuronal messenger in the nervous system. Most of the effects of NO are mediated by glutamate, although in high concentrations, may act as a neurotoxin. NO can react with superoxide anion to produce peroxinitrite, an even more potent oxidant associated with lipid peroxidation and cytotoxic effects, in part through the oxidizing of tissue sulfhydrils. Metabolic alterations in circulating blood cells are widely accepted as representative of similar central nervous system changes in human PD. Increased NO release of neutrophils and decreased catalase activity in erythrocytes were observed at the beginning of PD; H_2O_2 release by neutrophils and mitochondrial impaired function may be later signs in PD (Gatto et al., 1996).

1.3 Clinical evidence of oxidative stress and damage in Parkinson's disease

Human neurodegenerative diseases are characterized by cumulative neuronal damage that leads to neurological deficits when neuronal loss reaches a critical level. Actually, the clinical evolution of patients with neurological diseases is based on psychological tests. The current hypotheses are that brain oxidative stress and damage are involved in the pathogenesis of neurodegenerative diseases such as Alzheimer's and Parkinson's diseases and non-neurodegenerative vascular dementia. Involvement of oxidative stress in the pathogenesis of PD is supported both, by postmortem studies and by studies showing the increased level of oxidative stress in the *substantia nigra pars compacta* (Boveris & Navarro, 2008). Under normal conditions, the continuous generation of oxidants is compensated by the powerful action of protective enzymes: superoxide dismutase (SOD), catalase and glutathione peroxidase. Oxidative stress may be a consequence of reduced efficiency of these endogenous antioxidants that may render PD patients more susceptible to oxidative stress. Increases of pro-oxidants, as H_2O_2 and nitric oxide (NO), and decreases of antioxidants, either enzymatic or non enzymatic compounds, are considered an indication of oxidative stress. Oxidative damage is characterized by increases in the levels of the oxidation products of macromolecules, such as thiobarbituric acid reactive substances (TBARS), and protein carbonyls.

Oxidative stress, to which neurons are highly susceptible, is also known to induce oxidative changes in human red blood cells (RBCs), *in vivo* and *in vitro* (Gatto et al., 1996; Repetto & Llesuy, 2004, Repetto, 2008). Based on the hypothesis that oxidative changes are not organ specific, their activities may be evaluated in peripheral and red blood cells.

The situation of oxidative stress evaluated by the peripheral markers of oxidative stress in the blood of neurological patients, seem to provide a reflection of the brain condition. Brain oxidative stress, with oxygen free radicals being responsible for brain damage, signals to peripheral blood, at least, through the diffusible products of lipid peroxidation. The peripheral markers provide a useful tool to determine the evolution of brain oxidative stress in neurological patients (Repetto, 2008).

2. Materials and methods

2.1 Patients

The clinic diagnostic of PD is realized in accordance with the "United Kingdom Parkinson Disease Brain Bank Criteria". Patients (n = 15, age = 66 ± 4 years) were evaluated according to the Hoehn and Yahr's scale in stages 1 to 3, and required a history of positive response to levodopa therapy. No patient presented vascular lesions on CT scanning. The controls groups (Table 1 and Table 2) consisted of 75 and 80 healthy people of 58 ± 2 years and 71 ± 10 years, respectively.

2.2 Peripheral markers of oxidative stress

Blood was obtained by venipuncture and placed into glass tubes with heparinised syringes for separation of erythrocytes or mononuclear cells.

To determine tert-butyl hydroperoxide-initiated chemiluminescence (BOOH-CL), heparinised blood samples were centrifuged at 300 g for 10 min. The plasma fraction (supernatant) was separated for evaluation of the total reactive antioxidant potential (TRAP). Mononuclear cells were discarded by aspiration. Erythrocytes were suspended in saline solution 0.9 % P/V NaCl and were washed three times by centrifugation at 300 g with the same saline solution at 25 °C, and then diluted 1/10 in 1 mM acetic acid and 4 mM magnesium sulfate. The protein concentration was determines with the Folin reagent, using bovine serum albumin (grade III) as the standard.

The peripheral markers of oxidative stress assayed were:

2.2.1 Tert-butyl hydroperoxide initiated chemiluminescence (BOOH-CL)

The increased values of BOOH-CL indicate the occurrence of oxidative stress in the membrane of the erythrocytes due to consume of the endogenous antioxidants. The chemiluminescence associated to lipid peroxidation (BOOH-CL) was measured with a Packard Tricarb model 3355 liquid scintillation counter in the out-of-coincidence mode. This assay estimates indirectly and with high sensitivity the tissue levels of α-tocopherol by inhibition of the propagation step of lipid peroxidation, as discussed by González Flecha et al. (1991). Red blood cells were suspended in 4 mL of 120 mM KCl, 30 mM phosphate buffer, pH 7.40 at 0.1-0.2 mg protein/mL. Low-potassium glass vials of 25 mm diameter and 50 mm height filled with the sample suspension were used. Instrument background, in the absence of vials, was 2400 ± 60 counts per minutes (cpm) and the emission from the empty vials was 3000 ± 60 cpm. Chemiluminescence measurements were started by the addition of 3 mM tert-butyl hydroperoxide and the counting continued until a maximal level of emission was reached, usually after 20 minutes. Determinations were carried out at 30°C. The results are expressed as cpm/mg protein (González Flecha et al., 1991).

2.2.2 Plasma antioxidant capacity (TRAP)

The decreased values of TRAP in plasma indicate a reduction in the level of plasmatic hydrosoluble antioxidants (*i.e.*, GSH, uric acid, ascorbic acid and bilirubin). The total reactive antioxidant potential of plasma was measured by chemiluminescence. This assay determines total endogenous water soluble antioxidants, mainly glutathione, ascorbic acid, bilirubin and albumin uric acid in plasma. The addition of 10 μL of sample to 20 mM 2,2-azobis (2- amidinopropane) (ABAP) in 100 mM phosphate buffer, pH 7.40 and 40 μM luminol decreased the chemiluminescence to basal levels and prevented the spike of light emission for a period proportional to the amount of antioxidants present in the sample (induction time, δ). The system was calibrated with Trolox (a hydrosoluble vitamin E analogue). The results are expressed as μmoL Trolox per g of organ, or μM Trolox considering 1 g of tissue as 1 mL of water (Lissi et al., 1992).

2.2.3 Thiobarbituric acid reactive substances (TBARS)

The increase in TBARS results from augmented levels of systemic and neuronal hydroperoxides that lead to an increment in lipid peroxidation. TBARS was assayed by the spectrophotometric determination as described by Fraga et al. (1988). Thiobarbituric acid reacts with malondialdehyde, a product of lipid peroxidation, showing maximal absorbance at 535 nm. The reaction mixture consists of 1 mL of plasma, 1 mL of 120 mM KCl, 1 mL of 30 mM phosphate buffer, pH 7.40, 0.05 mL of buthylhydroxytoluene 4 % w/v in ethanol, 1 ml of thrichloroacetic acid 20 % w/v and 1 mL thiobarbituric acid 0.7 % w/v. The deproteinized mixture was heated at 100 °C for 20 minutes. Results ($E = 156$ mM^{-1}cm^{-1}) are expressed as nmol/L plasma (Fraga et al., 1988).

2.2.4 Cu–Zn superoxide dismutase (SOD)

An increase in the activity of the antioxidant enzyme SOD has been regarded as a marker of systemic oxidative stress, since the up-regulation of the antioxidant enzyme expression was considered as an adaptive response to the oxidative stress situation. SOD activity was determined by measuring the ability of red blood cells to inhibit the autoxidation of epinephrine at pH 10.2. The increase in absorbance at 480 nm was 0.025 U-min with no added SOD, and 50% inhibition was achieved by 46 ng/mL of bovine SOD. One unit of SOD activity was defined as the inhibition of the epinephrine oxidation rate by 50%. The inhibition was determined comparing the regression lines of autoxidation of epinephrine standard solutions against varying amounts of sample. Activity is expressed in U SOD/mg protein (Misra & Fridovich, 1972; Serra et al., 2000).

3. Results

The data given in Table 1 show the association of PD with oxidative stress. BOOH-CL was increased by 86% and TRAP values showed a decrease of 33% in PD, together with increases of 19% in TBARS and 55% in SOD, by comparison with the healthy controls (Serra et al., 2001; Repetto, 2008).

Variables	BOOH-CL (cpm/mg Hb) x 10^2	TRAP (μM Trolox)	TBARS (nmol MDA/mL)	SOD (U_{SOD}/mg prot.)
Parkinson's Disease	202 ± 10 $p < 0.001$ $n = 12$	242 ± 25 $p < 0.001$ $n = 12$	3.46 ± 0.18 $p < 0.05$ $n = 15$	15.83 ± 0.57 $p < 0.001$ $n = 15$

Table 1. BOOH-CL and TRAP in erythrocytes and plasma of patients with Parkinson's disease; TBARS in plasma and SOD in erythrocytes. Probabilities as compared against pooled healthy controls (n = 75) of comparable ages.

The concentration of non-enzymatic antioxidants decreases during oxidative damage. A lower level of antioxidants as a consequence of a previous situation of oxidative damage will correspond to a higher BOOH-CL, TBARS and SOD. These three increases are indicative of the occurrence of systemic oxidative stress.

Present results demonstrate that the BOOH-CL, TBARS, TRAP and SOD variables for determining oxidative stress and antioxidant status would be a useful tool for the biochemical and clinical evaluation of patients during the progression of the disease and clinical treatment (Repetto, 2008; Serra et al., 2009).

Chemiluminescence methods allow evaluating and quantifying the toxic oxygen species and antioxidant defenses in blood samples of the patients. They are: tert-butyl hydroperoxide initiated chemiluminescence (BOOH-CL) and total reactive antioxidant potential (TRAP).

Chemiluminescence occurs when a chemical reaction produces an electronically excited species which emits light on its return to the ground state. Singlet oxygen and triplet carbonyl compounds are the most important chemiluminescent species in lipid peroxidation of biological systems (Figure 1).

The experimental conditions defined here for BOOH-CL (Figure 1) and TRAP (Figure 2) may be used to evaluate oxidative stress in blood of patients in PD patients. The two assays appear as useful to evaluate the overall level of the non-enzymatic antioxidant defenses in the sample. The substances that constitute the non-enzymatic antioxidant defenses (α-tocopherol, ascorbic acid, retinal, uric acid, albumin, ceruloplasmin, glutathione, etc) decrease their concentration during oxidative stress due to their reaction with reactive oxygen or nitrogen species and, in consequence, their elimination.

The levels of methaemoglobin (Met-Hb) are regarded as an index of intracellular damage to the red cell, increased when α-tocopherol is consumed and the rate of lipid peroxidation is increased. Scavenging of free radicals by α-tocopherol is the first and the most critical step in defending against oxidative damage to the red cells. When α-tocopherol is adequate, GSH and ascorbic acid may complement the antioxidant functions of α-tocopherol by providing the reducing equivalents necessary for its recycling/regeneration.

On the other hand, when α-tocopherol is absent, GSH and ascorbic acid may release transitional metals from the bound forms and/or maintain metal ions in a catalytic state. Free radical generation catalyzed by transition metal ions can in turn initiate oxidative damage to cell membranes. Membrane damage leads to the release of heme compounds of the erythrocytes. The heme compounds released may further promote oxidative damage especially when reducing compounds are present.

The lower level of antioxidants as a consequence of the occurrence of oxidative stress is also sustained by higher values of chemiluminescence (Figures 1 and 2). The increase of BOOH-CL is indicative that α-tocopherol is the antioxidant consumed in erythrocytes and suggest that reactive oxygen species and lipid peroxidation catalyzed by reduced transition metals may be responsible for the onset of oxidative damage and the occurrence of systemic oxidative stress in patients suffering PD (Table 1).

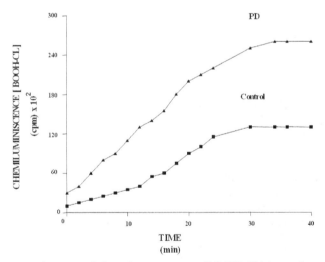

Fig. 1. Photoemission kinetics of chemiluminescence (BOOH-CL) in erythrocytes of a control subject and a PD patient.

The evolution of chemiluminescence shows that at 30 min of the beginning of the lipid peroxidation propagation step, the erythrocyte's BOOH-CL of PD patients were 3 fold greater than those observed in the control subject (control value: 100×10^2 cpm) (Figure 1). These results are in agreement with the consumption time of the endogenous hydrosoluble antioxidants in plasma, showing a 50% of decrease in the induction time in PD patients compared with control subject (control value: 4 min) (Figure 2).

As cell membranes and lipoproteins contain lipophilic antioxidants and plasma contains hydrophilic antioxidants, that are able to react with lipid peroxyl radicals, eventually terminating the chain reaction the chemiluminescence technique may be applied to study the antioxidant effect of many compounds or the presence of antioxidant molecules in a biological tissue. The reaction between a lipid and hydroperoxyl radicals with a molecule of antioxidant prevent the emission of light (González Flecha et al., 1991; Repetto, 2008).

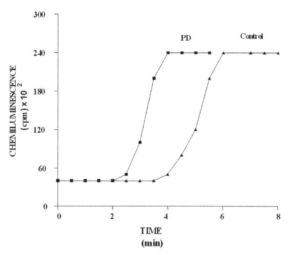

Fig. 2. Time profiles of luminol luminescence with plasma from a PD patient and a control subject.

The biological effects induced by free radicals are neutralized in vivo by antioxidative defense mechanisms, which include ascorbic acid, uric acid, α-tocopherol, carotenoids, glutathione and antioxidant enzymes. However, the extensive generation of oxygen reactive species in some pathological conditions appears to overwhelm natural defense mechanisms, thereby reducing dramatically the levels of endogenous antioxidants.

The non-enzymatic antioxidants decrease their concentration during oxidative damage. A lower level of antioxidants as a consequence of a previous situation of oxidative damage will correspond to a higher chemiluminescence. The increase of BOOH-CL is indicative of the occurrence of systemic oxidative stress.

Accordingly, there is a statistically significant decrease in the measured TRAP, suggesting that an enhanced susceptibility of erythrocytes to the oxidative stress correlates with a decrease in its antioxidant defenses (Figures 3 and 4).

Chemiluminescence is a simple method to providing tools to evaluate the clinical situation of patients, allowing quantification of the plasma antioxidant content, the correlation with the advance of the pathology, the effects of pharmacological treatments and the relative contribution of total endogenous antioxidants to the plasma.

Chemiluminescence is a collective term, which includes the emission of light by molecules which have been excited to a higher energy level as a result of a chemical reaction. Singlet oxygen or triplet carbonyl compounds are likely to be the most important chemiluminescent species in lipid peroxidation of biological systems; both of them can originate from recombination of two peroxyl radicals to a non-radical product according to Russell's mechanism by a number of chemical pathways.

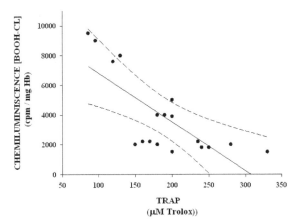

Fig. 3. Correlation between BOOH-CL in erythrocytes and TRAP in plasma of PD patients. Pearson's correlation coefficient was 0.790 ($p < 0.001$). The solid line is the linear regression ($r = -0.752$), dotted lines the 99% confidence intervals.

Although lipids in the cell are protected from autoxidation by a protein coat and/or by the presence of high concentration of antioxidants, it seems evident that some autoxidation of PUFA in cells must occur. Antioxidant status in biological samples is regarded as an indicator of oxidative stress, and in many cases low antioxidant capacity of tissue and body fluids is a consequence of increased oxidative processes (Halliwell & Gutteridge, 1984).

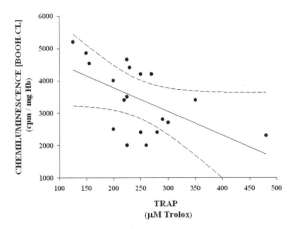

Fig. 4. Correlation between BOOH-CL in erythrocytes and TRAP in plasma of control group. Pearson's correlation coefficient was 0.600 ($p < 0.01$). The solid line is the linear regression ($r = -0.554$), dotted lines the 99% confidence intervals.

Close quantitative correspondences were found when TRAP and BOOH-CL were plotted against the Hoehn and Yahr's scale in Parkinson's patients (Figures 5 and 6).
The evidence linking neurodegenerative diseases with oxidative stress suggested that different substances might be involved in Parkinson's, Alzheimer's and Vascular diseases.

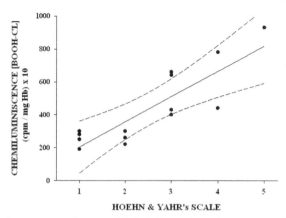

Fig. 5. Correlation between erythrocyte BOOH-CL and Hoehn and Yahr's clinical scale of PD patients (Pearson's correlation coefficient, r = 0.842, p < 0.001). The solid line is the linear regression (r = 0.857), dotted lines the 99% confidence intervals.

This hypothesis was tested using Discriminant Analysis in order to find if it is possible to separate PD, Alzheimer's disease patients (AD), Vascular dementia patients (VD) and healthy controls (C) based on the measured biochemical variables (Serra et al., 2001).
The first Discriminant Function (DF) obtained was: DF 1 = - 18.47 SOD - 1.21 CAT - 0.99 GSH - 3.42 TBARS + 2.42 TRAP - 1.12 Age + 30.23, where CAT and GSH are the values of the antioxidant enzyme catalase and the glutathione system respectively which, albeit not yielding significant differences *per se*, proved useful when included in the discriminant function.
The values assigned by this function to each observation resulted in the correct identification of 100% of PD, 94% of AD and 100% of VD as diseased subjects and 93% of the C group as healthy. It was also possible to discriminate between DAT and VD using the second DF:
DF 2 = - 1.16 SOD + 0.86 CAT + 1.34 GSH + 2.26 TBARS - 1.35 TRAP + 3.58 Age - 5.59, which correctly identified 88.9% of DAT and 73.3% of VD.

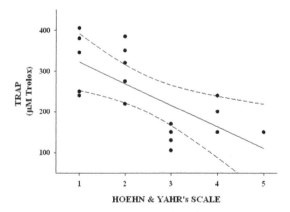

Fig. 6. Correlation between TRAP and Hoehn and Yahr's clinical scale of PD (Pearson's correlation coefficient, r = 0.890, p < 0.003). Solid line is the linear regression (r = -0.684), dotted lines the 99% confidence intervals.

The discriminant functions define four quadrants (Figure 7) with the healthy controls lying in the negative X (first Discriminant Function) region and all the diseased subjects in the positive X. The AD patients fall in the positive X and positive Y (second Discriminant Function) and the VD in the positive X and negative Y. The PD patients were not associated with any of the other groups of patients (9 were classified as AD and 6 as VD).

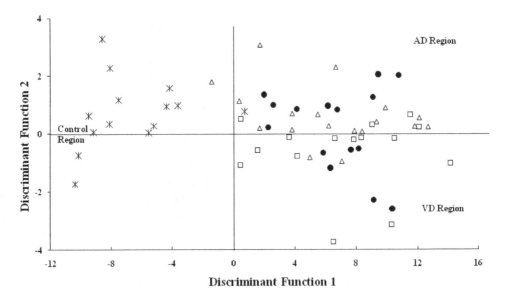

Fig. 7. Plot of pathological and control subjects on the two axes derived from Discriminant Functions. Clinical conditions are: PD patients (n = 15): Filled circles; AD Patients (n = 18): Empty triangles; VD Patients (n = 15): Empty squares; Healthy Controls (n = 14): Asterisks.

The Discriminant Function 2 correctly recognizes AD and VD, showing that these two groups might be considered as separate oxidative disorders (measured by biochemical variables of the peripheral oxidant/antioxidant system). The control and diseased regions are clearly separated, as well as AD and VD regions. PD patients are evenly distributed overlapping AD and VD, suggesting biochemical similarities with both diseases.

The peripheral antioxidant profile of PD shows a degree of overlap (already shown in Figure 7) with those of AD and VD. While dementias can be readily distinguished from each other, the PD profile might be described as intermediate between AD and VD. This might be explained noting that the main neuronal populations affected are different in each disease. Their identity (dopaminergic, noradrenergic, serotoninergic and cholinergic) is well established: mainly dopaminergic neurons die in PD and cholinergic neurons in AD patients; while VD doesn't present neuronal selectivity. The three diseases are associated with oxidative disorders predominating in different anatomical areas of the brain. An intermediate mechanism might be hypothesized for the PD patients (Serra et al., 2001).

Table 2 presents the values of the oxidant and antioxidant variables in the three neurological diseases and healthy controls studied obtained in a different protocol (Serra et al., 2009).

Group	TBARS nmol MDA/ml plasma	TRAP µM Trolox	SOD U_{SOD}/mg protein	CAT k'/ml RBC	GPx µM GPx/ml RBC
Parkinson's Disease n = 15	3.46 ± 0.18 p < 0.05	295 ± 26 p < 0.01	15.83 ± 0.57 p < 0.001	49.5 ± 3.4 N.S.	2.1 ± 0.3 N.S.
Alzheimer's Disease n = 112	3.61 ± 0.13 p < 0.001	277 ± 12 p < 0.001	17.75 ± 0.47 p < 0.001	43.9 ± 3.0 N.S.	1.8 ± 0.1 N.S.
Vascular Dementia n = 57	3.50 ± 0.12 p < 0.01	309 ± 18 p < 0.001	16.69 ± 0.61 p < 0.001	39.4 ± 3.8 N.S.	2.1 ± 0.2 N.S.
Healthy Controls n = 80	2.91 ± 0.08	410 ± 19	10.24 ± 0.28	45.8 ± 3.9	1.9 ± 0.2

Table 2. TBARS, TRAP measured in plasma, the enzymes SOD, CAT and GPx (glutathione peroxidase) measured in erythrocytes of patients with Parkinson's disease, Alzheimer's disease and Vascular dementia. Probabilities as compared against pooled healthy controls of comparable ages. RBC: Red blood cells; N.S.: non-significant differences.

As free radical stress results from an imbalance between free radical production and antioxidant system, it may be possible to measure the antioxidant levels separately or as a total global antioxidant capacity of a biological tissue. The reactive oxygen and nitrogen species are generated in living systems and oxidize a number of cellular constituents like lipids, proteins and DNA. As a consequence of this, antioxidants come into play and act as free radical scavengers, inhibit lipid peroxidation and other free radical mediated processes; they are able to protect the human body from several diseases attributed to the reaction of radicals.

Moreover, the present results show linearity between pairs of oxidative stress variables and the ordering of the neurological patients' diseases along the different regression lines pointing to the existence of an overall balance between oxidative insult, damage and protection (Table 2 and Figures 8 and 9) (Serra et al., 2009).

The linear correlations described between the three variables also include a significant negative linear correlation between plasma TRAP and erythrocyte SOD (r = -0.980, p < 0.001, not shown), which is implied by the other two relationships.

4. Conclusions

PD is a common neurodegenerative movement disorder, which affects increasing numbers of the elderly population. The disorder is characterized by a selective degeneration of dopaminergic neurons in the *substantia nigra*. Although the molecular mechanism associated with neurodegeneration in PD is not known, it is becoming increasingly evident that neuronal death in this disease is a multifactorial process that may involve monoamino oxidase-mediated abnormal dopamine metabolism, increase of iron levels, hydrogen peroxide generation, transition metal and α-synuclein dyshomeostasis, abnormal mitochondrial function and oxidative stress and damage. Free radicals have been postulated as involved

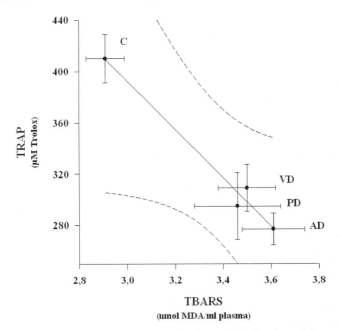

Fig. 8. Correlation between plasma TBARS and plasma TRAP values. Mean values (*points*) and standard error (*bars*), solid line is the linear regression (r = -0.989), dotted lines the 99% confidence intervals. C: healthy controls (n = 80); PD: Parkinson's disease patients (n = 15); AD: Alzheimer's disease patients (n = 112); VD: Vascular Dementia patients (n = 57) (Data from Serra et al., 2009).

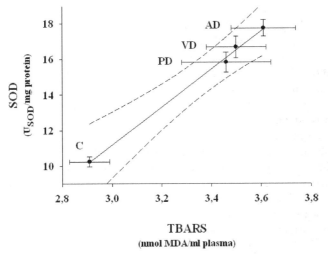

Fig. 9. Correlation between plasma TBARS and erythrocyte SOD values (r = 0.998). Statistics and abbreviations as in Figure 8 (Serra et al., 2009).

in PD disease. The concept of free radical involvement is supported by enhanced basal lipid peroxidation in *substantia nigra* (Navarro & Boveris, 2009) and plasma of PD patients, demonstrated by increased levels of TBARS and lipid peroxidation. The assay of oxidative stress parameters in plasma and red blood cells in humans is usually attempted through the determination of: a decreased in the level of antioxidants, and an increase in the by-products of free radical reactions. The increase of BOOH-CL and TBARS are indicative that α-tocopherol is the antioxidant consumed in erythrocytes and suggest that reactive oxygen species and lipid peroxidation catalyzed by reduced transition metals may be responsible for the onset of oxidative damage and the occurrence of systemic oxidative stress in PD. The levels of intracellular (GSH) and plasma antioxidants are reduced in PD patients, suggesting that changes in GSH homeostasis and metabolism are early component of the pathological process of PD. SOD increases point to the existence of oxidative insult and systemic oxidative stress, alongside with the differences indicated by markers representing conditions that change in a few days period, through a marker representing the homeostatic long term response of the bone marrow in the order of 60–80 days.

It is also interesting to note the coincidence resulting from the linear ordering of the responses in relation with the complexity of the pathologies (Figures 8 and 9), accordingly with the simple Sies scale model. *The steady-state formation of prooxidants in cells and organs is balanced by a similar rate of their consumption by antioxidants that are enzymatic and/or non-enzymatic. Oxidative stress results from imbalance in this prooxidant/antioxidant equilibrium in favor of the prooxidants* (Sies, 1991).

In pathological situations the reactive oxygen species are generated as a consequence of lipid peroxidation and may occur with α-tocopherol deficiency. In addition to containing high concentrations of polyunsaturated fatty acids and transitional metals, red blood cells are constantly being subject to various types of oxidative stress. However, red blood cells are protected by a variety of antioxidant systems, capable of preventing most of the adverse effects under normal conditions. Among the antioxidant systems, in the red cells, α-tocopherol possesses an important and unique role. α-tocopherol may protect the red cells from oxidative damage via a free radical scavenging mechanism or as a structural component of the cell membranes (Repetto, 2008).

Cellular oxidative stress and peroxidation of membrane lipids play a role in the pathogenesis of PD. A condition of systemic oxidative stress, determined in red blood cells by BOOH-CL and SOD activity, and in plasma by TBARS and TRAP, was identified in PD patients. Accordingly, there is a statistically significant decrease in the measured TRAP, suggesting that an enhanced susceptibility of erythrocytes to the oxidative stress correlates with a decrease in its antioxidant defenses. These results indicate that peripheral markers, likely reflecting neuronal conditions in red blood cells and plasma, BOOH-CL, TRAP, TBARS and SOD evaluated by the present procedures, could be a useful complementary measurement when assessing the oxidative stress condition in different clinical pathological situations. Oxidative stress is one of the risk factors, which can initiate and/or promote neurodegeneration in PD, and correlates with the severity of the disease. The concept that free radicals, lipid peroxidation and oxidative stress were involved in the neuronal abnormalities of PD was simultaneous with the recognition of complex I dysfunction in PD. The original idea of oxidative stress has been extended to oxidative and nitrative stress for the protein damage and loss of dopaminergic neurons in Parkinson's disease (Navarro et al., 2009).

5. Acknowledgment

This work was supported by grants from the University of Buenos Aires (B056) and from the PRALIB, CONICET (PIP 6320) from Argentina.

6. References

Bender, A.; Krishnan, K.J.; Morris, C.M.; Taylor, G.A.; Reeve, A.K. & Perry, R.H. (2006). High levels of mitochondrial DNA deletions in *substantia nigra* neurons in aging and Parkinson´s disease. *Nature Genetic*, Vol. 38, pp. 515-517, ISSN: 1061-4036, EISSN: 1546-1718

Boveris, A. & Navarro, A. (2008) Brain mitochondrial dysfunction in aging. *Life*, Vol. 60, No.5, pp. 308-314, ISSN: 1521-6543, EISNN: 1521-6551

Boveris, A.; Repetto, M.G.; Bustamante, J.; Boveris, A.D. & Valdez, L.B. (2008). The concept of oxidative stress in pathology. In: Álvarez, S.; Evelson, P. (ed.), *Free Radical Pathophysiology*, pp. 1-17, Transworld Research Network: Kerala, India, ISBN: 978-81-7895-311-3

Dalakas, M.C.; Fujii, M.; Li, M. & McElroy, B. (2000). The clinical spectrum of anti-GAD antibody-positive patients with stiff-person syndrome. *Neurology*, Vol. 55, pp. 1531–1535, ISSN: 1080-2371; EISSN: 1538-6899

Domínguez, R.O.; Marschoff, E.R.; Guareschi, E.M.; Repetto, M.G.; Famulari, A.L.; Pagano, M.A. & Serra, J.A. (2008). Insulin, glucose and glycated haemoglobin in Alzheimer´s and vascular dementia with and without superimposed Type II diabetes mellitus condition. *Journal of Neural Transmission*, Vol. 115, pp. 77-84, ISSN: 0300-9564, EISSN: 1435-1463

Fahn, S.; Elton, R.L. & UPDRS program members (1987). Unified Parkinson's disease Rating Scale. In: Fahn, S.; Marsden, C.D.; Goldstein, M.; Calne, D.B. (ed.). *Recent developments in Parkinson's disease*. Macmillan Healthcare Information: Florham Park, NJ, USA; Vol. 2, pp. 153–163

Famulari, A.; Marschoff, E.; Llesuy, S.; Kohan, S.; Serra, J.; Domínguez, R.; Repetto, M.G.; Reides, C. & Lustig, E.S. de (1996). Antioxidant enzymatic blood profiles associated with risk factors in Alzheimer's and vascular diseases. A predictive assay to differentiate demented subjects and controls. *Journal of the Neurological Sciences*, Vol. 141, pp. 69-78, ISSN: 0022-510X

Farooqui, T. & Farooqui, A. (2011) Lipid-mediated oxidative stress and inflammation in the pathogenesis of Parkinson´s disease. *Parkinson's disease*. DOI: 10.4061/2011/247467

Fiszman, M.; D´Eigidio, M.; Ricart, K.; Repetto, M.G.; Llesuy, S.; Borodinsky, L.; Trigo, R.; Riedstra, S.; Costa, P.; Saizar, R.; Villa, A. & Sica, R. (2003). Evidences of oxidative stress in Familial Amyloidotic Polyneuropathy Type 1. *Archives of Neurology*, Vol. 60, pp. 593-597, ISSN 0003-9942, EISSN 0375-8540

Fraga, C.; Leibovitz, B. & Tappel, A. (1988). Lipid peroxidation measured as thiobarbituric acid-reactive substances in tissue slices: characterization and comparison with homogenates and microsomes. *Free Radicals in Biology and Medicine*, Vol. 4, pp. 155-161, ISSN: 0891-5849

Friedlich, A.L.; Smith, M.A.; Zhu, X.; Takeda, A.; Nunomura, A.; Moreira, P. & Perry, G. (2009). Oxidative stress in Parkinson´s disease. *The Open Patholology Journal*, Vol. 3, pp. 38-42, ISSN: 1874-3757

Gatto, E.; Carreras, M.C.; Pargament, G.; Reides, C.; Repetto, M.G.; Llesuy, S.; Fernández
    Pardal, M. & Poderoso, J. (1996). Neutrophil function nitric oxide and blood
    oxidative stress in Parkinson's disease. *Movement Disorders*, Vol. 11, pp. 261-267,
    ISSN: 0885-3185

Gatto, E.; Carreras, C.; Pargament, G.; Riobó, N.; Reides, C.; Repetto, M.; Fernández Pardal,
    N.; Llesuy, S. & Poderoso, J. (1997). Neutrophyl function nitric oxide and blood
    oxidative stress in Parkinson´s Disease. *Focus Parkinson´s Disease*, Vol. 9, pp. 12-14

Gibb, W.R. & Lees, A.J. (1988). The relevance of the Lewy body to the pathogenesis of
    idiopathic Parkinson's disease. *Journal Neurology Neurosurgery Psychiatry*, Vol. 51,
    pp. 745-752, ISSN: 00223050. EISSN: 1468330X

González Flecha, B.; Llesuy, S. & Boveris, A. (1991). Hydroperoxide-initiated
    chemiluminescence: assay for oxidative stress in biopsies of heart, liver and muscle.
    Free Radicals in Biology and Medicine, Vol. 10, pp. 93-100, ISSN: 0891-5849

Halliwell, B. & Gutteridge, J.M.C. (1984). Oxygen toxicity, oxygen radicals, transition metals
    and disease. *Biochemical Journal*, Vol. 218, pp. 1-14, ISSN: 0264-6021

Hoehn, M.M. & Yahr, M.D. (1967). Parkinsonism: onset, progression and mortality.
    Neurology, Vol. 17, pp. 427–442, ISSN: 1080-2371; EISSN: 1538-6899

Hughes, A.J.; Ben-Shlomo, S.E.; Daniel, S.E. & Lees, A.J. (1992). What features improve the
    accuracy of clinical diagnosis in Parkinson's disease: a clinicopathological study?
    Neurology, Vol. 2, pp. 1142–1146, ISSN: 1080-2371; EISSN: 1538-6899

Kozlowski, H.; Janck-Klos, A.; Brasun, J.; Gaggelli, E.; Valensin D. & Valensin, G. (2009).
    Copper, iron, and Zinc ions homeostasis and their role in neurodegenerative
    disorders (metal uptake, transport, distribution and regulation). *Coordination
    Chemistry Review*, Vol. 253, pp. 2665-2685, ISSN: 0010- 8545

Lissi, E.; Pascual, C. & Del Castillo, M. (1992). Luminol luminescence induced by 2, 2'-Azo-
    bis (2-amidinopropane) thermolysis. *Free Radical Research Communications*, Vol. 17,
    pp. 299- 311, 1992, ISSN: 8755-0199

Lustig, E.S. de; Serra, J.A.; Kohan, S.; Canziani, G.A.; Famulari, A.L. & Domínguez, R.O.
    (1993). Copper zinc superoxide dismutase activity in red blood cells and serum in
    demented patients and in aging. *Journal of the Neurological Sciences*, Vol. 115, pp. 18-
    25, ISSN: 0022-510X

McNamara, P.; Durso, R. & Harris, E. (2007). "Machiavellianism" and frontal dysfunction:
    evidence from Parkinson's disease. *Cognitive neuropsychiatry*, Vol. 12, pp. 285-300,
    ISSN: 0264-3294, EISSN: 1464-0627

Misra, H. & Fridovich, I. (1972). The role of superoxide anion in the autooxidation of
    epinephrine and a simple assay for superoxide dismutase. *The Journal of Biological
    Chemistry*, Vol. 247, pp. 3170-3175, ISSN: ISSN 0021-9258, EISSN 1083-351X

Movement Disorder Society Task Force on Rating Scales for Parkinson's disease: The
    Unified Parkinson's Disease Rating Scale (UPDRS): status and recommendations
    (2003). *Movement Disorders*, Vol. 18, pp. 738-50, ISSN: 0885-3185

Navarro, A. & Boveris, A. (2004). Rat brain and liver mitochondria develop oxidative stress
    and lose enzymatic activities on aging. *American Journal of Physiology - Regulatory,
    Integrative and Comparative Physiology*, Vol. 287, pp. 1244-1249, ISSN: 0363-6119,
    EISSN: 1522-1490

Navarro, A.; Boveris, A.; Bández, M.J.; Sánchez-Pino, M.J.; Gómez, C.; Muntane, G. &
    Ferrer, I. (2009). Human brain cortex: mitochondrial oxidative damage and

adaptive response in Parkinson's disease and in dementia with Lewy bodies. *Free Radicals in Biology and Medicine*, Vol. 46, pp. 1574-1580, ISSN: 0891-5849

Navarro, A. & Boveris, A. (2009). Brain mitochondrial dysfunction and oxidative damage in Parkinson's disease. *Journal of Bioenergetics and Biomembranes*, Vol. 41, pp. 517-521. ISSN: 0145-479X. EISSN: 1573-6881

Navarro, A.; Bández, M.; Gómez, C.; Sánchez-Pino, M.; Repetto, M.G. & Boveris, A. (2010). Effects of rotenone and pyridaben on complex I electron transfer and on mitochondrial nitric oxide synthase functional activity. *Journal of Bioenergetics and Biomembranes*, Vol. 42, pp. 405-412, ISSN: 0145-479X. EISSN: 1573-6881

Opazo, C.; Barría, M.I.; Ruiz, F.H. & Inestrosa, N.C. (2003). Copper reduction by copper binding proteins and its relation to neurodegenerative diseases. *Biometals*, Vol. 16, pp. 91-98, ISSN: 0966-0844, EISSN: 1572-8773

Pardo Andreu, G.L; Inada, N.M.; Vercesi, A.E. & Curti, C. (2009). Uncoupling and oxidative stress in liver mitochondrial isolated from rats with acute iron overload. *Archives Toxicology*, Vol. 83, pp. 47-53, ISSN: 0340-5761, EISSN: 1432-0738

Petrozzi, L.; Ricci, G.; Giglioli, N.J.; Siciliano, G. & Mancuso, M. (2007). Mitochondria and neurodegeneration. *Bioscience Reports*, Vol. 27, pp. 87-104, ISSN: 0144-8463, EISSN: 1573-4935

Quinn N. (1989). Multiple system atrophy-the nature of the beast. *Journal Neurology Neurosurgery Psychiatry*, Vol. 52, pp. 78-89, ISSN: 00223050. EISSN: 1468330X

Repetto, M.G.; Reides, C.; Evelson, P.; Kohan, S.; Lustig, E.S. de & Llesuy, S. (1999). Peripheral markers of oxidative stress in probable Alzheimer patients. *European Journal of Clinical Investigation*, Vol. 29, pp. 643-649, ISSN: 0014-2972, EISSN: 1365-2362

Repetto, M.G. & Llesuy, S.F. (2004). Peripheral markers of oxidative stress in neurological patients. Reprinted from XIII Bienal Meeting of the Society for Free Radical Research International (SFRR). In: Boveris, A. (ed.), *Proceedings of the Society for Experimental Biology and Medicine*, John Wiley & Sons Inc Publisher: NJ, USA, pp. 251-255, ISSN: 0037-9727, EISSN: 1525-1373

Repetto, M.G. (2008). Clinical use of chemiluminescence assays for the determination of systemic oxidative stress. In: Álvarez, S.; Evelson P. (ed.), *Handbook of chemiluminescent methods in oxidative stress assessment.* Transworld Research Network: Kerala, India; pp. 163-194, ISBN: 978-81-7895-334-2

Repetto, M.G. & Boveris A. (2011). Transition metals: bioinorganic and redox reactions in biological systems. In: *Transition metals: uses and characteristics.* Nova Science Publishers Inc (ed.): New York, USA. In press, ISBN: 978-1-61761-110-0

Rossi, L.; Lombardo, M.; Ciriolo, M. & Rotilio, G. (2004). Mitochondrial dysfunction in neurodegenerative diseases associated with copper imbalance. *Neurochemical Research*, Vol. 29, pp. 493-504, ISSN: 0364-3190, EISSN: 1573-6903

Schrag, A.; Ben-Shlomo, Y. & Quinn, N. (2002). How valid is the clinical diagnosis of Parkinson's disease in the community? *Journal Neurology Neurosurgery Psychiatry*, Vol. 73, pp. 529-534, ISSN: 00223050. EISSN: 1468330X

Serra, J.A.; Marschoff, E.R.; Domínguez, R.O.; Lustig, E.S. de; Famulari, A.L.; Bartolomé, E.L. & Guareschi, E.M. (2000). Comparison of the determination of superoxide dismutase and antioxidant capacity in neurological patients using two different procedures. *Clinica Chimica Acta*, Vol. 301, pp. 87–102, ISSN: 0009-8981

Serra, J.A.; Domínguez, R.O.; Lustig, E.S. de; Guareschi, E.M.; Famulari, A.L.; Bartolomé, E.L. & Marschoff, E.R. (2001). Parkinson's disease is associated with oxidative stress: comparison of peripheral antioxidant profiles in living Parkinson's, Alzheimer's and vascular dementia patients. *Journal of Neural Transmission,* Vol. 108, pp. 1135–1148, ISSN/ISBN: 03009564

Serra, J.A.; Domínguez, R.O.; Marschoff, E.R.; Guareschi E.M.; Famulari, A.L. & Boveris, A. (2009) Systemic oxidative stress associated with the neurological diseases of aging. *Neurochemical Research,* Vol. 34, pp. 2122–2132, ISSN/ISBN: 03643190

Sies, H. (1991). Role of reactive oxygen species in biological processes. *Wiener Klinische Wochenschrift,* Vol. 69, pp. 965–968, ISSN: 1613-7671

Sigleton, A.B.; Farrer, M.; Johnson, J.; Singleton, A.; Hague, S.; Kachergus, J.; Hulihan, M.; Peuralinna, T.; Dutra, A.; Nussbaum, R.; Lincoln, S.; Crawley, A.; Hanson, M.; Maraganore, D.; Adler, C.; Cookson, M.R.; Muenter, M.; Baptista, M.; Miller, D.; Blancato, J.; Hardy, J. & Gwinn-Hardy, K. (2003). Alpha-synuclein locus triplication causes Parkinson's disease. *Science,* Vol. 302, pp. 841, ISSN: 0036-8075, EISSN 1095-9203

Spencer, W.; Jeyabalan, J.; Kichambre, S. & Gupta, R. (2011). Oxidatively generated DNA damage after Cu (II) catalysis of dopamine and related catecholamine neurotransmitters and neurotoxins: Role of reactive oxygen species. *Free Radicals in Biology and Medicine,* Vol. 50, pp. 139-147, ISSN: 0891-5849

5

Filterable Forms of *Nocardia*: An Infectious Focus in the Parkinsonian Midbrains

Shunro Kohbata[1], Ryoichi Hayashi[2],
Tomokazu Tamura[3] and Chitoshi Kadoya[4]
[1]*Gifu University,*
[2]*Shinshu University,*
[3]*Fuji National Hospital,*
[4]*Kamisone Hospital*
Japan

1. Introduction

Nocardia is a strictly aerobic gram-positive, partially acid-fast mycelial bacterium that superficially resembles the fungus (Beaman & Beaman, 1994). The bacterium causes L-dopa-responsive movement disorder accompanied by neuronal inclusions resembling Lewy bodies, suggesting a possible link between *Nocardia* and Parkinson's disease (PD) (Kohbata & Beaman, 1991). PD is a slowly progressive, acute monophasic neurological disorder with a lengthy prodromal phase before the onset and with longer duration of disease (Fearnley & Lees, 1991; Hawkes, 2008). It is characterized pathologically by neuronal loss, reactive gliosis, and Lewy bodies in the remaining neurons in the midbrain substantia nigra (Greenfield & Bosanquet, 1953). Spread of Lewy bodies occurs from the brainstem through midbrain and basal forebrain to the cerebral cortex (Braak et al., 2003). Furthermore, the transfer of the nigral lesion to fetal grafts in PD patients with fetal nigral transplantation happens (Braak & Tredici, 2008; Li, et al., 2008). The transfer experiment of the nigral lesion to experimental animals did not attain satisfactory results by using antibiotic-containing homogenizing buffer (Bethlem & Jager, 1960). PD is probably caused by an environmental agent rather than a hereditary factor. The environmental agent may be parasitic to midbrain nigral tissues and bacterial in nature. Heredity might play a role in predisposing certain individuals to PD cause.

Antibody to *Nocardia* is found in the serum of PD patients (Kohbata & Shimokawa, 1993). The 125 human brain specimen (including PD, Dementia with Lewy bodies, and other patients) is not positive for filamentous gram-positive nocardiae by Gram staining (Lu et al., 2005), though *Nocardia*-like beaded cells were present in the midbrain nigral lesions of two patients suffered from encephalitis with a parkinsonian syndrome (Bojinov, 1971 ; Kohbata & Beaman, 1991). On the other hand, an accumulation of acid-fast lipochrome bodies, morphologically identical to filterable forms of *Nocardia* (i.e., filterable nocardiae), within the neuroglia of midbrain nigral lesion is dense in the early stage of PD (Kohbata et al., 1998).

Filterable nocardiae are gram-negative, acid-fast, and PAS-positive granular cells. They are, in vitro & in vivo, morphologically characterized by gelatinous masses containing yellow-fluoresced granules under ultraviolet light when stained with acridine orange and grow to be cylindrical tubules such as that of mycelial bacterium in the presence of erythrocyte lysates. An experimental infection causes a late-onset movement disorder after a long incubation period. Filterable nocardiae, degeneratively generated from *Nocardia*, have a high predilection for erythrocytes and spread through neuroglia to neurons in the mouse brain as intracellular parasites (Kohbata et al., 2009). We attempted to investigate their isolation from the nigral tissues of patients with PD and to detect their presence in the midbrain.

2. Subjects and methods

2.1 Subjects
Six PD patients (aged 65 to 82 years; median age, 72 years) and four patients without neurological disorder (aged 60 to 70 years; median age, 65 years), serving as age-matched controls, were selected from the archives of the Department of Pathology, Chubu National

Subject	Age (yr)	Gender[a]	Duration[b] (yr)	Cause of death	Hoehn & Yahr[c]	Reference
Parkinson's disease						
PD1	65	m	2	Pneumonia	II	Kohbata et al., 1998
PD2	68	m	9	Suicidal attack	III	Kohbata et al., 1998
PD3	75	m	5	Pneumonia	V	This study
PD4	82	f	10	Leukemia	V	This study
PD5	68	f	19	Pneumonia	V	Kohbata et al., 1998
PD6	73	m	26	Choking	V	This study
Control						
C1	60	m	-	Pulmonary cancer	-	Kohbata et al., 1998
C2	61	m	-	Pulmonary cancer	-	Kohbata et al., 1998
C3	70	m	-	Pulmonary cancer	-	Kohbata et al., 1998
C4	70	m	-	Sepsis	-	This study

Table 1. Clinical characteristics in PD and control patients examined.
a, Gender; f = female, m = male.
b, Duration indicates the time from clinical diagnosis of PD to death. c, Hoehn & Yahr 1967.

Hospital (Aichi, Japan), Nagano Red-Cross Hospital (Nagano, Japan), Shinshu University (Nagano, Japan), and Fuji National Hospital (Shizuoka, Japan). Details concerning PD and control patients were shown in the Table. Two suspected PD patients (sPD; female, 78 years old, sPD2 male; 75 years old), in addition to that of PD patients 1 and 4 as shown in Table, were picked up to obtain several frozen midbrain samples of the nigral tissue. Informed consent was obtained from the patients and their family members. The privacy rights of all subjects were always observed. PD was diagnosed by neurologists on the basis of the results of neurological examinations (Kohbata et al., 1998). Paraffin-embedded tissues, serially sectioned into 5-µm sections, and then placed on glass slides according to an atlas (Haines, 1987). The sections at the level of the caudal substantia nigra were examined. The sections were stained with hematoxylin and eosin (H&E). All procedures were performed in compliance with relevant laws and institutional guidelines. The protocol was approved by the appropriate institutional committees.

2.2 Culturing of brain samples

Frozen midbrain samples, ca. one cubic cm in volume, were dissected into small pieces and inoculated into 50 ml of brain heart infusion supplemented with 0.4% (w/v) yeast extract (BYE). After one-day incubation at 37 °C with shaking (130 strokes per minute), the culture was centrifuged for 10 min at 5000 rpm. Supernatant was filtrated through a 0.45 µm and then through a 0.22 µm filter. Filtrate samples were transferred into equal volumes of BYE broth medium and incubated at 37 °C with shaking for two days. One hundred microliters of filtrate samples was inoculated into 50 ml of BYE broth medium with or without 1% (v/v) erythrocyte lysates to be incubated. Erythrocyte lysates were prepared as described previously (Kohbata et al., 2009). Culture samples at various incubation periods were applied to glass slides with a loop and fixed by heat. Samples were histochemically and immunohistochemically examined as described in 2.5. Light microscopy.

2.3 Detection of DNA in the culture samples

DNA was prepared as described previously (Kohbata, 1998; Kohbata et al., 2009). Briefly, five milliliters of extraction buffer (100 mM Tris-HCl, pH 9.0, 40 mM EDTA), 1 ml of 10% SDS, 3 ml of benzyl chloride were added to 10 ml of the culture samples or to 1 wet gram of filamentous gram-positive nocardiae within sterile tubes. For collection of filamentous gram-positive nocardiae, one milliliter of stock culture was transferred into 50 ml of BHI broth and incubated at 37 °C with rotational agitation (150 rpm) as described previously (Kohbata & Beaman, 1991). At 16 h after inoculation, the bacterial pellets were harvested by centrifugation for 15 min at 3000 rpm. The bacterial pellets were washed three times with sterile DW. The tube was vortexed and incubated at 50 °C for 30 min with shaking, ensure the two phases remained thoroughly mixed. Three milliliter of 3 M of sodium acetate, pH 5.0, was then added, and the tube was kept on ice for 15 min. After centrifugation at 5000 rpm at 4 °C for 30 min, the supernatant was collected, and DNA was precipitated with isopropanol. The samples were applied to the wells of a 0.8% gel run in TAE buffer (40 mM Tris, 20 mM acetate, 2 mM EDTA, pH 8.0). Bands were visualized by staining with ethidium bromide (1 µg/ml), destained with distilled water, and photographed. The procedure employed was as follows: A) PCR amplification. B) Restrictive digestion analysis of genome DNA. C) Subcloning of DNA. Amplification of gene fragments and polymerase chain reaction-mediated synthesis were performed as described previously (Kohbata et al., 2009). Genome

DNA was incubated for 1 hr at 37 °C in the presence of 5 U of *Eco*R1 or *Hin*d III (Nippon gene, Tokyo, Japan) according to the manufacture's instructions. The fragments produced were separated on a 0.8% gel run in TAE buffer. Several fragments were produced by complete *Hin*d III digestion. Eight fragments, each composed of nearly 1000 bases, were selected and inserted into a pUC118 (Takara, Tokyo, Japan) plasmid vector system. Purified plasmids were sequenced as described previously (Kohbata et al., 2009). Sequence analysis was performed through queries of GenBank using the Basic Local Alignment Search Tool (BLAST).

2.4 Light microscopy
Smear samples of broth cultures were Gram-stained. Via a PAS, smear samples or midbrain sections were stained. For immunostaining, smear samples or midbrain sections were stained with antiserum, the specificity of which has been already confirmed (Kohbata et al., 2009). Processing was performed according to conventional peroxidase-antiperoxidase complex or avidin-biotin complex protocols. 3, 3'-diaminobenzine was used as the chromogen. Midbrain sections of PD patients 1, 2, and 5 were stained with 0.1% acridine orange (AO, Polyscience Inc., PA., USA) in McIlvaine's buffer for 4 min. Several sections were stained with 10 µg/ml of 4, 6-diamidino-2-phenylindole (DAPI, Polyscience, PA, USA) and observed with an epifluorescence microscope (Fluorophoto VFR, Nikon, Japan) as described previously (Kohbata, 1998; Kohbata et al., 2009).

3. Results

3.1 Morphological and immunological features of filterable isolates
Several clusters composed of numerous gram-negative granules were observed in one-day cultures of PD patient 1 culture filtrates (Fig. 1A). In two-day cultures, the same granular cells were also seen. Many immunoreactive brilliant granules were present in the clusters (Fig. 1B). PAS-stained clusters were observed (Fig. 1C). Large globules composed of small red PAS-positive granules were seen in the smears from the one-day culture supplemented with erythrocyte lysates (Fig. 1D). Several clusters of gram-negative granules were also seen in one-day culture of PD patient 4 culture filtrates (Fig. 1E). In two-day cultures, similar gram-negative granules were observed. Numerous brilliant immunoreactive granules were present in brown clusters (Fig. 1F). Large globules composed of gram-negative granules were seen when supplemented with erythrocyte lysates. PAS-positive clusters were not seen. In one-day cultures from patient sPD1, many clusters of numerous gram-negative granules were observed (Fig. 1G). They were not reactive to the antiserum (Fig. 1H). Any gram-negative or gram-positive granules were not observed in one-day and two-day cultures of sPD patient 2 filtrates.

3.2 DNA genomic features of filterable isolates
Genomic DNA was detected in broth cultures PD4 (3 & 4 on Fig. 2A), but not in broth cultures PD1 (1 & 2 on Fig. 2A). PCR-mediated synthesis failed to amplify the 16S rDNA of filterable organisms. Genomic DNA digested with *Eco*R1 or *Hin*d III revealed a profile (4 & 5 on Fig. 2B) different from that of *Nocardia*. Eight fragment sequences were analyzed. The 4295-base genome was AT-rich, with a G+C content of 41%. G+C content in each fragment varied from 39 to 48%. Most fragments contained several A/T homopolymers. One of these fragments revealed that the genome was AT-rich with a G+C content of 40%; it contained six

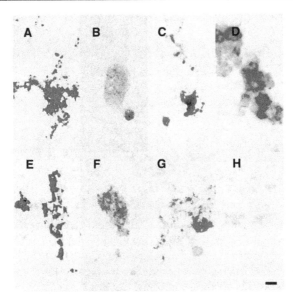

Fig. 1. Light micrographs of broth cultures. Gram-stained (A), immunostained (B), and PAS-stained (C) smears of BYE broth cultures at one day after inoculation of PD1 culture filtrates. PAS-stained smears of BYE broth medium inoculated with PD1 filtrates when supplemented with erythrocyte lysates (D). Gram-stained (E) and immunostained (F) smears of BYE broth cultures at one day after inoculation of PD4 culture filtrates. Gram-stained (G) and immunostained (H) smears of BYE broth cultures at one day after inoculation of suspected PD1 culture filtrates. Panel A through H are the same magnification (bar = 10 μm).

tetramers and three pentamers of adenine or thymine within its 679-base sequence. BLAST analysis indicated that each fragment sequence bore no similarity to genes found in any other sequenced organisms.

3.3 Eosinophilic and immunoreactive inclusion-bearing midbrain neurons of the VL pars compacta and central gray area of PD patient 1

Neurons harbored eosinophilic inclusions such as a peripheral halo with eosinophilic body (Fig. 3A), with small eosinophilic body (Fig. 3B), with eosinophilic body containing a dense center (Fig. 3C), and with double eosinophilic dense bodies (Fig. 3D). Each of next immunostained sections revealed reactive inclusion bodies (Fig. 3E), reactive granular inclusions (Fig. 3F), inclusion bodies with reactive peripheries (Fig. 3G), and tubule-like bodies with reactive peripheries (Fig. 3H). Inclusion bodies within midbrain neurons were negative on several sections stained with PAS.

3.4 Neurons harboring immunoreactive, PAS-positive inclusions and degenerative neurons in the pars compacta of PD patient 2

Immunoreactive and PAS-positive inclusions occupied one half of the neuronal cytoplasm (Figs. 4A & 4B). Immunoreactive corpora were composed of a deformed portion (arrowheads on Fig. 4A). Red inclusions within shrunken pigmented neurons and partially

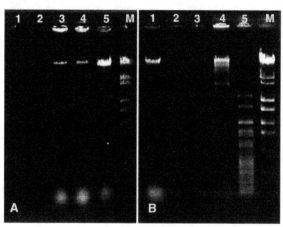

Fig. 2. Genome DNAs in the broth cultures. Detection of genomic DNA (A). 1; 1-day culture of PD1. 2; 2-day culture of PD1. 3; 1-day culture of PD4. 4; 2-day culture of PD4. 5; genomic DNA of *Nocardia*. M; marker 6 (Wako, Tokyo, Japan). Restrictive digestion analysis using *Eco*R1 and *Hind* III (B). 1; genomic DNA of *Nocardia*. 2; digested genomic DNA of *Nocardia* with *Eco*R1. 3; digested genomic DNA of *Nocardia* with *Hind* III. 4; digested genomic DNA of filterable organisms collected from patient PD4 with *Eco*R1. 5; digested genomic DNA of filterable organisms collected from patient PD4 with *Hind* III. M; marker 6. The preparation method is described in the text.

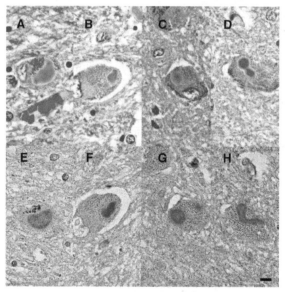

Fig. 3. Light micrograph of the VL pars compacta and the central gray area neurons of patient PD1. H&E-stained sections of the VL pars compacta (A) and of the central gray area (B, C, and D). Immunostained sections of the VL pars compacta (E) and of the central gray area (F, G, and H). Magnification of panels a through h is the same (bar = 10 μm).

red-colored ring-like inclusions within pigmented neurons were observed (Figs. 4C & 4D). The cytoplasm was filled with numerous brilliant brown granules. The same granules were deposited in neuroglia (Fig. 4E). Numerous brown granules were localized within the neuronal cytoplasm (Fig. 4F). One half of the cytoplasm was occupied by granule-containing gelatinous masses composed of a deformed portion (arrowheads on Fig. 4G).

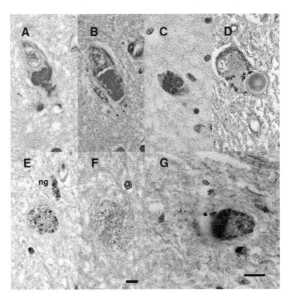

Fig. 4. Light micrographs of the VM and VL pars compacta neurons in PD patient 2. Immunostained (A) and PAS-stained next (B) sections of the VM pars compacta. PAS-stained sections (C) of the VM pars compacta and that (D) of the VL pars compacta. Immunostained sections (E and F) of the VL pars compacta. Magnification of panels a through f is the same (bar = 10 μm). H&E-stained section (G) of the VL pars compacta. Bar = 10 μm. ng; neuroglia.

3.5 Immunoreactive and PAS-positive corpora in the VM pars compacta of the substantia nigra of PD patients

The blue spots, probably identical to astroglia, were predominantly present in the VM pars compacta of PD patient 1 (Fig. 5A). In the same location, many PAS-positive spots were present among the blue spots (Fig. 5B). In higher magnification of the nigral region shown by an arrowhead on Fig. 5A or Fig. 5B, faintly immunoreactive (Fig. 5C) and PAS-positive (Fig. 5D) corpora were seen among the blue spots of which size was similar to that of corpora. An examination of other tissue section reveals that several immunoreactive (Fig. 5E) and many PAS-positive (Fig. 5F) spots were present. In higher magnification of the nigral region shown by an arrowhead on Fig. 5E or Fig. 5F, immunoreactive granule-containing (Fig. 5G) and PAS-positive corpora (Fig. 5H) were seen. Many immunoreactive (Fig. 6A & 6E) and PAS-variable (Fig. 6B) spots were seen in PD patient 2. In higher magnification of the nigral region shown by an arrowhead on Fig. 6A, 6E, 6B or 6F, immunoreactive (Fig. 6C & 6G) or PAS-positive (Fig. 6D) granule-containing corpora were observed. Faintly PAS-positive corpora were present (Fig. 6H). Several corpora were likely

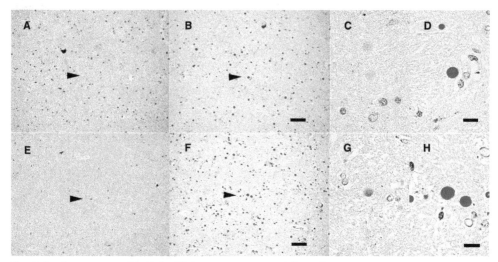

Fig. 5. Light micrographs of the VM pars compacta of the substantia nigra in PD patient 1. Immunostained sections (A, C, E, & G). PAS-stained sections (B, D, F, & H). Panels A, B, E, and F are the same magnification (bar = 50 μm). Panels C, D, G, and H are the same magnification (bar = 10 μm). The section composed of panels A through D is 120 μm-distant from other section of panels E through H in paraffin sections.

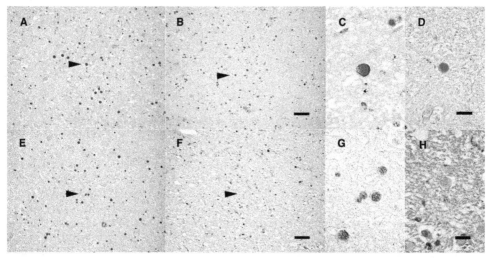

Fig. 6. Light micrographs of the VM pars compacta of the substantia nigra in PD patient 2. Immunostained sections (A, C, E & G). PAS-stained sections (B, D, F, & H). Panel A, B, E, and F are the same magnification (Bar = 50 μm). Panel C, D, G, and H are the same magnification (bar = 10 μm). The section composed of panels A through D is 285 m-distant from other section of panels E through H in paraffin sections.

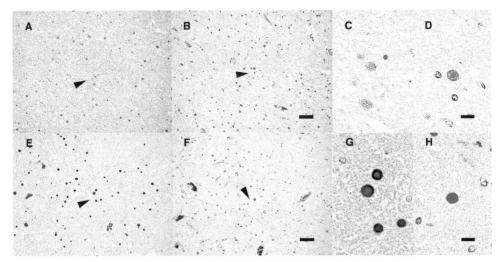

Fig. 7. Light micrographs of the VM pars compacta of the substantia nigra in PD patients 4 and 5. Immunostained sections of PD patients 4 (A & C) and 5 (E & G). PAS-stained sections of PD4 (B & D) and PD 5 (F & H). Panels A, B, E, and F are the same magnification (Bar = 50 µm). Panels C, D, G, and H are the same magnification (bar = 10 µm).

composed of immunoreactive granules. Many immunoreactive (Fig. 7A) and PAS-positive (Fig. 7B) spots were seen in PD patient 4. In higher magnification of the nigral region shown by an arrowhead on Figs. 7A or 7B, immunoreactive and PAS-positive granule-containing corpora were observed (Figs. 7 C & 7D). The same corpora were present in the VM compacta of PD patient 3. Many immunoreactive (Fig. 7E) and PAS-positive (Fig. 7F) spots were seen. In higher magnification of the nigral region shown by arrowhead on Fig, 7E or Fig. 7F, immunoreactive and PAS-positive corpora were observed (Figs. 7G & 7H). The same corpora were present in PD patient 6. A few immunoreactive spots were seen (Fig. 8A), but PAS-positive spots were not evident (Fig. 8B). In higher magnification of the nigral region shown by an arrowhead on Fig. 8A or Fig. 8B, immunoreactive (Fig. 8C) or pink-colored (Fig. 8D) corpora were present in control patient 1. In control patient 2, several immunoreactive (Fig. 8E) and PAS-positive (Fig. 8F) spots were seen. In higher magnification of the nigral region shown by an arrowhead on Fig. 8E or Fig. 8F, immunoreactive granule-containing (Fig. 8G) and pink-colored (Fig. 8H) corpora were observed. The same corpora were seen sparsely present in the substantia nigra of control patients 3 and 4.

3.6 PAS-positive corpora and gelatinous mass harboring acid-fast or AO-positive granules in the midbrain of PD patient 1

Many PAS-positive granule-bearing neuroglia (arrows on Fig. 9A), clusters of PAS-positive granules (Fig. 9B), PAS-positive large corpora (Fig. 9C), and acid-fast granule-containing gelatinous masses (Fig. 9D) were present in the VL pars compacta. When stained with AO, many fluorescent granules variable in size were seen within corpora (Fig. 9E). Near an autofluorescent granule-bearing neuron (an arrow in Fig. 9F), gelatinous masses were not autofluorescent. When stained with AO they fluoresced brilliantly nearby lipofuscin-bearing neuron (an arrow in Fig. 9G) and were found to be composed of fluorescent granules of similar size at higher magnification (Fig. 9H).

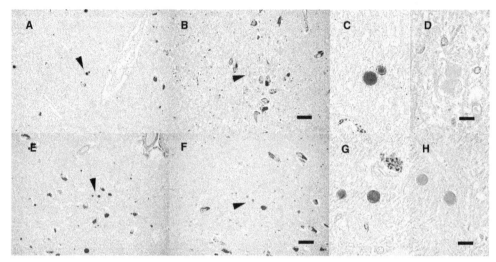

Fig. 8. Light micrographs of the VM pars compacta of the substantia nigra in control patients C1 and C2. Immunostained sections of control patients C1 (A & C) and C2 (E & G). PAS-stained sections of C1 (B & D) and C2 (F & H). Panels A, B, E, and F are the same magnification (Bar = 50 μm). Panels C, D, G, and H are the same magnification (bar = 10 μm).

3.7 Neurons connected to AO-positive gelatinous masses and degenerative neurons in the pars compacta of PD patient 1

The slide sections following that shown in Fig. 9G revealed gelatinous masses connected to the same lipofuscin-bearing neurons (arrowheads on Figs. 10A & 10B). Brilliantly yellow-fluorescent neuron-like bodies were present nearby several melanin-pigmented neurons (Fig. 10C). In H&E-stained sections, they appeared as invisible ghost cells (an arrow on Fig. 10D). Under higher magnification of the VL pars compacta shown by an arrow on Fig. 10D, they were observed as gelatinous masses containing many granules (Fig. 10E).

3.8 AO- and DAPI-positive granule-containing gelatinous masses and immunoreactive corpora connected with neurites in PD patients 2, 3, and 5

AO- and DAPI-positive granules were localized within gelatinous masses in the same section of PD patient 2 (Figs. 11A and 11B). In PD patient 5, gelatinous masses containing AO- and DAPI-positive granules were also observed. Immunoreactive corpora (Fig. 11C) were observed to be connected with neurites containing PAS-positive granules on the next section (an arrowhead on Fig. 11D). Immunoreactive corpora were composed of a deformed portion (an arrowhead on Fig. 11E) where PAS-positive granule-bearing neurites connected on the next section (an arrowhead on Fig. 11F).

4. Discussion

4.1 Isolation study of the nigral tissue samples

Gram-negative, immunoreactive, and PAS-positive granular cells were observed in broth cultures of PD patient 1 filtrates. Gram-negative and immunoreactive granular cells were

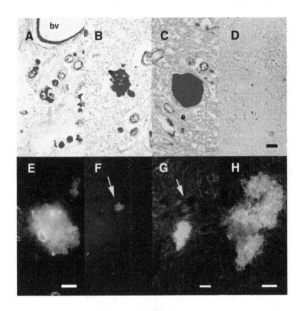

Fig. 9. Light micrographs of the VL and VM pars compacta and the central gray area of PD patient 1. PAS-stained sections (A, B, and C) and acid fast-stained section (D) of the VL pars compacta. Panels A through D are the same magnification (Bar = 10 μm). Acridine orange-stained sections from the central gray area under ultraviolet light (E). Bar = 10 μm. Unstained (F) and acridine orange-stained (G) sections from the VM pars compacta under ultraviolet light. Panels F and G are the same magnification (bar = 25 μm). Acridine orange-stained section from the VM pars compacta under ultraviolet light (H). Bar = 10 μm. bv; blood vessel.

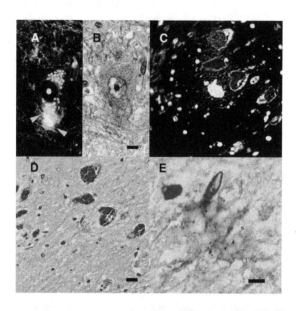

Fig. 10. Light micrographs of the different VM and VL pars compacta of PD patient 1. Acridine orange-stained (A) under ultraviolet light and H&E-stained (B) sections from the VM pars compacta. Panels A & B are the same magnification (Bar = 10 µm). Acridine orange-stained section under ultraviolet light (C) and H&E-stained (D) section from the pars compacta. Panels C and D are the same magnification (bar = 25 µm). H&E-stained section (E) from the pars compacta. Bar = 10 µm.

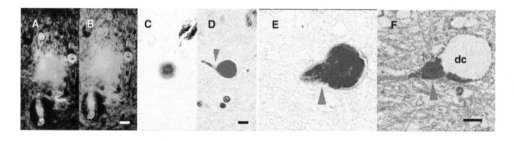

Fig. 11. Micrographs of the VM and VL pars compacta of PD patients2, 3, and 5. Acridine orange-stained (A) and DAPI-stained (B) sections of the VM pars compacta of PD2 under ultraviolet light. Panels A and B are the same magnification (bar = 10 µm). Immunostained (C) and PAS-stained (D) sections of the VM pars compacta in PD3. Panels C and D are the same magnification (bar = 10 µm). Immunostained (E) and PAS-stained (F) sections of the VL pars compacta in PD5. Panels E and F are the same magnification (bar = 10 µm). dc; detached corpora.

also observed in that of PD 4 filtrates. Both of the growth were enhanced by erythrocyte lysates supplemented. The two filterable organisms shared morphological, immunological, and physiological features with filterable nocardiae. One may postulate **first** that filterable nocardiae are likely born inside the cyst of *Nocardia* under aerated conditions and released into an environmental wind to colonize a preferable unknown site of infection (Kohbata, 1998; Kohbata et al., 2009). Filterable nocardiae may cause air-borne infection, localize within an as-yet unknown primary niche, and occupy erythrocytes as their preferred niche. Via erythrocyte, filterable nocardiae might infect other hosts horizontally or vertically. **Second**, intraerythrocytic pathogen may seed astroglia. After an invasion of astroglia, filterable nocardiae might produce cysts and preferentially multiply in the midbrain nigral tissues of PD patients, by lacking a cylindrical tubule formation. The primer, amplifying the 16S rDNA of *Nocardia*, was not effective in the detection of 16S rDNA of filterable organisms. The first trial aiming to detect of 16S rRNA, specific to gram-positive filamentous nocardiae (i.e., so-called *Nocardia*), in Lewy body-containing brain specimens did not attain satisfactory outcomes (Chapman et al., 2003; Lu et al., 2005). Filterable nocardiae might happen to be undergoing degeneration inside a new pathogenic niche.

4.2 Distribution and localization in control or PD patients

Immunoreactive and PAS-positive corpora were present in the substantia nigra of control patients. The observed corpora's morphological features are identical to those of corpora amylacea (i.e., astroglial PAS-positive inclusions). A literature reveals that corpora amylacea become microscopically detectable in the central nervous system in the first decade of life. After the age of 50, corpora amylacea increase numerous in the central nervous system (Cavanagh, 1999). Seropositivity for *Nocardia* is frequent in healthy aged as well as young subjects (Hubble et al., 1995, Kohbata & Shimokawa, 1993). Corpora amylacea are likely to be filterable nocardiae in origin. Filterable nocardiae form PAS-positive cysts at the tips of cylindrical tubules in the presence of erythrocyte lysates. Many corpora, morphologically & immunologically identical to filterable nocardiae cysts, were densely present in the substantia nigra of PD patients when compared with that of control patients. Several corpora were present in the VL pars compacta of PD patients. Gelatinous masses containing granules were connected with midbrain neurons (Figs. 10A & 10B) and present in perikarya (Fig. 4G). Immunoreactive and PAS-positive granules were present in neurites (Figs. 11C, 11D, 11E, & 11F) or perikarya (Figs. 4A & 4B). Filterable nocardiae may multiply inside astroglia, where they might invade neurons through astroglial-neuronal synapses. Immunoreactive granules were deposited in neuronal cytoplasm (Figs. 4E & 4F) as well as in various stages of Lewy body (Figs. 3E, 3F, 3G, & 3H). The gelatinous masses containing granules occupied ghost neurons (Fig. 10E). Filterable nocardiae may be involved not only in the neuronal loss but also in the Lewy body formation. Spread of Lewy bodies from the brainstem through midbrain and basal forebrain to the cerebral cortex might result from an invasion by filterable nocardiae through blood stream.

4.3 Host response to their presence

A comparison with the VL pars compacta of age-matched controls reveals that numerous melanin-pigmented neurons were absent from PD patients. The corpora in the VM pars compacta of PD patient 1 were faintly to weakly immunoreactive when compared with not only that of other PD patients but also that of control patients. In the early stage of PD, many dense clusters of acid-fast lipochrome bodies were observed. Many doughnut-like acid-fast pathogens are present on the surface or the inside of the mouse midbrain one week following the onset of movement disorder (Kohbata et al., 2009). Filterable nocardiae likely invade the midbrain substantia nigra, probably the VL pars compacta, on a massive scale from the disease onset to the early stage. Microglia, only protecting neuroglia against infection, may become activated to gather at and rapidly attack the site of infection (Verkhratsky & Butt, 2007). Faintly immunoreactive spots (Figs. 5A & 5E) may be subject to the host immune response. Filterable nocardiae's invasion and the host immune response might result in a severe loss of the VL pars compacta dopaminergic neurons, which could ensue and lead to the onset of disease. The substantia nigra of PD patients is likely to be under activated microglia in comparison to that of control patients (McGeer et al., 1998; Mirza et al., 2000). Filterable organisms, isolated from early stage PD patient 1, were PAS-positive and immunoreactive. The corpora were intensely PAS-positive and faintly immunoreactive. From the broth cultures of PAS-negative filterable organisms PD 4, sufficient amounts of genomic DNAs were obtained. Filterable organisms PD 1, under stressed conditions, were PAS-positive. The PAS-positive thick layers may inhibit yields of the genomic DNAs by using the extraction buffer.

4.4 Host intracellular digestive system

Immunoreactive and PAS-positive corpora, of which size was similar in the VM pars compacta, were different in their shape and size in the VL pars compacta. An electron microscopic study of AC-positive corpora, shown in Fig. 9E and measured as ca. 30 μm in diameter, revealed several wall-free prokaryotes measured as ca. 0.5 μm in diameter (Kohbata et al., 2005). Filterable nocardiae may penetrate perivascular astroglia, multiply to be clusters of granules with 1.0 μm in diameter and form large corpora of which diameter was 25 μm (Fig. 9C). The neuronal cytoplasm was occupied with numerous immunoreactive granules (Figs. 4E and 4F), granule-containing (Fig. 4G), and AC-positive gelatinous masses (Fig. 10E). Filterable nocardiae are not likely to be trapped into heterophagic vacuoles fused with lysosomes to be degraded, suggestive of intracellular digestive system not functional. Mutations in the glucocerebrosidase genes encoding lysosomal enzymes emerge as strong genetic determinants predisposing people to PD (Aharon-Peretz et al., 2004). Filterable organisms may be not degraded by lysosomal enzymes in astroglia as well as neurons. Corpora amylacea might be an infectious focus in the PD midbrains. Intraneuronal PAS-positive inclusions (i.e., Lafora bodies), resemble or identical with corpora amylacea, are pathologically hallmark of Lafora disease (Minassian, 2001). The digestive system of astroglia as well as neurons may be not functional by the genetic lesions including impaired autophagy and mutations in the lysosomal protein glucohydrolase (Aguado et al., 2010; Minassian el al., 2000). Lafora bodies are distributed throughout the central nervous system (Schwarz & Yanoff, 1965). Intraneuronal PAS-positive inclusions, shown in Figs. 4B & 4C, partially resemble Lafora bodies (Namba, 1968). Filterable nocardiae could potentially invade the substantia nigra, dentate nucleus, thalamus, globus pallidus, and the 3rd & 4th layers of the cerebral cortex.

4.5 Adaptation of filterable nocardiae

An intraerythrocytic pathogen may seed astroglia to form corpora amylacea through the blood-brain barrier. Ever since the first decade of life, filterable nocardiae might infect the central nervous system of normal subjects, but rapidly to be eliminated. PAS-positive granules were present within perivascular neuroglia (arrowheads on Fig. 9A). Gelatinous masses containing many acid-fast granules were present in the VL pars compacta (Fig. 9D). Acid-fast lipochrome bodies are abundantly present around blood vessels in the early stages of infection, but not in later (Kohbata et al., 1998). PAS-positive filterable nocardiae, present during all stages of PD, are likely to adapt to survive within midbrain astroglia as well as neurons. Dust-like DAPI-positive granules were present within gelatinous masses (Fig. 11B). The filterable nocardiae, as intracellular parasites, were likely to adapt and survive as PAS-, AO-, DAPI-positive, or immunoreactive small granules inside both astroglia and neurons in PD patients. DAPI staining is used for the detection of AT-rich endosymbiotic bacteria (Sun et al., 2009). *Nocardia*, closely related to *Mycobacterium*, belong to the high-G+C subdivision of gram-positive eubacteria (Woese, 1987). The leprosy-causing pathogen *Mycobacterium leprae* remains uncultivatable on artificial medium and shows a high predilection for neuroglia of the peripheral nervous system. *M. leprae* has undergone major deletions yielding a smaller genome size and lower G+C contents (Cole et al., 2001). Eight fragment sequences of filterable organisms were analyzed to be AT-rich with lower G+C contents. Most fragment contained several A/T homopolymers. The shift toward high A+T content that is common in host-restricted symbiotic bacteria leads to increased occurrence of A/T homopolymers (Moran et al., 2009). An intracellular lifestyle inside erythrocytes, astroglia, or neurons may lead to the genomic DNA degeneration by the retention of the morphological, immunological, and physiological features under host-restricted conditions. It was possible to isolate filterable organisms present in the nigral lesions for investigation of their morphological, immunological, physiological, and genomic DNA features. This will facilitate challenge and isolation studies of filterable organisms which may be a cause of PD.

5. Conclusion

An isolation study of filterable nocardiae from several frozen nigral tissue samples of PD patients was performed. A preferential site of their growth in the midbrain of six PD patients was histochemically and immunohistochemically assessed. Filterable organisms isolated from two PD patients shared the same morphological, antigenic, and physiological features with filterable nocardiae. PCR-mediated identification was not successful. The partial genomic DNAs were AT-rich with a G+C content of 41 %, containing several A/T homopolymers. Neuronal vacuoles, ghost, and shrunken nigral neurons occupied by immunoreactive, PAS-positive granules, or granule-containing gelatinous masses were present in patients with early stages of PD. Immunoreactive and PAS-positive corpora were densely distributed throughout the VM pars compacta of the substantia nigra in six PD patients. Gelatinous masses or immunoreactive corpora likely connected with midbrain neurons were observed. The results suggest that filterable organisms isolated from the nigral tissue samples likely originate from the degeneration of filterable nocardiae. Filterable nocardiae may multiply within astroglia, through which they might invade midbrain neurons, and could play a significant role in both neuronal loss and Lewy body formation.

6. Acknowledgements

We thank Dr. Ohara S (Matsumoto National Hospital, Matsumoto City, Nagano, Japan) for his help with the brain sampling. We appreciate the letter of support from European country peoples for the 0311 2011.

7. References

Aguado, C., Sarker, S., Korolchuk, VI., Criado, O., Vernia, S., Boya, P., Sanz, P., Rodriguez de Cordoba, S., Knecht, E. & Robinsztein, D.C. (2010). Laforin, the most common protein mutated in Lafora disease, regulates autophagy, *Hum Mol Genet*, Vol. 19, No. 14, pp. 2867-2876

Aharon-Peretz, J., Rosenbaum, H. & Gershoni-Baruch R. (2004). Mutations in the glucocerebrosidase gene and Parkinson's disease in Ashkenazi Jews, *New E J Med*, Vol. 351, No. 4, pp 1972-1977

Beaman, B.L. & Beaman, L. (1994). *Nocardia* species: host-parasite relationships, *Clin Microbiol Rev*, Vol. 7, No. 2, pp. 213-264

Bethlem, J. & Jager, D.H. (1960). The incidence and characteristics of Lewy bodies in idiopathic paralysis agitans (Parkinson's disease), *J Neurol Neurosurg Psychiat*, Vol. 23, pp. 74-80

Bojinov, S. (1971). Encephalitis with acute parkinsonian syndrome and bilateral inflammatory necrosis of the substantia nigra, *J Neurol Sci*, Vol. 12, No. 4, pp. 383-415

Braak, H. & Tredici, K.D. (2008). Assessing fetal nerve cell grafts in Parkinson's disease, *Nat Med*, Vol. 14, No. 5, pp. 483-485

Braak, H., Rub, U., Gai, WP. & Tredici, K.D. (2003). Idiopathic Parkinson's disease: possible routes by which vulnerable neuronal types may be subject to neuroinvasion by an unknown pathogen, *J Neural Transm*, Vol. 110, No. 5, pp. 517-536

Cavanagh, J.B. (1999). Corpora amylacea and the family of polyglucosan disease, *Brain Res Rev*, Vol 29, No. 2-3, pp. 265-95

Chapman, G., Beaman, B.L., Loeffler, D.A., Camp, D.M., Domino, E.F., Dickson, D.M., Ellis, W.G., Chen, I., Bachus, S.E. & LeWitt, P.A. (2003). In situ hybridization for detection of nocardial 16S rRNA: reactivity within intracellular inclusions in experimentally infected cynomolgus monkeys--and in Lewy body-containing human brain specimens, *Exp Neurol*, Vol. 184, No. 2, pp. 715-725

Cole, S.T., Eiglmeier, K., Parkhill, J., James, K.D., Thomson, N.R., Wheeler, P.R., Honore, N., Garnier, T., Churcher, C., Harris, D., Mungall, K., Basham, D., Brown, D., Chillingworth, T., Connor, R., Davies, R.M., Devlin, K., Duthoy, S., Feltwell, T., Fraser, A., Hamlin, N., Holroyd, S., Hornsby, T., Jagels, K., Lacroix, C., Maclean J., Moule, S., Murphy, L., Oliver, K., Quall, M.A., Rajandream, M.-A., Rutherford, K.M., Rutter, S., Seeger, K., Simon, S., Simmonds, M., Skelton, J., Squares, R., Squares, S., Stevens, K., Taylor, K., Whitehead, S., Woodward, J.R. & Barrel, B.G. (2001). Massive gene decay in the leprosy bacillus, *Nature*, Vol. 409, No. 6823, pp. 1007-1011

Fearnley, J.M. & Lees, A.J. (1991). Ageing and Parkinson's disease: substantia nigra regional selectivity, *Brain*, Vol. 114, Pt. 5, pp. 2283-2301

Greenfield, J.G. & Bosanquet, F.D. (1953). The brain-stem lesions in parkinsonism, *J Neurol Neurosurg Psychiat*, Vol. 16, No. 4, pp. 213-226

Haines, D.E. (1987). *Neuroanatomy; an atlas of structure, sections, and system* (2), Urban & Scwarzenberg, Baltimore-Munich

Hawkes, C.H. (2008). The prodromal phase of sporadic Parkinson's disease: dose it exist and is so how long is it?, *Mov Disord*, Vol. 23, No. 13, pp. 1799-1807

Hoehn, M.M. & Yahr, M.D. (1967). Parkinsonism: onset, progression, and mortality, *Neurology*, Vol. 17, No. 5, pp. 427-442

Hubble, J.P., Cao, T., Kjelstrom, J.A., Koller W.C. & Beaman, B.L. (1995). *Nocardia* species as an etiologic agent in Parkinson's disease: serological testing in a case-control study, *J Clin Microbiol*, Vol. 33, No. 10, pp. 2768-2769

Kohbata, S., Emura, S. & Kadoya, C. (2009). Filterable forms of *Nocardia*: a preferential site of infection in the mouse brain, *Microbes Infect*, Vol. 11, No. 8-9, pp. 744-752

Kohbata, S., Hayashi, R., Tamura, T., Hayashi, R. & Kadoya, C. (2005). Filterable nocardiae-like organism isolated from the midbrain nigral tissue in Parkinson's disease, *Abstracts of the 16th International Congress on Parkinson's Disease and related Disorders*, pp. 168-169, Berlin, Germany, June 5-9, 2005.

Kohbata, S., Tamura, T. & Hayashi, R. (1998). Accumulation of acid-fast lipochrome bodies in glial cells of the midbrain nigral lesion in Parkinson's disease, *Clin Diag Lab Immunol*, Vol. 5, No. 6, pp. 888-893

Kohbata, S. (1998). Tinctorial properties of spherical bodies in broth cultures of *Nocardia asteroides* GUH-2, *Microbiol Immunol*, Vol. 42, No. 3, pp. 151-157

Kohbata, S. & Shimokawa, K. (1993). Circulating antibody to *Nocardia* in the serum of patients with Parkinson's disease, *Adv Neurol*, Vol. 60, pp. 355-357

Kohbata, S. & Beaman, B.L. (1991). L-Dopa-responsive movement disorder caused by *Nocardia asteroides* localized in he brains of mice, *Infect Immunit*, Vol. 59, No. 1, pp. 181-191

Li, J-Y., Englund, E., Holton, J.L., Soulet, D., Hagell, P., Lees, A.J., Lashley, T., Quinn, N.P., Rehncrona, S., Bjorklund A., Widner, H., Revesz, T., Lindvall, O. & Brundin P. (2008). Lewy bodies in grafted neurons in subjects with Parkinson's disease suggest host to-graft disease propagation, *Nat Med*, Vol. 14, No. 5, pp. 501-503

Lu, L., Camp, D.M., Loeffler, D.A. & LeWitt, P.A. (2005). Lack of evidence for *Nocardia asteroides* in brain specimens from Lewy body-containing disorders, *Microbial Pathogenesis*, Vol. 39, No. 5-6, pp. 205-211

McGeer, P.L., Itagaki, S., Akiyama, H. & McGeer, E.G. (1988). Rate of cell death in parkinsonism indicates active neuropathological process, *Ann Neurol*, Vol. 24, No.4, pp. 574-576

Minassian, B.A. (2001). Lafora's disease: towards a clinical, pathologic, and molecular synthesis, *Pediatr Neurol*, Vol. 25, No. 1, pp. 21-29

Minassian, B.A., Ianzano L., Meloche, M., Andermann, E., Rouleau, G.A., Delgado-Escueta, A.V. & Scherer, S.W. (2000). Mutation spectrum and predicted function of laforin in Lafora's progressive myoclonus epilepsy, *Neurology*, Vol. 55, No. 3, pp. 341-346

Mirza, B., Hadberg, H., Thomsen, P. & Moos, T. (2000). The absence of reactive astrocytosis is indicative of a unique process in Parkinson's disease, *Neuroscience*, Vol. 95, No. 2, pp. 425-432

Moran, N.A., McLaughlin, H.J. & Sorek, R. (2009). The dynamics and time scale of ongoing erosion in symbiotic bacteria, *Science*, Vol. 323, No. 5912, pp. 379-382

Namba, M. (1968). Lafora disease, *Nousinkei*, Vol. 20, PP. 6-13 (in japanese).

Schwarz, G.A. & Yanoff, M. (1965). Lafora's disease, *Arch Neurol*, Vol. 12, pp. 172-188

Sun, H.Y., Noe, J., Barber, J., Coyne, R.S., Cassidy-Hanley, D., Clark, T.G., Findley, R.C. & Dickerson, H.W. (2009). Endosymbiotic bacteria in the parasitic ciliate *Ichthyophthirius*, *Appl Environ Microbiol*, Vol. 75, No. 23, pp. 7445-7452

Verkhratsky, A. & Butt, A. (2007). *Glial Neurobiology*, John Wiley & Sons, West Sussex, England

Woese, C.R. (1987). Bacterial evolution, *Microbiol Rev*, Vol. 51, No. 2, pp. 221-271

6

The Execution Step in Parkinson's Disease – On the Vicious Cycle of Mitochondrial Complex I Inhibition, Iron Dishomeostasis and Oxidative Stress

Marco T. Núñez, Pamela Urrutia,
Natalia Mena and Pabla Aguirre
University of Chile
Chile

1. Introduction

The evidence for the participation of redox-active iron and reactive oxygen species (ROS) in a number of neurodegenerative diseases, including, Huntington's disease, Alzheimer's disease, Friedreich's ataxia, Amyotrophic lateral sclerosis (ALS) and Parkinson's disease is by now unquestionable.

In particular, in the case of Parkinson's disease (PD) iron accumulation has been demonstrated in the dopaminergic neurons of the substantia nigra pars compacta and neuronal death in this area is prevented by pharmacological agents with iron chelating capacity. Other pathognomonic signs of PD include inhibition of mitochondrial complex I and decreased glutathione (GSH) content. In this chapter we will discuss the effects of complex I inhibition on Fe-S cluster synthesis and iron homeostasis, and the positive feedback loop between iron, glutathione and ROS that ends in cell death. We will also discuss the possible role of hepcidin as a mediator of inflammatory stimuli that trigger iron dishomeostasis.

2. Iron homeostasis and dishomeostasis - the role of iron transporters on iron accumulation

2.1 Iron homeostasis

The components of neuronal iron homeostasis are shown in Figure 1. The scheme includes transferrin and transferrin receptor (TfR), inflow (DMT1; SLC11A2) and efflux (ferroportin 1, FPN1) iron transporters, the iron storage protein ferritin, the ferrireductase Dcytb, responsible for the reduction of extracellular Fe^{3+} to Fe^{2+} prior to transport by DMT1, and the ferroxidase ceruloplasmin, responsible for the oxidation of Fe^{2+} after transport by FPN1 and prior to the binding by apoTf. Transferrin-bound iron uptake starts with the binding of transferrin to surface receptors, followed by internalization into the endosomal system, release of iron mediated by the acidification of the endosome, reduction possibly mediated by Steap3, and transport into the cytosol by endosomal DMT1. Once in the cytoplasm, Fe^{2+}

becomes part of the labile or reactive iron pool where it distributes to mitochondria, neuromelanin and ferritin or engages in electron exchange reactions (Kakhlon & Cabantchik, 2002; Kruszewski, 2003). All the components described in Figure 1 have been detected in the brain (Haeger et al., 2010; Moos et al., 2007; Rouault et al., 2009), with the exception of Steap3, described in erythroid precursor cells (Ohgami et al., 2005).

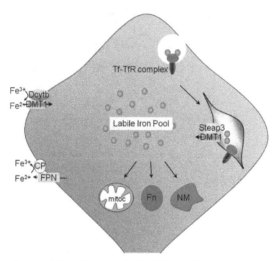

Fig. 1. **Components of neural iron homeostasis.** The molecular components comprise the transferrin-transferrin receptor complex, inflow (DMT1) and efflux (ferroportin, FPN1) iron transporters, the iron storage protein ferritin, the ferrireductase Dcytb, responsible for the reduction of Fe^{3+} prior to transport by DMT1 and the ferroxidase ceruloplasmin, responsible for the oxidation of Fe^{2+} after transport by FPN1 and prior to Fe^{3+} binding to apoTf.

The mammalian DMT1 gene undergoes alternative splicing. The 1A and 1B mRNA DMT1 variants originate from alternative splicing at the 5′ end (exons 1A and 1B), while the +IRE or –IRE variants originate from splicing on the 3′ end (exons 16/16A and 17) (Hubert & Hentze, 2002). These variants give raise to four DMT1 protein isoforms, all of them active in Fe^{2+} transport (Ludwiczek et al., 2007).

It is generally accepted that the two +IRE isoforms are post-transcriptionally regulated by the IRE/IRP system, which regulates translation of iron homeostasis proteins, which include the TfR, DMT1 and ferritin, in response to the concentration of reactive iron in the cytoplasm (Garrick & Garrick, 2009). Knowledge of differential transcriptional regulation of DMT1 expression is emerging. Both the inflammatory cytokine nuclear factor kappa B (NFκB) and the nuclear factor Y regulate DMT1(1B) expression in embryonic carcinoma cells (Paradkar & Roth, 2006). In contrast, hypoxia up regulates expression of the DMT1(1A) isoform, presumably through activation of hypoxia inducible factor 1b (HIF1b) (Lis et al., 2005; Wang et al., 2010a).

2.2 Iron essentiality in the brain

Iron is an essential element for the development of early cognitive functions. Late fetal and early postnatal iron deficiency causes learning and memory disabilities in humans that persist following iron repletion (Lozoff et al., 1996; Grantham-McGregor & Ani, 2001; Beard & Connor, 2003; Felt et al., 2006). In animal models, nutritional iron deficiency interferes with hippocampus-depending learning (McEchron & Paronish, 2005; Ranade et al., 2008) and synaptic plasticity (Jorgenson et al., 2005). These functional failings have been ascribed to the iron requirements of metabolic pathways involved in neurotransmitter synthesis and myelin formation. Enzymes involved in neurotransmitter synthesis that contain iron as a prosthetic group are recognized targets of iron deficiency (Kwik-Uribe et al., 2000; Taneja et al., 1986; Youdim et al., 1980). Tryptophan hydroxylase, required for serotonin synthesis, tyrosine hydroxylase, required for dopamine and norepinephrine synthesis, monoamine oxidases A and B involved in dopamine catabolism, glutamate decarboxylase , involved in gamma-aminobutyric acid synthesis and glutamate transaminase, involved in L-glutamate synthesis, belong to this group.

Current understanding of the molecular mechanisms underlying the essential role of iron in neuronal function is in large part unknown. Just of late, a role for iron in synaptic plasticity and the associated postsynaptic Ca^{2+} signals has begun to emerge (Hidalgo et al., 2007; Hidalgo & Núñez, 2007). Recent work has shown that in hippocampal neurons, iron chelation with desferrioxamine blocks NMDA-induced calcium signals and the ensuing ERK1/2 activation (Muñoz et al., 2011). Moreover, iron chelation decreases basal synaptic transmission and inhibits iron-induced synaptic stimulation in hippocampal slices, and also impairs sustained long-term potentiation (LTP) induced by strong stimulation. Together, these results suggest that upon NMDA receptor stimulation, iron is required for the generation of calcium signals which in turn promote ERK1/2 activation, an essential step of sustained LTP.

Iron concentration in cerebrospinal fluid (CSF) ranges between 0.2 and 1.1 μM whereas transferrin concentration is around 0.24 μM (Symons & Gutteridge, 1998; Moos & Morgan, 1998). Thus, CSF iron often exceeds the binding capacity of transferrin, and non transferrin bound iron (NTBI) uptake is expected to occur in neurons that express DMT1.

In the brain, DMT1 is expressed in hippocampal pyramidal and granule cells, cerebellar granule cells, pyramidal cells of the piriform cortex, substantia nigra and the ventral portion of the anterior olfactory nucleus, striatum, cerebellum, hippocampus and thalamus, as well as in vascular cells throughout the brain and ependymal cells in the third ventricle (Gunshin et al., 1997; Williams et al., 2000; Burdo et al., 2001).

The pervasive presence of DMT1 in neurons suggests that this transporter is necessary for their regular function (Hidalgo & Núñez, 2007; Wright & Baccarelli, 2007; Pelizzoni et al., 2011; Muñoz et al., 2011). Hippocampal neurons express the 1B, but not the 1A, isoform (Haeger et al., 2010). Since expression of the IB isoform responds to NFkB, regulation of neuronal DMT1 levels by inflammatory stimuli is possible.

2.3 Iron toxicity

Iron is an intrinsic ROS producer. When one or more of its six ligand binding sites is not tightly bound iron becomes redox-active and capable to engage in one-electron exchange reactions producing free radicals (Graf et al., 1984). This is due to the occurrence of the Haber-Weiss and Fenton reactions. The thermodynamic balance of these reactions indicates that in the reductive environment of the cell, iron, in the presence of oxygen, catalyzes the consumption of GSH and the production of the hydroxyl radical (Halliwell, 2006b; Bórquez et al., 2008). In dopaminergic cells, another source of free radicals derives from the non-enzymatic oxidation of dopamine mediated by redox-active iron, resulting in semiquinones and H_2O_2 production (Zoccarato et al., 2005). Thus, iron, both through the Fenton reaction or by dopamine oxidation, is a dangerous pro-oxidant agent.

Overwhelming evidence indicates that iron accumulation is a common feature of a number of neurodegenerative disorders of the central nervous system that include Huntington's disease, Alzheimer's disease, Friedreich's ataxia, Amyotrophic lateral sclerosis (ALS) and Parkinson's disease (Jellinger, 1999; Sayre et al., 2000; Bartzokis et al., 2000; Perry et al., 2003; Zecca et al., 2004; Berg & Youdim, 2006; Wilson, 2006; Weinreb et al., 2011).

Iron accumulation has been demonstrated in the dopaminergic neurons of the substantia nigra pars compacta (Youdim et al., 1989; Hirsch et al., 1991; Gorell et al., 1995; Vymazal et al., 1999). Interestingly, 1-methyl-4-phenyl-1,2,3,6-tetrahydropyridine (MPTP), a drug that causes experimental Parkinson's disease up regulates DMT1(+IRE) protein expression in mice ventral mesencephalon, where it increases neuronal death presumably through abnormal increases in cellular iron content (Salazar et al., 2008; Jiang et al., 2010). Additionally, DMT1(-IRE) mediates L-DOPA neurotoxicity in primary cortical neurons (Du et al., 2009).

The position of iron dishomeostasis in the progression of events leading to neuronal death is unknown, since iron accumulation has been detected in tissue from patients who have died after the final steps of the pathology. Nevertheless, since neuronal death caused by MPTP or 6-hydroxydopamine intoxication is blocked by pharmacologic or genetic chelation of iron (Kaur et al., 2003; Shachar et al., 2004; Youdim et al., 2004; Youdim & Buccafusco, 2005; Zheng et al., 2010) or by dysfunction of the iron transporter DMT1 (Salazar et al., 2008), it is possible that iron dishomeostasis takes place in the late stages of the disease as part of a vicious cycle resulting in uncontrolled oxidative damage and cell death. A recent study in mecencephalic dopaminergic neurons shows that low (0.25-0.5 μM) concentrations of MPP+, the active metabolite of MPTP and a potent mitochondrial complex I inhibitor, induces neuritic tree collapse without loss of cell viability (Gómez et al., 2010). This collapse was effectively prevented by decreasing iron supply or by the addition of antioxidants. Thus, it seems plausible that increased intracellular iron is involved in the early steps of dopaminergic neuron dysfunction.

Iron toxicity is not restricted to dopaminergic neurons. Neurotoxic concentrations of NMDA induces iron-induced the NO-Dexras1-PAP7 signaling cascade in glutamatergic PC12 cells. Upon activation, PAP7 binds to intracellular DMT1 and relocates it to the plasma membrane. Increased intracellular iron, the physiological function of DMT1, increases the production of hydroxyl radicals. Thus, the DMT1-iron uptake-hydroxyl radical signaling pathway appears to mediate NMDA neurotoxicity (Cheah et al., 2006).

3. Decreased mitochondrial Fe-S cluster synthesis as a consequence of complex I dysfunction

3.1 Mitochondrial complex I inhibition in PD

Decreased activity of mitochondrial complex I, found in post-mortem tissue of PD patients (Schapira et al., 1990; Tretter et al., 2004; Banerjee et al., 2009; Hattingen et al., 2009), is probably a founding event in neuronal death. Interestingly, this phenotype is replicated in experimental PD induced by MPTP intoxication, which induces parkinsonian symptoms in mice, primates and humans. Inhibition of complex I leads to impaired mitochondrial ATP production and an accelerated production ROS (Langston et al., 1983; Singer & Ramsay, 1990; Scotcher et al., 1990; Noll et al., 1992).

The association between complex I inhibition and PD is further supported by the observation that rats intoxicated with the selective inhibitor of complex I rotenone, develop a syndrome similar to PD, characterized by neuronal degeneration and the formation of inclusion bodies rich in alpha-synuclein (Betarbet et al., 2000). Likewise, inhibition of glutaredoxin 2, an enzyme involved in Fe-S synthesis, produced an alteration in iron metabolism in a model of Parkinson's disease (Lee et al., 2009). Additionally, mutations in mitochondrial proteins PINK-1 and DJ-1 result in a genetic form of PD, leading further support for an important role of mitochondria in PD neurodegeneration (Bonifati et al., 2003; Valente et al., 2004; Blackinton et al., 2005).

ROS seem to have a negative effect on complex I activity. Experiments with isolated synaptosomal mitochondria revealed that low concentrations of H_2O_2 decrease complex I activity by 10%. This relatively minor effect of H_2O_2 was additive to partial inhibition of complex I induced by low (5 nM-1 μM) concentrations of rotenone (Chinopoulos & Adam-Vizi, 2001). Similarly, sub-mitochondrial particles exposed to O_2^-, H_2O_2, or $\cdot OH$ presented decreased activity of NADH dehydrogenase, a marker of complex I activity (Zhang et al., 1990). Thus, an initial inhibition of complex I could generate a positive loop between ROS generation and further complex I inhibition.

3.2 Mitochondrial iron-sulfur cluster synthesis

By being the locus of heme and iron-sulfur (Fe-S) clusters synthesis, the mitochondria is an essential organelle for cell iron homeostasis (Rouault & Tong, 2005). Fe-S clusters, formed by the tetrahedral coordination of sulfur groups with Fe atoms, are small inorganic cofactors believed to be the first catalysts in the evolution of macromolecules. In eukaryotes the most common species of Fe-S clusters are the 2Fe-2S and 4Fe-4S forms (Rouault & Tong, 2005; Lill & Muhlenhoff, 2008; Ye & Rouault, 2010). Today, Fe-S clusters are found as prostetic groups of a wide range of proteins. In mitochondria, proteins such as NADH dehydrogenase (complex I), succinate dehydrogenase (complex II), cytochrome c reductase (complex III) and aconitase contain Fe-S clusters. Fe-S clusters are also exported to cytosol for incorporation into cytoplasmic proteins that require them, such as aconitase, xanthine oxidase, glutamine phosphoribosyl pyrophosphate amidotransferase and nuclear proteins involved in DNA repair (Martelli et al., 2007). For a compendium of Fe-S clusters see The Prosthetic Groups and Metal Ions in Protein Active Sites (PROMISE) http://metallo.scripps.edu/promise/MAIN.html).

The biogenesis of Fe-S clusters in mitochondria has been proposed as a sensor of the cellular Fe status, being high Fe-S cluster levels indicative of high intracellular iron concentrations and vice versa (Rouault & Tong, 2005). Additionally, the loss of function of proteins involved in mitochondrial biogenesis of the clusters or in cluster export to the cytoplasm, has been associated with deregulation of cytoplasmic Fe metabolism, mitochondrial accumulation of Fe and clinical manifestations such as sideroblastic microcytic anemia, myopathy and ataxia (Rouault & Tong, 2008). Recent data from our laboratory indicate that inhibition of complex I by rotenone results in decreased synthesis of Fe-S clusters, as shown by the decreased activity of the Fe-S cluster-containing enzymes cytosolic aconitase, mitochondrial aconitase, xanthine oxidase and glutamyl phosphoribosyltransferase as well as the activation of cytosolic Iron Regulatory Protein 1 (IRP1) (Mena et al., 2011). We think that as a consequence of decrease synthesis of Fe-S complexes, and the consequent activation of IRP1, a decreased activity of complex I results in a false "low iron" signal that activates the iron uptake system.

In consequence, diminished Fe-S cluster synthesis could play a fundamental role in promoting the accumulation of iron observed in PD. Future research is needed to evaluate its participation in neurodegenerative diseases in which iron accumulation is observed.

4. Cell death in PD: necrosis, apoptosis or necroptosis?

The two main pathways of cell death in neurodegenerative and other ROS-related disorders are apoptosis and necrosis. Apoptosis, also termed "programmed cell death" is understood as a regulated process consisting in the activation of caspases by endogenous or external stress signals. Necrosis, morphologically characterized by a gain in cell volume, plasma membrane rupture and subsequent loss of intracellular contents, is considered as an uncontrolled form of cell death. Lately, evidence is accumulating indicating that necrotic death may be also regulated by a set of signal transduction pathways (Kroemer et al., 2009). A third cell death pathway is "necroptosis" or programmed necrosis. Necroptosis death begins by activation of death receptors and its execution involves the active disintegration of mitochondrial, lysosome and plasma membranes. Necroptosis participates in the pathogenesis of several diseases, including ischemic injury, neurodegeneration and viral infection (Vandenabeele et al., 2010). The execution step of necroptosis includes mitochondrial dysfunction, decreased ATP levels, increased oxidative stress and increased labile iron pool mediated by increased ferritin degradation (Vandenabeele et al., 2010).

While the evidence that iron overload in the brain causes necrotic death is scanty (Lobner & Ali, 2002; Maharaj et al., 2006), overwhelming evidence points to apoptosis as the most common pathway of death (Wang et al., 1998; Zaman et al., 1999; Barzilai et al., 2000; Kuperstein & Yavin, 2003; Liu et al., 2003; Zheng et al., 2005; Kooncumchoo et al., 2006; Xu et al., 2008; Kupershmidt et al., 2009; Shi et al., 2010; Ziv et al., 1997). The possible participation of necroptosis in neurodegenerative processes has not been explored but the common characteristics of redox-active iron, oxidative stress and mitochondrial dysfunction, all of which contribute to the execution of necroptosis, make possible that necroptosis may be involved in iron-associated neuronal death.

5. Inflammation and hepcidin – a nexus to iron dishomeostasis

In addition to iron accumulation, other event strongly associated with neuronal death in PD and other neurodegenerative disorders is the presence of inflammatory processes characterized by the occurrence of reactive microglia and the massive production of proinflammatory cytokines. Although both phenomena have been studied as independent events leading to the progression of disease, the recent identification in central nervous system of hepcidin, a hormone that mediates the relationship between systemic iron homeostasis and inflammation, might change our views.

5.1 Hepcidin, the master regulator of iron homeostasis

Hepcidin is a cationic peptide of 25 amino acids secreted into blood circulation by the liver. The mature peptide derives from a precursor of 84 amino acids that after two successive proteolytic cleavages generates the mature peptide. Hepcidin was initially described as a peptide with antimicrobial activity (Krause et al., 2000), however further studies revealed that it also acts as a major regulator of circulating iron levels (Nicolas et al., 2001; Pigeon et al., 2001).

Two processes contribute to the levels of circulating iron, the recycling of senescent red blood cells (RBC) and intestinal iron absorption. The recycling by spleen macrophages of heme iron from senescent RBC is the main contributor of iron to the circulation, providing about 95% of daily turnover. The recycling of RBC iron comprise the phagocytosis of senescent RBC, the release of the iron in the heme moiety of hemoglobin by heme oxygenase-1 and the subsequent release of this iron into the plasma mediated by FPN1 (De Domenico et al., 2008; Kovtunovych et al., 2010).

The physiological function of hepcidin is to down-regulate the levels of circulating iron. It does so by down-regulation of the iron exotransporter FPN1 in macrophages. The binding of hepcidin to FPN1 present in the plasma membrane of splenic macrophages induces the endocytosis of the complex and the subsequent degradation of FPN1 in the lysosome (Nemeth et al., 2004). The decreased levels of FPN1 lead to the accumulation of iron in macrophages and the decrease of circulating iron (Ganz, 2006).

Hepcidin synthesis is regulated by multiple stimuli that have an effect in the regulation of circulating iron levels: (i) increased iron levels induce an increase in hepcidin synthesis in the liver through a mechanism that depends on transferrin receptor 1 and 2, the hemochromatosis protein (HFE) and hemojuvelin/BMP (De Domenico et al., 2007; Gao et al., 2010); (ii) erythropoietin, a hormone that stimulates red blood cell production. Erythropoietin blocks hepcidin synthesis in order to increase circulating levels of iron necessary for hemoglobin synthesis (Wrighting & Andrew, 2006; Pinto et al., 2008); (iii) inflammatory stimuli, mainly the cytokine IL-6, that through stimulation of hepcidin synthesis reduces circulating levels of iron, preventing its use for the proliferation of pathogens (Wrighting & Andrews, 2006) and (iv) hypoxia, that through activation of the hypoxia inducible factor I down-regulates the synthesis of hepcidin in order to increase blood iron levels required for the synthesis of heme in new red blood cells, to counteract oxygen deprivation (Peyssonnaux et al., 2007).

The interaction of hepcidin with FPN1 generates an antiinflammatory response. Binding of hepcidin to FPN1 induces the recruitment and activation of the tyrosine kinase Janus kinase 2 (JAK-2) (De Domenico et al., 2009), which phosphorylates FPN1 in 2 adjacent tyrosines present in a cytosolic loop. Activation of JAK-2 allows for the phosphorylation and translocation to the nucleus of signal transducer and activator of transcription 3 (STAT-3), which induces the expression of genes that encode for proteins whose role is to suppress the inflammatory response (De Domenico et al., 2010a). Within them are the receptor for interleukin 17, a cytokine with antiinflammatory properties and the suppressor of cytokine signaling 3 (SOCS-3) (De Domenico et al., 2010b), a modulator that inhibits the transduction pathways associated with receptors for proinflammatory cytokines IL-6 and tumor necrosis factor-alpha (Croker et al., 2008).

5.2 Hepcidin expression in the CNS

Hepcidin shows a wide distribution in the CNS, most notably in the midbrain, with a clear presence in the superior colliculus, the geniculate nucleus, some fiber bundles of the substantia nigra pars reticulata and the substantia nigra pars compacta (Zechel et al., 2006) and the striatum (Wang et al., 2010b). Hepcidin is expressed mainly in glial cells, as well as in neurons and endothelial cells of choroid plexus (Zechel et al., 2006; Marques et al., 2009).

Hepcidin expression changes with age: increased mRNA levels of hepcidin in cortex, striatum and hippocampus have been observed with aging (Wang et al., 2010b).

As stated above, hepcidin synthesis is induced by inflammatory stimuli. Bacterial lipopolisaccharide (LPS), a potent inflammatory agent, induces liver hepcidin expression. LPS also increases hepcidin expression in the brain. After an intraperitoneal injection of LPS, a transient transcription of the gene for hepcidin ensues in the choroid plexus, which correlates with increased levels of pro-hepcidin in the cerebrospinal fluid (Marques et al., 2009). The highest hepcidin expression was observed at 3 hours returning to baseline levels 24 hours after the injection. Interestingly, LPS treatment induces a 10-fold increase in hepcidin expression in the substantia nigra (Wang et al., 2008), which correlates with a marked increase in iron levels observed in this region in PD.

5.3 FPN1 expression in the CNS
As described above, the iron transporter FPN1 is the receptor for hepcidin. The expression of this transporter-receptor in mouse brain is quite ubiquitous; it is present in oligodendrocytes, microglia, astrocytes and neurons (Song et al., 2010). Space-temporal expression of FPN1 in neurons is variable (Moos & Rosengren Nielsen, 2006). In young brain a high immunoreactivity is found in the neurons of the hippocampus and striatum (cell bodies and in projection fibers), a mild expression in the substantia nigra pars compacta and the superior colliculus and low expression in the substantia nigra pars reticulata (Boserup et al., 2011). In the adult brain, FPN1 immunoreactivity is lower in the projections of the striatum, but no differences have been found in neuronal cell bodies (Moos & Rosengren Nielsen, 2006).

An interesting fact is that the spatial distribution of FPN1 and hepcidin are similar. Although the effects of hepcidin on FPN1 levels can differ according to cell type (Chaston et al., 2008), the injection of hepcidin in mice lateral cerebral ventricle, causes a decrease in the levels of FPN1 in the cerebral cortex, hippocampus and striatum (Wang et al., 2010b), suggesting that their cellular targets in the brain generate the same response than that observed in macrophages, that is, iron retention inside the cells. This conclusion is strengthened by the fact that high doses of hepcidin produce an increase in the iron storage protein ferritin, thus indicating increased cellular iron concentration in these brain areas.

Unexpected for a high cell iron situation, in the hippocampus and cortex of rats treatment with hepcidin induces the decrease of both FPN1 protein and mRNA and an increase in total DMT1 (Li et al., 2011), a situation that should drive further iron accumulation.

Hippocampal neurons in culture treated with hepcidin also show a decrease in the expression of FPN1, which is reflected in a reduction of the iron released from these cells (Wang et al., 2010b). There are no studies in other cell types, however, and it is possible that the response in glial cells should be similar to neurons and macrophages, particularly since microglia cells derive from the same precursor cells that give rise to macrophages (Ginhoux et al., 2010).

5.4 Hepcidin - a nexus between inflammation and iron accumulation in PD
Reports of some cases of PD associated with head trauma (Lees, 1997) and encephalitis (Jang et al., 2009) strongly suggest that inflammation can promote this neurodegenerative disease. Currently, there is a growing array of evidences describing inflammatory properties in the parkinsonian brain. Indeed, many cases of PD are accompanied by general inflammation of the brain, with a dramatic proliferation of reactive amoeboid macrophages and microglia HLA-DR+ in the substantia nigra (McGeer et al., 1988). In the striatum, macrophage

proliferation is accompanied by high expression of pro-inflammatory cytokines such as
TNF-α, IL-1β, IFN-γ and IL-6 (Mogi et al., 1994; Muller et al., 1998), which are expressed by
glial cells (Hirsch et al., 1998). Particularly, the presence of IL-1β, IL-6 and TNF-α has been
observed in cerebrospinal fluid and the basal ganglia of patients with PD (Nagatsu, 2002). In
addition to increased expression of inflammatory cytokines by activated microglia, factors
released by dead dopaminergic cells appear to increase the neuroinflammatory and immune
response, leading to irreversible destruction of these cells (Orr et al., 2002).

In general, pro-inflammatory cytokines such as TNF-α and IL-1 have neurotoxic effects,
while anti-inflammatory molecules are neuroprotective (Allan & Rothwell, 2001).
Intriguingly, IL-6, a classical proinflammatory cytokine, has a dual effect, at low
concentrations it protects for neuronal death while at larger concentrations it is highly toxic
(Li et al., 2009).

It is not completely understood how the inflammatory response is generated in PD. It has been
proposed that the inflammatory response is a product of the oxidative load induced by the
metabolism of dopamine (DA). Deamination of DA by monoamine oxidase generates
hydrogen peroxide (Gotz et al., 1994), whereas the not enzymatic auto-oxidation produces
additionally DA quinones and semiquinones (Stokes et al., 1999). These metabolites, in
conjunction with the highly toxic hydroxyl radical generated through the Fenton reaction, are
likely to alter protein structure and decrease glutathione levels by generating increased
oxidative stress (Halliwell, 2006a), which could lead to activation of an inflammatory response
(Park et al., 1999; Di Loreto et al., 2004). In fact, antioxidants such as green tea polyphenols are
strong inhibitors of the inflammatory response (Conner and Grisham, 1996; Singh et al., 2010),
and may reduce the incidence of dementia, AD, and PD (Mandel et al., 2011).

An inflammatory component has also been observed in several animal models of PD: the
injection of 6-hydroxydopamine, MPTP and rotenone generates microglial activation,
astrogliogenesis and secretion of inflammatory cytokines (Barnum & Tansey, 2010). The
injection of LPS, a potent inducer of inflammation, has also been used as a model of PD.
Stereotaxic injection of LPS in the nigro-striatal pathway induced a strong
macrophage/microglial reaction in substantia nigra, being the substantia nigra more
responsive than the striatum to the inflammatory stimulus (Herrera et al., 2000).
Furthermore, no detectable damage to either the GABAergic or the serotoninergic neurons
was observed, a demonstration of the particular sensitivity sustantia nigra pars compacta
neurons to inflammatory stimuli.

The abundant evidence for the existence of inflammatory processes in PD, and the induction
of hepcidin synthesis by cytoquines such as IL-6, suggest that brain hepcidin levels should
be higher in inflammatory processes. Hepcidin should induce differential iron accumulation
in the diverse cell types present in the brain, based in the different levels of expression of its
receptor, FPN1. In the adult brain, the expression of FPN1 is lower in neurons than in glia,
thus hepcidin would induce a redistribution of iron, accumulating it mainly in the glial cells,
which would act as an "iron sponge". Additionally, the activation of the signal transduction
pathway associated with the binding of hepcidin to FPN1, could reduce the inflammatory
response generated during neurodegeneration. Alternatively, the decrease in FPN1 induced
by hepcidin binding in neurons could result in increased iron accumulation and oxidative
stress, which could accelerate the death of these cells.

Future studies on the participation of hepcidin on the disregulation of iron homeostasis in
glia and neurons as a response to inflammation, will provide valuable information about its
protective or deleterious role in the progress of neurodegenerative diseases.

6. Glutathione metabolism in PD – a cause or a consequence of increased ROS and increased iron content?

The tripeptide glutathione (γ-L-glutamyl-L-cysteinylglycine) is the most abundant and the main antioxidant agent in the central nervous system, where it reaches mM concentrations (Meister & Anderson, 1983; Dringen et al., 2000). In its redox cycling, glutathione is present either in its reduced (GSH) form or its oxidized disulfide (GSSG) form, the ratio GSH/GSSG being faithful reflection of the redox state of the cell (Schafer & Buettner, 2001).

Early post-mortem studies revealed decreased levels of GSH in degenerating substantia nigra of PD patients (Perry et al., 1982; Sofic et al., 1988; Sian et al., 1994), the observation implicating that GSH depletion may play a major role in the neurodegenerative process. The question arises whether GSH depletion is an early event during the progression of the disease or a reflection of increased oxidative stress resulting, for example, from mitochondrial complex I inhibition or from iron accumulation.

Chronic sub-maximal inhibition of GSH synthesis in N27 dopaminergic cells results in about 50% inhibition of mitochondrial electron transport chain complex I without ensuing cell death, inhibition that was reversed upon removal of the inhibitor (Chinta & Andersen, 2006). Thus, increased oxidative stress generated by complex I inhibition should result in decreased GHS levels and further inhibition of complex I. Conversely, a decrease in GSH levels, provoked by unknown causes, could result in inhibition of complex I activity.

Iron induces the consumption of GSH. After exposure to increasing concentrations of iron, SH-SY5Y dopaminergic cells undergo sustained iron accumulation and a biphasic change in intracellular GSH levels, increasing at low (1-5 μM) Fe and decreasing thereafter. Indeed, cell exposure to high iron concentrations (20-80 μM) markedly decreases the GSH / GSSG molar ratio and the GSH half-cell reduction potential, which associated with loss of cell viability (Núñez et al., 2004).

It is therefore possible that a decrease in GSH levels is a consequence of the increased oxidative load produced by the increase in intracellular Fe. Nevertheless, increased iron and decreased GSH may be intertwined in a positive feedback loop, since in dopaminergic neurons the pharmacological reduction of GSH levels results in increased levels of TfR and an increased labile iron pool (Kaur et al., 2009). Thus, the question remains as to which of the three processes initiates the oxidative spiral, but a reasonable assumption is that if one of them ensues the others will follow.

7. A positive feedback loop in the death of neurons

We propose that inhibition of mitochondrial complex I by endogenous and/or exogenous toxins, and inflammatory processes produced by trauma or other causes, result in a vicious cycle of increased oxidative stress, increased iron accumulation and decreased GSH content (Figure 2). In this scheme, neuronal death linked to complex I dysfunction is brought about by a positive feedback loop in which complex I inhibition results in decreased Fe-S cluster synthesis, IRP1 activation, increased DMT1 and TfR expression and iron accumulation. Complex I dysfunction and increased cellular iron result in decreased GSH levels. Both increased oxidative stress and low GSH levels further inhibit complex I activity. Central to this scheme is the deregulation of iron homeostasis since iron chelators effectively block cell death and prevent early events in neurodegeneration such as neuritic tree shortening. Another input to this cycle is brought about by inflammatory cytoquines that induce hepcidin synthesis which, by inducing FPN1 degradation, results in increased cellular iron.

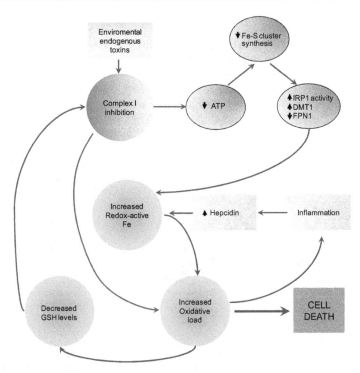

Fig. 2. **A positive feedback loop resulting in uncontrolled oxidative load.** Complex I
inhibition results in decreased levels of ATP and decreased Fe-S synthesis (see text).
Decreased Fe-S cluster synthesis results in activation of IRP1 that needs a 4Fe-4S cluster to
acquire its inactive state. Increased IRP1 activity results in increased DMT1 and transferrin
receptor and decreased FPN1 synthesis, which results in increased iron accumulation.
Increased iron induces increased oxidative stress and GSH consumption. Both increased
oxidative stress and decreased GSH produce further complex I inhibition.

8. Conclusion

Diminished activity of mitochondrial complex I, iron accumulation, oxidative stress and
inflammation are common pathognomonic signs of sporadic PD. It is possible that the
initiation of any one of these processes will initiate or enhance the others, through the
generation of positive feedback loops that will produce apoptotic neuronal death.
Intervention of these positive loops should result in prolonged life of the affected neurons.
Still unanswered is the question of why substantia nigra pars compacta neurons are so
particular prone to this disregulation.

9. Acknowledgment

This work was financed by grant 1100599 from Fondo Nacional de Ciencia y Tecnología
Chile, (FONDECYT) and by project ICM-P05-001-F from the Millennium Scientific Initiative,
Ministerio de Economía, Chile.

10. References

Allan, S. M. & Rothwell, N. J. (2001). Cytokines and acute neurodegeneration. *Nat Rev Neurosci*, Vol. 2, No. 10, (October 2001), pp. 734-744, ISSN 1471-003X

Banerjee, R., Starkov, A. A., Beal, M. F. & Thomas, B. (2009). Mitochondrial dysfunction in the limelight of Parkinson's disease pathogenesis. *Biochim Biophys Acta*, Vol. 1792, No. 7, (Decembre 2008), pp. 651-663, ISSN 0006-3002

Barnum, C. J. & Tansey, M. G. (2010). Modeling neuroinflammatory pathogenesis of Parkinson's disease. *Prog Brain Res*, Vol. 184, (October 2010), pp. 113-132, ISSN 1875-7855

Bartzokis, G., Sultzer, D., Cummings, J., Holt, L. E., Hance, D. B., Henderson, V. W. & Mintz, J. (2000). In vivo evaluation of brain iron in Alzheimer disease using magnetic resonance imaging. *Arch Gen Psychiatry*, Vol. 57, No. 1, (January 2000), pp. 47-53, ISSN 0003-990X.

Barzilai, A., Zilkha-Falb, R., Daily, D., Stern, N., Offen, D., Ziv, I., Melamed, E. & Shirvan, A. (2000). The molecular mechanism of dopamine-induced apoptosis: identification and characterization of genes that mediate dopamine toxicity. *J Neural Transm Suppl*, Vol. 60, (February 2001), pp. 59-76, ISSN 0303-6995

Beard, J. L. & Connor, J. R. (2003). Iron status and neural functioning. *Annu Rev Nutr*, Vol. 23, (April 2003), pp. 41-58, ISSN 0199-9885

Berg, D. & Youdim, M. B. (2006). Role of iron in neurodegenerative disorders. *Top Magn Reson Imaging*, Vol. 17, No. 1, (December 2006), pp. 5-17, ISSN 0899-3459

Betarbet, R., Sherer, T. B., MacKenzie, G., Garcia-Osuna, M., Panov, A. V. &Greenamyre, J. T. (2000). Chronic systemic pesticide exposure reproduces features of Parkinson's disease. *Nat Neurosci*, Vol. 3, No. 12, (December 2000), pp. 1301-1306, ISSN 1097-6256.

Blackinton, J., Ahmad, R., Miller, D. W., van der Brug, M. P., Canet-Aviles, R. M., Hague, S. M., Kaleem, M. & Cookson, M. R. (2005). Effects of DJ-1 mutations and polymorphisms on protein stability and subcellular localization. *Brain Res Mol Brain Res*, Vol. 134, No. 1, (March 2005), pp. 76-83, ISSN 0169-328X.

Bonifati, V., Rizzu, P., van Baren, M. J., Schaap, O., Breedveld, G. J., Krieger, E., Dekker, M. C., Squitieri, F., Ibanez, P., Joosse, M., van Dongen, J. W., Vanacore, N., van Swieten, J. C., Brice, A., Meco, G., van Duijn, C. M., Oostra, B. A. & Heutink, P. (2003). Mutations in the DJ-1 gene associated with autosomal recessive early-onset parkinsonism. *Science*, Vol. 299, No. 5604, (November 2002), pp. 256-259, ISSN 1095-9203.

Bórquez, D., Valdés, P. & Nuñéz, M.T. (2008). Iron Toxicity: A critical Review on its Role in Parkinson´s Disease, In: *Neurodegenerative Diseases: From Molecular Concepts to Therapeutic Targets*, Von Bernhardi, R. & Inestrosa, N., pp. 189-204, Nova Science Publishers, ISBN 978-160-4561-67-8, New York, USA.

Boserup, M. W., Lichota, J., Haile, D. & Moos, T. (2011). Heterogenous distribution of ferroportin-containing neurons in mouse brain. *Biometals*, (January 2011), ISSN 1572-8773.

Burdo, J. R., Menzies, S. L., Simpson, I. A., Garrick, L. M., Garrick, M. D., Dolan, K. G., Haile, D. J., Beard, J. L. & Connor, J. R. (2001). Distribution of divalent metal transporter 1 and metal transport protein 1 in the normal and Belgrade rat. *J Neurosci Res*, Vol. 66, No. 6, (December 2002), pp. 1198-1207, ISSN 0360-4012.

Chaston, T., Chung, B., Mascarenhas, M., Marks, J., Patel, B., Srai, S. K. & Sharp, P. (2008). Evidence for differential effects of hepcidin in macrophages and intestinal epithelial cells. *Gut*, Vol. 57, No. 3, (October 2007), pp. 374-382, ISSN 1468-3288.

Cheah, J. H., Kim, S. F., Hester, L. D., Clancy, K. W., Patterson, S. E., 3rd, Papadopoulos, V. & Snyder, S. H. (2006). NMDA receptor-nitric oxide transmission mediates neuronal iron homeostasis via the GTPase Dexras1. *Neuron*, Vol. 51, No. 4, (August 2006), pp. 431-440, ISSN 0896-6273.

Chinopoulos, C. & Adam-Vizi, V. (2001). Mitochondria deficient in complex I activity are depolarized by hydrogen peroxide in nerve terminals: relevance to Parkinson's disease. *J Neurochem*, Vol. 76, No. 1, (January 2001), pp. 302-306, ISSN 0022-3042.

Chinta, S. J. & Andersen, J. K. (2006). Reversible inhibition of mitochondrial complex I activity following chronic dopaminergic glutathione depletion in vitro: implications for Parkinson's disease. *Free Radic Biol Med*, Vol. 41, No. 9, (October 2006), pp. 1442-1448, ISSN 0891-5849.

Conner, E. M. &Grisham, M. B. (1996). Inflammation, free radicals, and antioxidants. *Nutrition*, Vol. 12, No. 4, (April 1996), pp. 274-277, ISSN 0899-9007.

Croker, B. A., Kiu, H. & Nicholson, S. E. (2008). SOCS regulation of the JAK/STAT signalling pathway. *Semin Cell Dev Biol*, Vol. 19, No. 4, (August 2008), pp. 414-422, ISSN 1084-9521.

De Domenico, I., Lo, E., Ward, D. M. & Kaplan, J. (2009). Hepcidin-induced internalization of ferroportin requires binding and cooperative interaction with Jak2. *Proc Natl Acad Sci U S A*, Vol. 106, No. 10, (February 2009), pp. 3800-3805, ISSN 1091-6490.

De Domenico, I., Lo, E., Ward, D. M. & Kaplan, J. (2010a). Human mutation D157G in ferroportin leads to hepcidin-independent binding of Jak2 and ferroportin down-regulation. *Blood*, Vol. 115, No. 14, (February 2010), pp. 2956-2959, ISSN 1528-0020.

De Domenico, I., McVey Ward, D. & Kaplan, J. (2008). Regulation of iron acquisition and storage: consequences for iron-linked disorders. *Nat Rev Mol Cell Biol*, Vol. 9, No. 1, (November 2007), pp. 72-81, ISSN 1471-0080.

De Domenico, I., Ward, D. M. & Kaplan, J. (2007). Hepcidin regulation: ironing out the details. *J Clin Invest*, Vol. 117, No. 7, (July 2007), pp. 1755-1758, ISSN 0021-9738.

De Domenico, I., Zhang, T. Y., Koening, C. L., Branch, R. W., London, N., Lo, E., Daynes, R. A., Kushner, J. P., Li, D., Ward, D. M. & Kaplan, J. (2010b). Hepcidin mediates transcriptional changes that modulate acute cytokine-induced inflammatory responses in mice. *J Clin Invest*, Vol. 120, No. 7, (June 2010), pp. 2395-2405, ISSN 1558-8238.

Di Loreto, S., Caracciolo, V., Colafarina, S., Sebastiani, P., Gasbarri, A. & Amicarelli, F. (2004). Methylglyoxal induces oxidative stress-dependent cell injury and up-regulation of interleukin-1beta and nerve growth factor in cultured hippocampal neuronal cells. *Brain Res*, Vol. 1006, No. 2, (March 2004), pp. 157-167, ISSN 0006-8993.

Dringen, R., Gutterer, J. M. & Hirrlinger, J. (2000). Glutathione metabolism in brain metabolic interaction between astrocytes and neurons in the defense against reactive oxygen species. *Eur J Biochem*, Vol. 267, No. 16, (August 2000), pp. 4912-4916, ISSN 0014-2956.

Du, F., Qian, Z. M., Zhu, L., Wu, X. M., Yung, W. H., Tsim, T. Y. & Ke, Y. (2009). L-DOPA neurotoxicity is mediated by up-regulation of DMT1-IRE expression. *PLoS One*, Vol. 4, No. 2, (February 2009), pp. e4593, ISSN 1932-6203.

Felt, B. T., Beard, J. L., Schallert, T., Shao, J., Aldridge, J. W., Connor, J. R., Georgieff, M. K. & Lozoff, B. (2006). Persistent neurochemical and behavioral abnormalities in adulthood despite early iron supplementation for perinatal iron deficiency anemia in rats. *Behav Brain Res*, Vol. 171, No. 2, (May 2006), pp. 261-270, ISSN 0166-4328.

Ganz, T. (2006). Hepcidin and its role in regulating systemic iron metabolism. *Hematology Am Soc Hematol Educ Program*, (November 2006), pp. 29-35, 507, ISSN 1520-4391.

Gao, J., Chen, J., De Domenico, I., Koeller, D. M., Harding, C. O., Fleming, R. E., Koeberl, D. D. & Enns, C. A. (2010). Hepatocyte-targeted HFE and TFR2 control hepcidin expression in mice. *Blood*, Vol. 115, No. 16, (February 2010), pp. 3374-3381, ISSN 1528-0020.

Garrick, M. D. & Garrick, L. M. (2009). Cellular iron transport. *Biochim Biophys Acta*, Vol. 1790, No. 5, (April 2009), pp. 309-325, ISSN 0006-3002.

Ginhoux, F., Greter, M., Leboeuf, M., Nandi, S., See, P., Gokhan, S., Mehler, M. F., Conway, S. J., Ng, L. G., Stanley, E. R., Samokhvalov, I. M. & Merad, M. (2010). Fate mapping analysis reveals that adult microglia derive from primitive macrophages. *Science*, Vol. 330, No. 6005, (October 2010), pp. 841-845, ISSN 1095-9203.

Gomez, F. J., Aguirre, P., Gonzalez-Billault, C. & Núñez, M. T. (2010). Iron mediates neuritic tree collapse in mesencephalic neurons treated with 1-methyl-4-phenylpyridinium (MPP+). *J Neural Transm*, (October 2) [Epub ahead of print], ISSN 1435-1463.

Gorell, J. M., Ordidge, R. J., Brown, G. G., Deniau, J. C., Buderer, N. M. & Helpern, J. A. (1995). Increased iron-related MRI contrast in the substantia nigra in Parkinson's disease. *Neurology*, Vol. 45, No. 6, (June 1995), pp. 1138-1143, ISSN 0028-3878.

Gotz, M. E., Kunig, G., Riederer, P. & Youdim, M. B. (1994). Oxidative stress: free radical production in neural degeneration. *Pharmacol Ther*, Vol. 63, No. 1, (January 1994), pp. 37-122, ISSN 0163-7258.

Graf, E., Mahoney, J. R., Bryant, R. G. & Eaton, J. W. (1984). Iron-catalyzed hydroxyl radical formation. Stringent requirement for free iron coordination site. *J Biol Chem*, Vol. 259, No 6, (March 1984), pp. 3620-3624, ISSN 0021-9258.

Grantham-McGregor, S. & Ani, C. (2001). A review of studies on the effect of iron deficiency on cognitive development in children. *J Nutr*, Vol. 131, No. 2S-2, (February 2001), pp. 649S-666S; discussion 666S-668S, ISSN 0022-3166.

Gunshin, H., Mackenzie, B., Berger, U. V., Gunshin, Y., Romero, M. F., Boron, W. F., Nussberger, S., Gollan, J. L. & Hediger, M. A. (1997). Cloning and characterization of a mammalian proton-coupled metal-ion transporter. *Nature*, Vol. 388, No. 6641, (July 1997), pp. 482-488, ISSN 0028-0836.

Haeger, P., Alvarez, A., Leal, N., Adasme, T., Núñez, M. T. & Hidalgo, C. (2010). Increased hippocampal expression of the divalent metal transporter 1 (DMT1) mRNA variants 1B and +IRE and DMT1 protein after NMDA-receptor stimulation or spatial memory training. *Neurotox Res*, Vol. 17, No. 3, (August 2009), pp. 238-247, ISSN 1476-3524.

Halliwell, B. (2006a). Oxidative stress and neurodegeneration: where are we now? *J Neurochem*, Vol. 97, No. 6, (June 2006), pp. 1634-1658, ISSN 0022-3042.

Halliwell, B. (2006b). Reactive species and antioxidants. Redox biology is a fundamental theme of aerobic life. *Plant Physiol*, Vol. 141, No. 2, (June 2006), pp. 312-322, ISSN 0032-0889.

Hattingen, E., Magerkurth, J., Pilatus, U., Mozer, A., Seifried, C., Steinmetz, H., Zanella, F. & Hilker, R. (2009). Phosphorus and proton magnetic resonance spectroscopy demonstrates mitochondrial dysfunction in early and advanced Parkinson's disease. *Brain*, Vol. 132, No. Pt 12, (December 2009), pp. 3285-3297, ISSN 1460-2156).

Herrera, A. J., Castano, A., Venero, J. L., Cano, J. & Machado, A. (2000). The single intranigral injection of LPS as a new model for studying the selective effects of inflammatory reactions on dopaminergic system. *Neurobiol Dis*, Vol. 7, No. 4, (August 2000), pp. 429-447, ISSN 0969-9961.

The Execution Step in Parkinson's Disease – On the Vicious Cycle of Mitochondrial Complex I Inhibition, Iron
Dishomeostasis and Oxidative Stress

133

Hidalgo, C., Carrasco, M. A., Muñoz, P. & Núñez, M. T. (2007). A role for reactive
oxygen/nitrogen species and iron on neuronal synaptic plasticity. *Antioxid Redox
Signal*, Vol. 9, No 2, (November 2006), pp. 245-255, ISSN 1523-0864.

Hidalgo, C. & Núñez, M. T. (2007). Calcium, iron and neuronal function. *IUBMB Life*, Vol.
59, No. 4-5, (May 2007), pp. 280-285, ISSN 1521-6543.

Hirsch, E. C., Brandel, J. P., Galle, P., Javoy-Agid, F. & Agid, Y. (1991). Iron and aluminum
increase in the substantia nigra of patients with Parkinson's disease: an X-ray
microanalysis. *J Neurochem*, Vol. 56, No. 2, (February 1991), pp. 446-451, ISSN 0022-
3042.

Hirsch, E. C., Hunot, S., Damier, P. & Faucheux, B. (1998). Glial cells and inflammation in
Parkinson's disease: a role in neurodegeneration? *Ann Neurol*, Vol. 44, No. 3 Suppl
1, (September 1998), pp. S115-120, ISSN 0364-5134.

Hubert, N. & Hentze, M. W. (2002). Previously uncharacterized isoforms of divalent metal
transporter (DMT)-1: implications for regulation and cellular function. *Proc Natl
Acad Sci U S A*, Vol. 99, No. 19, (September 2002), pp 12345-12350, ISSN 0027-8424.

Jang, H., Boltz, D. A., Webster, R. G. & Smeyne, R. J. (2009). Viral parkinsonism. *Biochim
Biophys Acta*, Vol. 1792, No. 7, (September 2008), pp. 714-721, ISSN 0006-3002.

Jellinger, K. A. (1999). The role of iron in neurodegeneration: prospects for pharmacotherapy
of Parkinson's disease. *Drugs Aging*, Vol. 14, No. 2, (March 1999), pp. 115-140, ISSN
1170-229X.

Jiang, H., Song, N., Xu, H., Zhang, S., Wang, J. & Xie, J. (2010). Up-regulation of divalent
metal transporter 1 in 6-hydroxydopamine intoxication is IRE/IRP dependent. *Cell
Res*, Vol. 20, No. 3, (February 2010), pp. 345-356, ISSN 1748-7838.

Jorgenson, L. A., Sun, M., O'Connor, M. & Georgieff, M. K. (2005). Fetal iron deficiency
disrupts the maturation of synaptic function and efficacy in area CA1 of the
developing rat hippocampus. *Hippocampus*, Vol. 15, No. 8, (September 2005), pp.
1094-1102, ISSN 1050-9631.

Kakhlon, O. & Cabantchik, Z. I. (2002). The labile iron pool: characterization, measurement,
and participation in cellular processes(1). *Free Radic Biol Med*, Vol. 33, No. 8,
(October 2002), pp. 1037-1046, ISSN 0891-5849.

Kaur, D., Lee, D., Ragapolan, S. & Andersen, J. K. (2009). Glutathione depletion in
immortalized midbrain-derived dopaminergic neurons results in increases in the
labile iron pool: implications for Parkinson's disease. *Free Radic Biol Med*, Vol. 46,
No. 5, (January 2009), pp. 593-598, ISSN 1873-4596.

Kaur, D., Yantiri, F., Rajagopalan, S., Kumar, J., Mo, J. Q., Boonplueang, R., Viswanath, V.,
Jacobs, R., Yang, L., Beal, M. F., DiMonte, D., Volitaskis, I., Ellerby, L., Cherny, R.
A., Bush, A. I. & Andersen, J. K. (2003). Genetic or pharmacological iron chelation
prevents MPTP-induced neurotoxicity in vivo: a novel therapy for Parkinson's
disease. *Neuron*, Vol. 37, No. 6, (April 2003), pp. 899-909, ISSN 0896-6273.

Kooncumchoo, P., Sharma, S., Porter, J., Govitrapong, P. & Ebadi, M. (2006). Coenzyme
Q(10) provides neuroprotection in iron-induced apoptosis in dopaminergic
neurons. *J Mol Neurosci*, Vol. 28, No. 2, (May 2006), pp. 125-141, ISSN 0895-8696.

Kovtunovych, G., Eckhaus, M. A., Ghosh, M. C., Ollivierre-Wilson, H. & Rouault, T. A.
(2010). Dysfunction of the heme recycling system in heme oxygenase 1-deficient
mice: effects on macrophage viability and tissue iron distribution. *Blood*, Vol. 116,
No. 26, (September 2010), pp. 6054-6062, ISSN 1528-0020.

Krause, A., Neitz, S., Magert, H. J., Schulz, A., Forssmann, W. G., Schulz-Knappe, P. & Adermann, K. (2000). LEAP-1, a novel highly disulfide-bonded human peptide, exhibits antimicrobial activity. *FEBS Lett*, Vol. 480, No. 2-3, (October 2000), pp. 147-150, ISSN 0014-5793.

Kroemer, G., Galluzzi, L., Vandenabeele, P., Abrams, J., Alnemri, E. S., Baehrecke, E. H., Blagosklonny, M. V., El-Deiry, W. S., Golstein, P., Green, D. R., Hengartner, M., Knight, R. A., Kumar, S., Lipton, S. A., Malorni, W., Núñez, G., Peter, M. E., Tschopp, J., Yuan, J., Piacentini, M., Zhivotovsky, B., Melino, G. & Nomenclature Committee on Cell, D. (2009). Classification of cell death: recommendations of the Nomenclature Committee on Cell Death 2009. *Cell Death Differ*, Vol. 16, No. 1, (October 2008), pp. 3-11, ISSN 1476-5403.

Kruszewski, M. (2003). Labile iron pool: the main determinant of cellular response to oxidative stress. *Mutat Res*, Vol. 531, No. 1-2, (November 2003), pp. 81-92, ISSN 0027-5107.

Kupershmidt, L., Weinreb, O., Amit, T., Mandel, S., Carri, M. T. & Youdim, M. B. (2009). Neuroprotective and neuritogenic activities of novel multimodal iron-chelating drugs in motor-neuron-like NSC-34 cells and transgenic mouse model of amyotrophic lateral sclerosis. *FASEB J*, Vol. 23, No. 11, (July 2009), pp. 3766-3779, ISSN 1530-6860.

Kuperstein, F. & Yavin, E. (2003). Pro-apoptotic signaling in neuronal cells following iron and amyloid beta peptide neurotoxicity. *J Neurochem*, Vol. 86, No. 1, (June 2003), pp. 114-125, ISSN 0022-3042.

Kwik-Uribe, C. L., Gietzen, D., German, J. B., Golub, M. S. & Keen, C. L. (2000). Chronic marginal iron intakes during early development in mice result in persistent changes in dopamine metabolism and myelin composition. *J Nutr*, Vol. 130, No. 11, (October 2000), pp. 2821-2830, ISSN 0022-3166.

Langston, J. W., Ballard, P., Tetrud, J. W. & Irwin, I. (1983). Chronic Parkinsonism in humans due to a product of meperidine-analog synthesis. *Science*, Vol. 219, No. 4587, (February 1983), pp. 979-980, ISSN 0036-8075.

Lee, D. W., Kaur, D., Chinta, S. J., Rajagopalan, S. & Andersen, J. K. (2009). A disruption in iron-sulfur center biogenesis via inhibition of mitochondrial dithiol glutaredoxin 2 may contribute to mitochondrial and cellular iron dysregulation in mammalian glutathione-depleted dopaminergic cells: implications for Parkinson's disease. *Antioxid Redox Signal*, Vol. 11, No. 9, (March 2009), pp. 2083-2094, ISSN 1557-7716.

Lees, A. J. (1997). Trauma and Parkinson disease. *Rev Neurol (Paris)*, Vol. 153, No. 10, (July 1998), pp. 541-546, ISSN 0035-3787.

Li, L., Holscher, C., Chen, B. B., Zhang, Z. F. & Liu, Y. Z. (2011). Hepcidin Treatment Modulates the Expression of Divalent Metal Transporter-1, Ceruloplasmin, and Ferroportin-1 in the Rat Cerebral Cortex and Hippocampus. *Biol Trace Elem Res*, (January 2011), ISSN 1559-0720.

Li, X. Z., Bai, L. M., Yang, Y. P., Luo, W. F., Hu, W. D., Chen, J. P., Mao, C. J. & Liu, C. F. (2009). Effects of IL-6 secreted from astrocytes on the survival of dopaminergic neurons in lipopolysaccharide-induced inflammation. *Neurosci Res*, Vol. 65, No. 3, (August 2009), pp. 252-258, ISSN 1872-8111.

Lill, R. & Muhlenhoff, U. (2008). Maturation of iron-sulfur proteins in eukaryotes: mechanisms, connected processes, and diseases. *Annu Rev Biochem*, Vol. 77, (March 2008), pp. 669-700, ISSN 0066-4154.

Lis, A., Paradkar, P. N., Singleton, S., Kuo, H. C., Garrick, M. D. & Roth, J. A. (2005). Hypoxia induces changes in expression of isoforms of the divalent metal transporter (DMT1) in rat pheochromocytoma (PC12) cells. *Biochem Pharmacol*, Vol. 69, No. 11, (May 2005), pp. 1647-1655, ISSN 0006-2952.

Liu, R., Liu, W., Doctrow, S. R. & Baudry, M. (2003). Iron toxicity in organotypic cultures of hippocampal slices: role of reactive oxygen species. *J Neurochem*, Vol. 85, No. 2, (April 2003), pp. 492-502, ISSN 0022-3042.

Lobner, D. & Ali, C. (2002). Mechanisms of bFGF and NT-4 potentiation of necrotic neuronal death. *Brain Res*, Vol. 954, No. 1, (October 2002), pp. 42-50, ISSN 0006-8993.

Lozoff, B., Wolf, A. W. & Jimenez, E. (1996). Iron-deficiency anemia and infant development: effects of extended oral iron therapy. *J Pediatr*, Vol. 129, No. 3, (September 1996), pp. 382-389, ISSN 0022-3476.

Ludwiczek, S., Theurl, I., Muckenthaler, M. U., Jakab, M., Mair, S. M., Theurl, M., Kiss, J., Paulmichl, M., Hentze, M. W., Ritter, M. & Weiss, G. (2007). Ca2+ channel blockers reverse iron overload by a new mechanism via divalent metal transporter-1. *Nat Med*, Vol. 13, No 4, (February 2007), pp. 448-454, ISSN 1078-8956.

Maharaj, D. S., Maharaj, H., Daya, S. & Glass, B. D. (2006). Melatonin and 6-hydroxymelatonin protect against iron-induced neurotoxicity. *J Neurochem*, Vol. 96, No. 1, (November 2005), pp. 78-81, ISSN 0022-3042.

Mandel SA, Amit T, Weinreb O, Youdim MB. (2011). Understanding the Broad-Spectrum Neuroprotective Action Profile of Green Tea Polyphenols in Aging and Neurodegenerative Diseases. *J Alzheimers Dis*. Mar 2. [Epub ahead of print], ISSN ISSN:1387-2877.

Marques, F., Falcao, A. M., Sousa, J. C., Coppola, G., Geschwind, D., Sousa, N., Correia-Neves, M. & Palha, J. A. (2009). Altered iron metabolism is part of the choroid plexus response to peripheral inflammation. *Endocrinology*, Vol. 150, No. 6, (February 2009), pp. 2822-2828, ISSN 1945-7170.

Martelli, A., Wattenhofer-Donze, M., Schmucker, S., Bouvet, S., Reutenauer, L. & Puccio, H. (2007). Frataxin is essential for extramitochondrial Fe-S cluster proteins in mammalian tissues. *Hum Mol Genet*, Vol. 16, No. 22, (June 2007), pp. 2651-2658, ISSN 0964-6906.

McEchron, M. D. & Paronish, M. D. (2005). Perinatal nutritional iron deficiency reduces hippocampal synaptic transmission but does not impair short- or long-term synaptic plasticity. *Nutr Neurosci*, Vol. 8, No. 5-6, (May 2006), pp. 277-285, ISSN 1028-415X.

McGeer, P. L., Itagaki, S., Boyes, B. E. & McGeer, E. G. (1988). Reactive microglia are positive for HLA-DR in the substantia nigra of Parkinson's and Alzheimer's disease brains. *Neurology*, Vol. 38, No. 8, (August 1988), pp. 1285-1291, ISSN 0028-3878.

Meister, A. & Anderson, M. E. (1983). Glutathione. *Annu Rev Biochem*, Vol. 52, (January 1983), pp. 711-760, ISSN 0066-4154.

Mena, N., Hirsch, E. & Núñez, M.T. (2011). Inhibition of mitochondrial complex I results in decreased synthesis of iron-sulfur clusters. In revision, *Biochim Biophys Res Comm*.

Mogi, M., Harada, M., Kondo, T., Riederer, P., Inagaki, H., Minami, M. &Nagatsu, T. (1994). Interleukin-1 beta, interleukin-6, epidermal growth factor and transforming growth factor-alpha are elevated in the brain from parkinsonian patients. *Neurosci Lett*, Vol. 180, No. 2, (October 1995), pp. 147-150, ISSN 0304-3940.

Moos, T. & Morgan, E. H. (1998). Evidence for low molecular weight, non-transferrin-bound iron in rat brain and cerebrospinal fluid. *J Neurosci Res*, Vol. 54, No. 4, (November 1998), pp. 486-494, ISSN 0360-4012.

Moos, T. & Rosengren Nielsen, T. (2006). Ferroportin in the postnatal rat brain: implications for axonal transport and neuronal export of iron. *Semin Pediatr Neurol*, Vol. 13, No. 3, (November 2006), pp. 149-157, ISSN 1071-9091.

Moos, T., Rosengren Nielsen, T., Skjorringe, T. & Morgan, E. H. (2007). Iron trafficking inside the brain. *J Neurochem*, Vol. 103, No. 5, (October 2007), pp. 1730-1740, ISSN 1471-4159.

Muller, T., Blum-Degen, D., Przuntek, H. & Kuhn, W. (1998). Interleukin-6 levels in cerebrospinal fluid inversely correlate to severity of Parkinson's disease. *Acta Neurol Scand*, Vol. 98, No. 2, (September 1998), pp. 142-144, ISSN 0001-6314.

Muñoz, P., Humeres, A., Elgueta, C., Kirkwood, A., Hidalgo, C. & Núñez, M. T. (2011). Iron mediates N-methyl-D-aspartate receptor-dependent stimulation of calcium-induced pathways and hippocampal synaptic plasticity. *J Biol Chem*, (February 2011), ISSN 1083-351X.

Nagatsu, T. (2002). Parkinson's disease: changes in apoptosis-related factors suggesting possible gene therapy. *J Neural Transm*, Vol. 109, No. 5-6, (July 2002), pp. 731-745, ISSN 0300-9564.

Nemeth, E., Tuttle, M. S., Powelson, J., Vaughn, M. B., Donovan, A., Ward, D. M., Ganz, T. & Kaplan, J. (2004). Hepcidin regulates cellular iron efflux by binding to ferroportin and inducing its internalization. *Science*, Vol. 306, No. 5704, (October 2004), pp. 2090-2093, ISSN 1095-9203.

Nicolas, G., Bennoun, M., Devaux, I., Beaumont, C., Grandchamp, B., Kahn, A. & Vaulont, S. (2001). Lack of hepcidin gene expression and severe tissue iron overload in upstream stimulatory factor 2 (USF2) knockout mice. *Proc Natl Acad Sci U S A*, Vol. 98, No. 15, (July 2001), pp. 8780-8785, ISSN 0027-8424.

Noll, T., Koop, A. & Piper, H. M. (1992). Mitochondrial ATP-synthase activity in cardiomyocytes after aerobic-anaerobic metabolic transition. *Am J Physiol*, Vol. 262, No. 5 Pt 1, (May 1992), pp. C1297-1303, ISSN 0002-9513.

Núñez, M. T., Gallardo, V., Muñoz, P., Tapia, V., Esparza, A., Salazar, J. & Speisky, H. (2004). Progressive iron accumulation induces a biphasic change in the glutathione content of neuroblastoma cells. *Free Radic Biol Med*, Vol. 37, No. 7, (September 2004), pp. 953-960, ISSN 0891-5849.

Ohgami, R. S., Campagna, D. R., Greer, E. L., Antiochos, B., McDonald, A., Chen, J., Sharp, J. J., Fujiwara, Y., Barker, J. E. & Fleming, M. D. (2005). Identification of a ferrireductase required for efficient transferrin-dependent iron uptake in erythroid cells. *Nat Genet*, Vol. 37, No. 11, (October 2005), pp. 1264-1269, ISSN 1061-4036.

Orr, C. F., Rowe, D. B. & Halliday, G. M. (2002). An inflammatory review of Parkinson's disease. *Prog Neurobiol*, Vol. 68, No. 5, (January 2003), pp. 325-340, ISSN 0301-0082.

Paradkar, P. N. & Roth, J. A. (2006). Nitric oxide transcriptionally down-regulates specific isoforms of divalent metal transporter (DMT1) via NF-kappaB. *J Neurochem*, Vol. 96, No. 6, (March 2006), pp. 1768-1777, ISSN 0022-3042.

Park, L. C., Zhang, H., Sheu, K. F., Calingasan, N. Y., Kristal, B. S., Lindsay, J. G. &Gibson, G. E. (1999). Metabolic impairment induces oxidative stress, compromises inflammatory responses, and inactivates a key mitochondrial enzyme in microglia. *J Neurochem*, Vol. 72, No. 5, (April 1999), pp. 1948-1958, ISSN 0022-3042.

Pelizzoni, I., Macco, R., Morini, M. F., Zacchetti, D., Grohovaz, F. & Codazzi, F. (2011). Iron handling in hippocampal neurons: activity-dependent iron entry and mitochondria-mediated neurotoxicity. *Aging Cell*, Vol. 10, No. 1, (November 2010), pp. 172-183, ISSN 1474-9726.

Perry, G., Taddeo, M. A., Petersen, R. B., Castellani, R. J., Harris, P. L., Siedlak, S. L., Cash, A. D., Liu, Q., Nunomura, A., Atwood, C. S. & Smith, M. A. (2003). Adventiously-bound redox active iron and copper are at the center of oxidative damage in Alzheimer disease. *Biometals*, Vol. 16, No. 1, (February 2003), pp. 77-81, ISSN 0966-0844.

Perry, T. L., Godin, D. V. & Hansen, S. (1982). Parkinson's disease: a disorder due to nigral glutathione deficiency? *Neurosci Lett*, Vol. 33, No. 3, (December 1982), pp. 305-310, ISSN 0304-3940.

Peyssonnaux, C., Zinkernagel, A. S., Schuepbach, R. A., Rankin, E., Vaulont, S., Haase, V. H., Nizet, V. & Johnson, R. S. (2007). Regulation of iron homeostasis by the hypoxia-inducible transcription factors (HIFs). *J Clin Invest*, Vol. 117, No. 7, (June 2007), pp. 1926-1932, ISSN 0021-9738.

Pigeon, C., Ilyin, G., Courselaud, B., Leroyer, P., Turlin, B., Brissot, P. & Loreal, O. (2001). A new mouse liver-specific gene, encoding a protein homologous to human antimicrobial peptide hepcidin, is overexpressed during iron overload. *J Biol Chem*, Vol. 276, No. 11, (December 2000), pp. 7811-7819, ISSN 0021-9258.

Pinto, J. P., Ribeiro, S., Pontes, H., Thowfeequ, S., Tosh, D., Carvalho, F. & Porto, G. (2008). Erythropoietin mediates hepcidin expression in hepatocytes through EPOR signaling and regulation of C/EBPalpha. *Blood*, Vol. 111, No. 12, (March 2008), pp. 5727-5733, ISSN 1528-0020.

Ranade, S. C., Rose, A., Rao, M., Gallego, J., Gressens, P. & Mani, S. (2008). Different types of nutritional deficiencies affect different domains of spatial memory function checked in a radial arm maze. *Neuroscience*, Vol. 152, No. 4, (March 2008), pp. 859-866, ISSN 0306-4522.

Rouault, T. A. & Tong, W. H. (2005). Iron-sulphur cluster biogenesis and mitochondrial iron homeostasis. *Nat Rev Mol Cell Biol*, Vol. 6, No. 4, (April 2005), pp. 345-351, ISSN 1471-0072.

Rouault, T. A. & Tong, W. H. (2008). Iron-sulfur cluster biogenesis and human disease. *Trends Genet*, Vol. 24, No. 8, (July 2008), pp 398-407, ISSN 0168-9525.

Rouault, T. A., Zhang, D. L. & Jeong, S. Y. (2009). Brain iron homeostasis, the choroid plexus, and localization of iron transport proteins. *Metab Brain Dis*, Vol. 24, No. 4, (October 2009), pp. 673-684, ISSN 1573-7365.

Salazar, J., Mena, N., Hunot, S., Prigent, A., Alvarez-Fischer, D., Arredondo, M., Duyckaerts, C., Sazdovitch, V., Zhao, L., Garrick, L. M., Núñez, M. T., Garrick, M. D., Raisman-Vozari, R. & Hirsch, E. C. (2008). Divalent metal transporter 1 (DMT1) contributes to neurodegeneration in animal models of Parkinson's disease. *Proc Natl Acad Sci U S A*, Vol. 105, No. 47, (November 2008), pp. 18578-18583, ISSN 1091-6490.

Salazar, J., Mena, N. & Núñez, M. T. (2006). Iron dyshomeostasis in Parkinson's disease. *J Neural Transm Suppl*, No. 71, (April 2007), pp. 205-213, ISSN 0303-6995.

Sayre, L. M., Perry, G., Atwood, C. S. & Smith, M. A. (2000). The role of metals in neurodegenerative diseases. *Cell Mol Biol (Noisy-le-grand)*, Vol. 46, No. 4, (June 2000), pp. 731-741, ISSN 0145-5680.

Schafer, F. Q. & Buettner, G. R. (2001). Redox environment of the cell as viewed through the redox state of the glutathione disulfide/glutathione couple. *Free Radic Biol Med*, Vol. 30, No. 11, (May 2005), pp. 1191-1212, ISSN 0891-5849.

Schapira, A. H., Cooper, J. M., Dexter, D., Clark, J. B., Jenner, P. & Marsden, C. D. (1990). Mitochondrial complex I deficiency in Parkinson's disease. *J Neurochem*, Vol. 54, No. 3, (March 1990), pp. 823-827, ISSN 0022-3042.

Scotcher, K. P., Irwin, I., DeLanney, L. E., Langston, J. W. & Di Monte, D. (1990). Effects of 1-methyl-4-phenyl-1,2,3,6-tetrahydropyridine and 1-methyl-4-phenylpyridinium ion on ATP levels of mouse brain synaptosomes. *J Neurochem*, Vol. 54, No. 4, (April 1990), pp. 1295-1301, ISSN 0022-3042.

Shachar, D. B., Kahana, N., Kampel, V., Warshawsky, A. & Youdim, M. B. (2004). Neuroprotection by a novel brain permeable iron chelator, VK-28, against 6-hydroxydopamine lession in rats. *Neuropharmacology*, Vol. 46, No. 2, (December 2003), pp. 254-263, ISSN 0028-3908.

Shi, Z. H., Nie, G., Duan, X. L., Rouault, T., Wu, W. S., Ning, B., Zhang, N., Chang, Y. Z. & Zhao, B. L. (2010). Neuroprotective mechanism of mitochondrial ferritin on 6-hydroxydopamine-induced dopaminergic cell damage: implication for neuroprotection in Parkinson's disease. *Antioxid Redox Signal*, Vol. 13, No. 6, (February 2010), pp. 783-796, ISSN 1557-7716.

Sian, J., Dexter, D. T., Lees, A. J., Daniel, S., Agid, Y., Javoy-Agid, F., Jenner, P. & Marsden, C. D. (1994). Alterations in glutathione levels in Parkinson's disease and other neurodegenerative disorders affecting basal ganglia. *Ann Neurol*, Vol. 36, No. 3, (September 1994), pp. 348-355, ISSN 0364-5134.

Singer, T. P. & Ramsay, R. R. (1990). Mechanism of the neurotoxicity of MPTP. An update. *FEBS Lett*, Vol. 274, No. 1-2, (November 1990), pp. 1-8, ISSN 0014-5793.

Singh, R., Akhtar, N. & Haqqi, T. M. (2010). Green tea polyphenol epigallocatechin-3-gallate: inflammation and arthritis. *Life Sci*, Vol. 86, No. 25-26, (May 2010), pp. 907-918, ISSN 1879-0631.

Sofic, E., Riederer, P., Heinsen, H., Beckmann, H., Reynolds, G. P., Hebenstreit, G. & Youdim, M. B. (1988). Increased iron (III) and total iron content in post mortem substantia nigra of parkinsonian brain. *J Neural Transm*, Vol. 74, No. 3, (January 1988), pp. 199-205, ISSN 0300-9564.

Song, N., Wang, J., Jiang, H. & Xie, J. (2010). Ferroportin 1 but not hephaestin contributes to iron accumulation in a cell model of Parkinson's disease. *Free Radic Biol Med*, Vol. 48, No. 2, (November 2009), pp. 332-341, ISSN 1873-4596.

Stokes, A. H., Hastings, T. G. & Vrana, K. E. (1999). Cytotoxic and genotoxic potential of dopamine. *J Neurosci Res*, Vol. 55, No. 6, (April 1999), pp. 659-665, ISSN 0360-4012.

Symons, M.C.R & Gutteridge, J.M.C. (1998). *Free Radicals And Iron: Chemistry, Biology And Medicine*. Oxford University Press, ISBN 019-8558-92-9, New York, USA.

Taneja, V., Mishra, K. & Agarwal, K. N. (1986). Effect of early iron deficiency in rat on the gamma-aminobutyric acid shunt in brain. *J Neurochem*, Vol. 46, No. 6, (June 1986), pp. 1670-1674, ISSN 0022-3042.

Tretter, L., Sipos, I. & Adam-Vizi, V. (2004). Initiation of neuronal damage by complex I deficiency and oxidative stress in Parkinson's disease. *Neurochem Res*, Vol. 29, No. 3, (March 2004), pp. 569-577, ISSN 0364-3190.

Valente, E. M., Abou-Sleiman, P. M., Caputo, V., Muqit, M. M., Harvey, K., Gispert, S., Ali, Z., Del Turco, D., Bentivoglio, A. R., Healy, D. G., Albanese, A., Nussbaum, R.,

The Execution Step in Parkinson's Disease – On the Vicious Cycle of Mitochondrial Complex I Inhibition, Iron
Dishomeostasis and Oxidative Stress

139

Gonzalez-Maldonado, R., Deller, T., Salvi, S., Cortelli, P., Gilks, W. P., Latchman, D. S., Harvey, R. J., Dallapiccola, B., Auburger, G. & Wood, N. W. (2004). Hereditary early-onset Parkinson's disease caused by mutations in PINK1. *Science*, Vol. 304, No. 5674, (April 2004), pp. 1158-1160, ISSN 1095-9203.

Vandenabeele, P., Galluzzi, L., Vanden Berghe, T. & Kroemer, G. (2010). Molecular mechanisms of necroptosis: an ordered cellular explosion. *Nat Rev Mol Cell Biol*, Vol. 11, No. 10, (October 2010), pp. 700-714, ISSN 1471-0080.

Vymazal, J., Righini, A., Brooks, R. A., Canesi, M., Mariani, C., Leonardi, M. & Pezzoli, G. (1999). T1 and T2 in the brain of healthy subjects, patients with Parkinson disease, and patients with multiple system atrophy: relation to iron content. *Radiology*, Vol. 211, No. 2, (May 1999), pp. 489-495, ISSN 0033-8419.

Wang, D., Wang, L. H., Zhao, Y., Lu, Y. P. & Zhu, L. (2010a). Hypoxia regulates the ferrous iron uptake and reactive oxygen species level via divalent metal transporter 1 (DMT1) Exon1B by hypoxia-inducible factor-1. *IUBMB Life*, Vol. 62, No. 8, (August 2010), pp. 629-636, ISSN 1521-6551.

Wang, Q., Du, F., Qian, Z. M., Ge, X. H., Zhu, L., Yung, W. H., Yang, L. & Ke, Y. (2008). Lipopolysaccharide induces a significant increase in expression of iron regulatory hormone hepcidin in the cortex and substantia nigra in rat brain. *Endocrinology*, Vol. 149, No. 8, (May 2008), pp. 3920-3925, ISSN 0013-7227.

Wang, S. M., Fu, L. J., Duan, X. L., Crooks, D. R., Yu, P., Qian, Z. M., Di, X. J., Li, J., Rouault, T. A. & Chang, Y. Z. (2010b). Role of hepcidin in murine brain iron metabolism. *Cell Mol Life Sci*, Vol. 67, No. 1, (November 2009), pp. 123-133, ISSN 1420-9071.

Wang, Z. J., Lam, K. W., Lam, T. T. & Tso, M. O. (1998). Iron-induced apoptosis in the photoreceptor cells of rats. *Invest Ophthalmol Vis Sci*, Vol. 39, No. 3, (March 1998), pp. 631-633, ISSN 0146-0404.

Weinreb, O., Mandel, S., Bar-Am, O. & Amit, T. (2011). Iron-chelating backbone coupled with monoamine oxidase inhibitory moiety as novel pluripotential therapeutic agents for Alzheimer's disease: a tribute to Moussa Youdim. *J Neural Transm*, (March 2011), ISSN 1435-1463.

Williams, K., Wilson, M. A. & Bressler, J. (2000). Regulation and developmental expression of the divalent metal-ion transporter in the rat brain. *Cell Mol Biol (Noisy-le-grand)*, Vol. 46, No. 3, (July 2000), pp. 563-571, ISSN 0145-5680.

Wilson, R. B. (2006). Iron dysregulation in Friedreich ataxia. *Semin Pediatr Neurol*, Vol. 13, No. 3, (November 2006), pp. 166-175, ISSN 1071-9091.

Wright, R. O. & Baccarelli, A. (2007). Metals and neurotoxicology. *J Nutr* Vol. 137, No. 12, (November 2007), pp. 2809-2813, ISSN 1541-6100.

Wrighting, D. M. & Andrews, N. C. (2006). Interleukin-6 induces hepcidin expression through STAT3. *Blood*, Vol. 108, No. 9, (July 2006), pp. 3204-3209, ISSN 0006-4971.

Xu, Q., Kanthasamy, A. G. & Reddy, M. B. (2008). Neuroprotective effect of the natural iron chelator, phytic acid in a cell culture model of Parkinson's disease. *Toxicology*, Vol. 245, No. 1-2, (February 2008), pp. 101-108, ISSN 0300-483X.

Ye, H. & Rouault, T. A. (2010). Erythropoiesis and iron sulfur cluster biogenesis. *Adv Hematol* 2010, (September 2010), ISSN 1687-9112.

Youdim, M. B., Ben-Shachar, D. & Riederer, P. (1989). Is Parkinson's disease a progressive siderosis of substantia nigra resulting in iron and melanin induced neurodegeneration? *Acta Neurol Scand Suppl*, Vol. 126, (January 1989), pp. 47-54, ISSN 0065-1427.

Youdim, M. B. & Buccafusco, J. J. (2005). Multi-functional drugs for various CNS targets in the treatment of neurodegenerative disorders. *Trends Pharmacol Sci*, Vol. 26, No. 1, (January 2005), pp. 27-35, ISSN 0165-6147.

Youdim, M. B., Green, A. R., Bloomfield, M. R., Mitchell, B. D., Heal, D. J. & Grahame-Smith, D. G. (1980). The effects of iron deficiency on brain biogenic monoamine biochemistry and function in rats. *Neuropharmacology*, Vol. 19, No. 3, (March 1980), pp. 259-267, ISSN 0028-3908.

Youdim, M. B., Stephenson, G. & Ben Shachar, D. (2004). Ironing iron out in Parkinson's disease and other neurodegenerative diseases with iron chelators: a lesson from 6-hydroxydopamine and iron chelators, desferal and VK-28. *Ann N Y Acad Sci*, Vol. 1012, (April 2004), pp. 306-325, ISSN 0077-8923.

Zaman, K., Ryu, H., Hall, D., O'Donovan, K., Lin, K. I., Miller, M. P., Marquis, J. C., Baraban, J. M., Semenza, G. L. & Ratan, R. R. (1999). Protection from oxidative stress-induced apoptosis in cortical neuronal cultures by iron chelators is associated with enhanced DNA binding of hypoxia-inducible factor-1 and ATF-1/CREB and increased expression of glycolytic enzymes, p21(waf1/cip1), and erythropoietin. *J Neurosci*, Vol. 19, No. 22, (November 1999), pp. 9821-9830, ISSN 1529-2401.

Zecca, L., Youdim, M. B., Riederer, P., Connor, J. R. & Crichton, R. R. (2004). Iron, brain ageing and neurodegenerative disorders. *Nat Rev Neurosci*, Vol. 5, No. 11, (October 2004), pp. 863-873, ISSN 1471-003X.

Zechel, S., Huber-Wittmer, K. & von Bohlen und Halbach, O. (2006). Distribution of the iron-regulating protein hepcidin in the murine central nervous system. *J Neurosci Res*, Vol. 84, No. 4, (August 2006), pp. 790-800, ISSN 0360-4012.

Zhang, Y., Marcillat, O., Giulivi, C., Ernster, L. & Davies, K. J. (1990). The oxidative inactivation of mitochondrial electron transport chain components and ATPase. *J Biol Chem*, Vol. 265, No. 27, (September 1990), pp. 16330-16336, ISSN 0021-9258.

Zheng, H., Youdim, M. B. & Fridkin, M. (2010). Site-activated chelators targeting acetylcholinesterase and monoamine oxidase for Alzheimer's therapy. *ACS Chem Biol*, Vol. 5, No. 6, (May 1990), pp. 603-610, ISSN 1554-8937.

Zheng, H., Youdim, M. B., Weiner, L. M. & Fridkin, M. (2005). Novel potential neuroprotective agents with both iron chelating and amino acid-based derivatives targeting central nervous system neurons. *Biochem Pharmacol*, Vol. 70, No. 11, (October 2005), pp. 1642-1652, ISSN 0006-2952.

Ziv, I., Barzilai, A., Offen, D., Nardi, N. & Melamed, E. (1997). Nigrostriatal neuronal death in Parkinson's disease--a passive or an active genetically-controlled process? *J Neural Transm Suppl*, Vol. 49, (January 1997), pp. 69-76, ISSN 0303-6995.

Zoccarato, F., Toscano, P. & Alexandre, A. (2005). Dopamine-derived dopaminochrome promotes H(2)O(2) release at mitochondrial complex I: stimulation by rotenone, control by Ca(2+), and relevance to Parkinson disease. *J Biol Chem*, Vol. 280, No. 16, (February 2005), pp. 15587-15594, ISSN 0021-9258.

7

Cyclin-Dependent Kinase 5 – An Emerging Player in Parkinson's Disease Pathophysiology

Zelda H. Cheung and Nancy Y. Ip

Division of Life Science, State Key Laboratory of Molecular Neuroscience and Molecular Neuroscience Center, Hong Kong University of Science and Technology, Clear Water Bay, Kowloon, Hong Kong, China

1. Introduction

Parkinson's disease (PD) is the most common neurodegenerative movement disorder that affects 1% of the general population at age 65, with the prevalence rising to 4-5% by age 85 (de Rijk *et al.* 1997). Symptoms of PD include muscle rigidity, resting tremor, bradykinesia, postural instability, speech impediment and cognitive decline. At the cellular level, PD is characterized by selective degeneration of dopaminergic neurons in the substantia nigra, and the presence of cytoplasmic inclusions known as Lewy bodies in the brains of PD patients (Levy *et al.* 2009). Despite the prevalence of PD, therapeutic agents that slow or halt disease progression are lacking. Current treatments for PD are highly limited and focus predominantly on symptomatic relief. For example, the most effective treatment for ameliorating PD symptoms is administration of levodopa, a precursor that is converted to dopamine in the brain, to restore dopamine levels in PD patients. Nonetheless, the efficacy of levodopa wears off with prolonged treatment, in addition to triggering dyskinesia as a side effect (Obeso *et al.* 2010, Poewe *et al.* 2010). There is thus an urgent need to elucidate the cellular mechanism underlying PD pathology for the development of more effective treatments.

The etiopathology of PD has remained largely enigmatic. Majority of the PD cases are idiopathic, although familial cases of PD with identifiable mutations also account for about 5% of all PD cases (Dauer and Przedborski 2003). Prior to the identification of these missense mutations, nonetheless, scientists have predominantly focused on the two known cellular hallmarks of PD, namely the degeneration of dopaminergic neurons and the presence of Lewy bodies. Since majority of the motor deficits exhibited by PD patients is reversed by elevating dopamine levels in the brain, it is believed that the motor symptoms of PD are due mostly to the loss of dopaminergic neurons in the substantia nigra (Obeso et al. 2010). This has sparked extensive research aimed at elucidating the mechanisms implicated in the degeneration of these neurons. Abnormality in various cellular processes have been linked to neuronal loss in PD, such as oxidative stress, mitochondrial dysfunction, aberrant proteasomal degradation and deregulation of the autophagy pathway (Levy et al. 2009). On the other hand, the precise role of Lewy bodies has become a little controversial. While protein aggregates and the presence of cytoplasmic inclusions have long been considered as toxic, recent evidence suggests that the aggregates may also exhibit neuroprotective roles by serving as traps for the toxic oligomeric forms (Rubinsztein 2006).

With the dawn of the molecular era, knowledge on the pathogenic mechanisms also shifted from detection of aberrant cellular processes to the identification of molecules implicated in the pathological pathways. Importantly, unraveling of mutations associated with familial cases of PD enabled the mapping of genes and signaling pathways to the dysfunction of various cellular processes. A number of genes were found to be mutated in familial PD, including α-synuclein, Parkin, PINK1, DJ-1, leucine rich repeated kinase 2 (LRRK2), ubiquitin-C-terminal hydrolase-L1 (UCH-L1), synphilin-1 and HtrA2/Omi (Schulz 2008). These studies also led to the identification of α-synuclein as the main constituent of Lewy bodies (Levy et al. 2009). This new wave of information prompted scientists to address the signaling events that are upstream of the elimination of the diseased neurons. Among the long list of molecules that were found to contribute to PD pathology, cyclin-dependent kinase 5 (Cdk5) has emerged as an important player through its implication in multiple cellular events that are altered in PD.

Cdk5 is a serine/threonine kinase that is essential for the migration, survival and differentiation of developing neurons (Cheung and Ip 2007, Dhavan and Tsai 2001). Activated through binding to its activator p35 or p39, Cdk5/p35 activity is important for the regulation of neuronal survival during physiological and pathological states (Cheung and Ip 2004). Cdk5 was first implicated in dopaminergic neuron loss in PD when injection of MPTP, a neurotoxin that selectively eliminates neurons in the substantia nigra, was demonstrated to increase Cdk5 activity (Smith et al. 2003). Inhibition of Cdk5 activity markedly attenuates MPTP-induced degeneration of dopaminergic neurons, thus revealing the involvement of Cdk5 in PD pathogenesis (Smith et al. 2003). Interestingly, Cdk5 expression is also associated with Lewy bodies (Takahashi et al. 2000). Since then, accumulating studies have identified additional Cdk5 substrates that may contribute to PD pathology. These findings revealed that Cdk5 regulates neuronal death through modulating multiple signaling pathways and cellular events in PD, and suggests that Cdk5 may emerge as a suitable target for development of PD therapeutics.

2. Cdk5 – a multi-faceted kinase

Cdk5 was identified based on sequence homology to cell cycle regulator cdc2 as a cdc2-related kinase (Lew *et al.* 1992, Meyerson *et al.* 1992) and also as a tau kinase (Kobayashi *et al.* 1993). Cdk5 is not activated by cyclins despite its structural similarity with other cyclin-dependent kinases. Rather, it is activated upon binding to activators p35 or p39. Cdk5 is ubiquitously expressed, but its activity is mostly limited to the nervous system due to the predominantly neural-specific expression of p35 and p39. Nonetheless, accumulating evidence demonstrates that Cdk5 activity can also be detected outside the nervous system, such as at the neuromuscular junction, pancreatic cells, adipose tissue and myeloid cells (Fu *et al.* 2001, Lilja *et al.* 2001, Choi *et al.* 2010, Arif *et al.* 2011). The importance of p35 and p39 as Cdk5 activators is further demonstrated by the comparable phenotype exhibited by Cdk5-deficient mice and p35/p39 double knock-out mice. Both exhibit perinatal death and severe cortical lamination defects (Ohshima *et al.* 1996, Ko *et al.* 2001). This is in contrast to single knock-out animals lacking p35 or p39, which survive through adulthood. In addition, aberrant cortical lamination was observed only in p35 knock-out mice (Ohshima *et al.* 1996, Ko *et al.* 2001, Chae *et al.* 1997). These observations indicate that while there is some redundancy, p35 and p39 are critical for the function of Cdk5.

2.1 Regulation of Cdk5 activity

Given the pivotal role of p35 and p39 in Cdk5 activation, changes in the expression level of p35 and p39 constitute one of the major mechanisms by which Cdk5 activity is regulated. Interestingly, Cdk5 activity is also regulated by calpain-mediated cleavage of p35 and p39 into p25 and p29, respectively. These fragments retain Cdk5-activating capability but exhibit significantly longer half-lives than p35 and p39, which are rather short-lived proteins (Patrick et al. 1999, Patzke and Tsai 2002). Cdk5 itself was found to contribute to the short half-life of p35 through phosphorylation of p35, which promotes its degradation by the proteasome pathway (Patrick et al. 1998). In addition, cleavage by calpain removes the myristoylation signal from p35 and p39, thus resulting in a redistribution of Cdk5 activity within the cell. Since p25 generation has been associated with excessive Cdk5 activation and neuronal loss in neurodegenerative disease (Patrick et al. 1999, Cruz and Tsai 2004), it has been speculated that Cdk5-p25 may be catalytically more active than Cdk5-p35. Nonetheless, a recent study demonstrated that the activity of Cdk5 is comparable regardless of whether it is associated with p35 or p25 (Peterson et al. 2010). These findings collectively suggest that the aberrant Cdk5 activity associated with p25 generation is likely due to prolonged activation of Cdk5, and not an elevated Cdk5 catalytic activity.

Aside from the regulation of p35 or p39 expression, and their degradation or cleavage, direct phosphorylation of Cdk5 also modulates its activity. Phosphorylation of Cdk5 at Tyr15 has been demonstrated to enhance Cdk5 activity (Sasaki et al. 2002, Fu et al. 2007, Cheung et al. 2007). This mechanism is particularly important for trophic factor-mediated regulation of Cdk5 activity, as a number of trophic factor receptors are receptor tyrosine kinases. Ligand binding triggers tyrosine kinase activation, which directly phosphorylates Cdk5 at Tyr15 to enhance Cdk5 activity. This phosphorylation was found to be crucial for the effect of Cdk5 on the signaling of trophic factors such as Ephrin A1 and BDNF (Cheung et al. 2007, Fu et al. 2007). Interestingly, S-nitrosylation of Cdk5 was also recently demonstrated to reduce Cdk5 activity (Zhang et al. 2010b). These findings indicate that post-translational modification of Cdk5 also constitutes an important mechanism for controlling Cdk5 activity.

2.2 Cdk5 as a regulator of neuronal survival

Despite being a member of the cyclin-dependent kinase family, Cdk5 is unique in several aspects. Not only is its mechanism of activation different, but its action in cell cycle regulation is also distinct from other cyclin-dependent kinases. Cyclin-dependent kinases are important enzymes that ensure the proper progression of cell cycle (Nguyen et al. 2002). The lack of Cdk5 expression in proliferating cells led to the conclusion that Cdk5 is not involved in the regulation of cell cycle progression (Tsai et al. 1993). Nonetheless, recent evidence indicates that Cdk5 also takes part in cell cycle control, acting as a suppressor of cell cycle re-entry in post-mitotic neurons (Zhang and Herrup 2008). Through the identification of a myriad of Cdk5 substrates, Cdk5 has been implicated in multiple aspects of neuronal development and neuronal functions. Aside from an obvious role of Cdk5 in neuronal migration as revealed by the severe cortical lamination defects in Cdk5-deficient mice (Ohshima et al. 1996), Cdk5 is also involved in neuronal differentiation and synapse formation during development (Cheung and Ip 2007). Furthermore, emerging evidence indicates that Cdk5 plays a critical role in synaptic function, synaptic plasticity and learning (Lai and Ip 2009, Hawasli and Bibb 2007).

The role of Cdk5 in neuronal survival is slightly more complex, and accumulating evidence suggests that Cdk5 functions as a double-edged sword. Following the identification of Cdk5 as a tau kinase (Kobayashi et al. 1993), deregulation of Cdk5 activity was found to contribute to neuronal loss in Alzheimer's disease (Patrick et al. 1999). Elevation of Cdk5 activity that is accompanied by p25 generation leads to neuronal death (Patrick et al. 1999). Although conflicting data have been obtained regarding the increase in p25 levels in post-mortem samples of Alzheimer's disease patients (Patrick *et al.* 1999, Li *et al.* 2003b, Tandon *et al.* 2003), subsequent studies have demonstrated augmented p25 expression and Cdk5 activity in response to a large number of pro-apoptotic agents or cell death stimuli, including MPTP (reviewed in Cheung and Ip 2004). These observations collectively establish a death-inducing role of Cdk5-p25. Interestingly, a pro-survival role of Cdk5 is also gaining recognition. Indeed, nuclear margination and cell swelling were observed in brainstem and spinal cord neurons in Cdk5-deficient brains (Ohshima et al. 1996). In addition, knock-down of Cdk5 expression alone results in apoptosis in developing retinal neurons (Cheung et al. 2008). Several mechanisms likely mediate the survival-maintaining property of Cdk5. For example, Cdk5 has been reported to be required for neuregulin-induced elevation of survival signaling pathway PI3K/Akt (Li et al. 2003a). In addition, phosphorylation of Bcl-2 at Ser70 by Cdk5 is essential for its anti-apoptotic property, which is pivotal for the maintenance of neuronal survival during development (Cheung et al. 2008). Cdk5 has also been demonstrated to exhibit a neuroprotective role through suppression of cell cycle re-entry, which is associated with cell death in post-mitotic neurons (Zhang et al. 2010a).

How Cdk5 manages to mediate both cell death and survival signals is incompletely understood. It is generally believed that while basal level of Cdk5 activity is required for neuronal survival, excessive activation, particularly in the presence of p25, leads to neuronal death. In addition, recent studies suggest that the subcellular localization of Cdk5 activity may also determine whether it serves a protective or detrimental role. Cdk5 activity has been demonstrated in the cytoplasm and nucleus. Myristoylation of p35 and p39 has been shown to regulate the distribution of Cdk5, with non-myristoylated p35 and p39 preferentially accumulated in the nucleus (Asada et al. 2008). Previously it has been suggested that nuclear Cdk5 may be selectively associated with neuronal loss, while cytoplasmic Cdk5 activity is linked to neuroprotection (O'Hare et al. 2005). Nonetheless, recent studies indicate that both cytoplasmic and nuclear Cdk5 activity can contribute to neuronal loss (Rashidian et al. 2009) or neuronal survival (Zhang et al. 2010a). It appears that the differential distribution of Cdk5 in the cytoplasm and nucleus, and their respective functions, depend on the types of insults that are being inflicted. Additional studies will be required to further delineate the precise involvement of nuclear and cytoplasmic Cdk5 in the regulation of neuronal survival.

3. Cdk5 in PD pathology

In agreement with the essential role of Cdk5 as a regulator of neuronal survival, Cdk5 is also implicated in neuronal loss in PD, with elevation of Cdk5 consistently associated with cell death in different PD models. Cdk5 was first linked to PD when inhibition of Cdk5 activity reduces neuronal loss in MPTP-injected mice (Smith et al. 2003). MPTP injection increases Cdk5 activity and p25 levels in the substantia nigra of the injected mice, and attenuating this increase with Cdk5 inhibitor or adenovirus-mediated overexpression of dominant-negative Cdk5 attenuates dopaminergic neuronal loss (Smith et al. 2003). Although treatment with

MPP+, the metabolized form of MPTP in the brain, has also been demonstrated to reduce Cdk5 activity through proteasome-dependent degradation of p35 (Endo et al. 2009), majority of the studies reported increase in Cdk5 activity following MPTP injection or MPP+ treatment (Smith *et al.* 2003, Wong *et al.* 2011, Smith *et al.* 2006, Qu *et al.* 2007, Huang *et al.* 2010), possibly due to the use of different toxin dosages. Interestingly, additional studies aimed at elucidating the mechanisms by which Cdk5 regulates neuronal loss implicate Cdk5 in multiple cellular processes that were found to be altered in PD. Here we summarize the role of Cdk5 in several pathogenic mechanisms postulated to contribute to PD pathology.

3.1 Autophagy deregulation

Autophagy, a homeostatic process for the turnover of cytoplasmic content and organelles, is increasingly implicated in neurodegenerative diseases. Currently three types of autophagy are identified based on the mechanisms by which cargo is delivered, namely macroautophagy, microautophagy and chaperone-mediate autophagy (CMA). Macroautophagy is initiated with the formation of autophagosome, a double-membraned vesicle that is formed through the extension of isolation membrane (also known as phagophore), to encircle part of the cytoplasm for degradation. Subsequent fusion of autophagosome with lysosome leads to the formation of autolysosome, where the cargo of the autophagosome is degraded by lysosomal enzymes (Mizushima 2007). Microautophagy also entails bulk sequestration of cytoplasmic content, but instead of acting through the formation of autophagosomes, it is directly sequestered into lysosomes. CMA, on the other hand, involves selective translocation of soluble target proteins, which usually contain the KFERQ motif, to the lysosomes. Heat-shock cognate 70 (hsc70) and lysosomes-associated membrane protein 2A (LAMP2A) are important chaperones for selective transport of cargo into the CMA pathway (Cheung and Ip 2009, Mizushima *et al.* 2008, Rubinsztein 2006).

While autophagy has long been regarded as a homeostatic cellular event, recent studies revealed that deregulation of the autophagic pathway also contributes to neurodegeneration. Transgenic animals lacking Atg5 or Atg7, genes that are critical for macroautophagy, develop neurodegeneration (Hara *et al.* 2006, Komatsu *et al.* 2006). In addition, activation of macroautophagy in a drosophila model of Huntington's disease significantly reduces huntingtin toxicity (Ravikumar et al. 2004), consistent with a role of macroautophagy in the clearance of protein aggregates. Deregulation of the autophagic pathway is also demonstrated in PD (Cheung and Ip 2009). For example, accumulation of autophagosomes is evident in post-mortem brains of PD patients (Mizushima et al. 2008). In addition, both CMA and macroautophagy were implicated in the regulation of α-synuclein level, the major constituent of Lewy body. In particular, CMA is required for the degradation of wildtype soluble α-synuclein (Cuervo *et al.* 2004, Vogiatzi *et al.* 2008, Webb *et al.* 2003). Interestingly, A53T and A30P mutants of α-synuclein, which are associated with familial PD, inhibit CMA-mediated degradation of wildtype α-synuclein. These mutants are in turn degraded by macroautophagy (Cuervo et al. 2004). Furthermore, inhibition of CMA by A53T α-synuclein mutant also impairs degradation of pro-survival transcription factor MEF2D (Yang et al. 2009). Reduced degradation of MEF2D results in accumulation of MEF2D in the cytoplasm and inhibition of MEF2D activity, leading to cell death (Yang et al. 2009). Interestingly, Cdk5 has been demonstrated to phosphorylate MEF2D at S444 to inhibit its activity and facilitate its cleavage by caspases (Tang *et al.* 2005, Gong *et al.* 2003), and is required for neuronal loss triggered by MPTP injection (Smith et al. 2006). It will be interesting to examine whether phosphorylation of MEF2D by Cdk5 plays a role in its degradation by CMA. Moreover, we have recently demonstrated that overexpression of A53T α-synuclein increases Cdk5 activity (Wong et al. 2011). It is tempting to speculate that in addition to the inhibition of CMA-mediated degradation of MEF2D by α-synuclein expression, elevated phosphorylation of MEF2D by Cdk5 may also contribute to cell loss triggered by α-synuclein expression. Studies aimed at addressing this possibility will provide important insights regarding the pathogenic mechanisms of PD.

It should be noted that overexpression of A53T and A30P mutants of α-synuclein also induces activation of macroautophagy (Wong *et al.* 2011, Cuervo *et al.* 2004, Vogiatzi *et al.* 2008). While induction of macroautophagy may facilitate clearance of these mutant α-synucleins, several studies suggest that elevation of macroautophagy in response to A53T α-synuclein expression or MPP$^+$ treatment may be associated with neuronal loss (Wong *et al.* 2011, Yang *et al.* 2009, Xilouri *et al.* 2009, Stefanis *et al.* 2001, Kirik *et al.* 2002, Choubey *et al.* 2011). Whether this induction serves a protective or detrimental role in PD thus remains unresolved. We have recently discovered a role of Cdk5 in the regulation of macroautophagy through its phosphorylation of lipid-binding protein endophilin B1 (Wong et al. 2011). Endophilin B1, also known as Bax-interacting factor 1 (Bif-1), was previously implicated in autophagy induction in fibroblasts through its association with autophagy machinery UVRAG and Beclin 1 (Takahashi et al. 2007). We demonstrated that Cdk5-mediated phosphorylation of endophilin B1 at T145 is required for starvation-induced macroautophagy in neurons. More importantly, our findings revealed that this phosphorylation event is critical for the activation of macroautophagy in response to MPP$^+$ stimulation or overexpression of A53T α-synuclein (Wong et al. 2011). Attenuation of macroautophagy induction significantly reduces neuronal loss in these PD models, suggesting that activation of macroautophagy in PD may contribute to neuronal loss. Remarkably, inhibition of Cdk5 activity or endophilin B1 T145 phosphorylation concomitantly reduces macroautophagy activation or neuronal loss (Wong et al. 2011). Collectively, our findings reveal that macroautophagy activation in PD may serve a detrimental role, with Cdk5 and endophilin B1 being the essential mediators of this induction.

Deregulation of autophagy in PD also occurs in the form of impaired mitophagy, the removal of mitochondria through macroautophagy (Youle and Narendra 2011). Recent evidence reveals that two genes that are mutated in cases of familial PD, PINK1 and Parkin, are critical for mitophagy (Narendra *et al.* 2008, Geisler *et al.* 2010, Lee *et al.* 2010, Jin *et al.* 2010, Ziviani *et al.* 2010). PINK1, a serine/threonine kinase that is expressed on the outer membrane of the mitochondria, is constitutively degraded in healthy mitochondria in a voltage-dependent manner. The high level of PINK1 on damaged mitochondria will then result in the recruitment of Parkin, a ubiquitin E3 ligase, to the mitochondria. Subsequent ubiquitination of the damage mitochondria, Parkin itself and VDAC is required for the removal of damaged mitochondria via mitophagy (Narendra *et al.* 2010, Geisler *et al.* 2010, Lee *et al.* 2010, Jin *et al.* 2010). Importantly, various PD-associated missense mutations have been demonstrated to trigger different extent of mitophagy impairment (Lee et al. 2010), suggesting that aberrant mitophagy may represent one of the mechanisms by which these mutations lead to PD. Interestingly, Cdk5 has been demonstrated to phosphorylate Parkin at S131 to reduce its E3 ubiquitin ligase activity, with the S131A mutant of Parkin more prone to accumulate into inclusions (Avraham et al. 2007). In addition, phosphorylation of Parkin by Cdk5 and casein kinase I also augments its aggregation and inactivation (Rubio de la Torre et al. 2009). It will be interesting to examine whether Cdk5-mediated inhibition of Parkin activity affects the mitophagy of damaged mitochondria in PD models.

3.2 Oxidative stress

Oxidative stress has long been demonstrated to play an essential role in PD pathogenesis. Lipid peroxidation, DNA damage and protein oxidation are all evident in PD brains (Levy et al. 2009). In support of the involvement of oxidative stress in PD, familial PD-associated missense mutations were identified in DJ-1, an atypical peroxiredoxin-like peroxidase with antioxidant activity (Andres-Mateos et al. 2007). In addition, mitochondrial dysfunction, which could directly lead to generation of reactive oxygen species, is also detected in PD. These findings collectively suggest that preserving the anti-oxidative machinery in PD will be critical for limiting PD pathology.

Interestingly, an anti-oxidative peroxidase peroxiredoxin 2 (Prx2) was found to be phosphorylated by Cdk5 in response to MPTP toxicity (Qu et al. 2007). Phosphorylation of Prx2 at T89 by Cdk5 reduces its peroxidase activity. In addition, treatment with MPP+ increases Cdk5 activity and phospho-T89 Prx2 level, while concomitantly decreasing Prx2 peroxidase activity. Importantly, the protective effect of Prx2 against MPP+-induced cell death is attenuated when a T89 phospho-mimetic mutant of Prx2 is expressed, suggesting that phosphorylation of Prx2 at T89 abrogates its protective effect (Qu et al. 2007). These observations collectively revealed that Cdk5 may contribute to neuronal loss in PD through inhibiting the peroxidase activity of Prx2, thus rendering the cells more susceptible to oxidative stress.

DNA damage is a frequent consequence of oxidative stress and is a known factor for triggering cell death. A recent study revealed that Cdk5 also mediates neuronal loss in PD through phosphorylation of apurinic/apyrimidinic endonuclease 1 (Ape1), an enzyme implicated in DNA repair (Huang et al. 2010). Cdk5-mediated phosphorylation of Ape1 at T232 reduces its endonuclease activity and abolishes its neuroprotective effect against MPP+-triggered neuronal death (Huang et al. 2010). Interestingly, another enzyme implicated in DNA damage response, ataxia telangiectasia mutated (ATM), is also identified as a Cdk5 substrate (Tian et al. 2009). ATM is a phosphoinositide-3-kinase related kinase that plays critical role in the mediation of DNA damage signals, and has been implicated in neuronal loss triggered by DNA damage (Herzog *et al.* 1998, Kruman *et al.* 2004, Lee *et al.* 2001). Elevation of Cdk5 activity in response to DNA damage results in phosphorylation of ATM at S1981, an event that is critical for the activation of ATM. Interestingly, inhibition of Cdk5 activity attenuates neuronal loss induced by DNA damaging agent camptothecin (Tian et al. 2009). Although whether ATM phosphorylation is triggered in PD models remains unexplored, given the implication of DNA damage and the potential induction of Cdk5 activity in PD, it will be interesting to further dissect the precise role of Cdk5 in regulating the anti-oxidative machinery of the cells.

3.3 Mitochondrial dysfunction

Mitochondrial dysfunction has emerged as an important pathogenic mechanism in PD. Reduced mitochondrial complex I activity was detected in PD patients (Levy et al. 2009). In addition, MPTP was demonstrated to inhibit complex I of the mitochondrial respiratory chain (Levy et al. 2009). More importantly, gene products of a number of the familial PD-associated missense mutations are found to be localized to the mitochondria, including PINK1, Parkin, LRRK2, DJ-1 and HtrA2/Omi (Knott et al. 2008). In particular, recent studies revealed PINK1 and Parkin as important regulators of mitochondrial morphology through facilitating mitochondrial fission (Cho et al. 2010). Given the association of neuronal apoptosis with elevated mitochondrial fission, regulation of mitochondrial fusion/fission event by PINK1 and Parkin may also contribute to neuronal loss in PD. In addition, as mentioned above, PINK1 and Parkin are also required for the selective mitophagy of mitochondria with low membrane potential (Youle and Narendra 2011). With Parkin identified as a Cdk5 substrate (Avraham et al. 2007) and the observed expression of Cdk5 and p35 in the mitochondrial fraction of cortical neurons (Cheung et al. 2008), it is tempting to speculate that Cdk5 may also regulate mitochondrial homeostasis during PD through controlling mitochondrial fission/fusion or mitophagy. In support of this possibility, Cdk5 has also been implicated in mitochondrial fission during apoptosis (Meuer et al. 2007). In addition, another Cdk5 substrate endophilin B1 is also demonstrated to regulate mitochondrial morphology (Wong *et al.* 2011, Karbowski *et al.* 2004). It is therefore important to further delineate the role of Cdk5 in mitochondrial morphogenesis and mitophagy in PD models.

Aside from being the powerhouse of the cell and a potential source of reactive oxygen species, the mitochondria also plays a central role in the intrinsic apoptotic pathway. Release of cytochrome c from the intermembrane space of mitochondria triggers caspase activation and apoptosis (Bredesen et al. 2006). Indeed, neuronal loss in PD has been attributed at least in part to the apoptotic pathway (Levy et al. 2009). Identification of Bcl-2, a key anti-apoptotic regulator of cytochrome c release from the mitochondria, as a Cdk5 substrate suggests that Cdk5 may also regulate neuronal loss in PD through phosphorylation of Bcl-2 (Cheung et al. 2008). Furthermore, Cdk5 substrate endophilin B1, being an interacting protein of pro-apoptotic Bcl-2 family member Bax (Wong *et al.* 2011, Cuddeback *et al.* 2001), has also been demonstrated to play a role in apoptosis. Inhibition of endophilin B1 expression attenuates cytochrome c release and caspase-3 activation in HeLa cells (Takahashi et al. 2005). Although whether endophilin B1 similarly regulates apoptosis in neurons remains to be explored, these observations suggest that Cdk5-mediated phosphorylation of endophilin B1 and Bcl-2 may regulate the mitochondrial apoptotic pathway in PD. Additional studies will be required to address this hypothesis.

3.4 Proteasomal pathway anomaly

The proteasome pathway has also been demonstrated to contribute to degradation of α-synuclein (Webb *et al.* 2003, Rubinsztein 2006), suggesting that reduction in proteasomal activity may contribute to α-synuclein aggregation. Strikingly, a 40% decrease in proteasome activity has been demonstrated in the substantia nigra of PD patients post-mortem brains (McNaught and Jenner 2001). Indeed, mutation in E3 ubiquitin ligase Parkin and ubiquitin-C-terminal hydrolase-L1 (UCH-L1), a protein implicated in the degradation of poly-ubiquitin chains, are evident in familial PD cases (Kitada *et al.* 1998, Leroy *et al.* 1998). Familial PD-associated missense mutation of Parkin reduces its enzyme activity (Shimura et al. 2000). With Cdk5-mediated phosphorylation of Parkin also demonstrated to reduce its E3 ubiquitin ligase activity, it will be important to investigate if Cdk5 is involved in the deregulation of the proteasomal pathway in PD.

4. Future perspectives

It has become increasingly clear that Cdk5 plays a pivotal role in neuronal loss in PD. Using both *in vivo* and *in vitro* cell-based systems, inhibition of Cdk5 consistently attenuates neuronal loss in various PD models. The identification of multiple Cdk5 substrates that directly participates in known pathogenic mechanisms of PD has provided the much needed mechanistic insights regarding the alteration of these processes in PD, and the precise involvement of Cdk5 (Figure 1). Nonetheless, our understanding is far from complete. In particular, in light of the convergence of several pathogenic mechanisms onto the mitochondria and the identification of a number of mitochondria-associated proteins as Cdk5 substrates, it is important to further delineate how Cdk5 regulates the signaling cascades at the mitochondria during PD. In addition, Cdk5 has also been demonstrated to

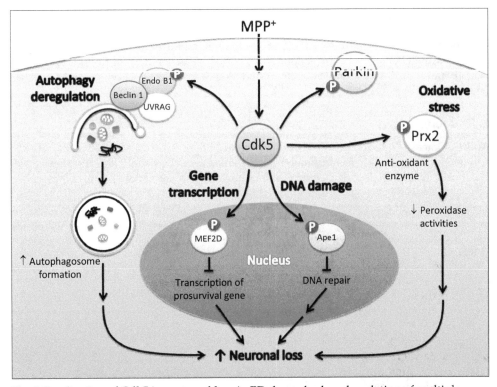

Fig. 1. Implication of Cdk5 in neuronal loss in PD through phosphorylation of multiple substrates. MPTP injection or MPP+ treatment elevates Cdk5 activity, which in turn phosphorylates a number of cellular proteins. Phosphorylation of endophilin B1 by Cdk5 is required for macroautophagy induction in PD models, which contributes to neuronal loss. Cdk5 also phosphorylates pro-survival transcription factor MEF2D and DNA repair enzyme Ape1 to inhibit their activities, thereby leading to cell death. Phosphorylation of anti-oxidant enzyme Prx2 by Cdk5 attenuates its peroxidase activity, leaving the cell more prone to oxidative stress. Cdk5-mediated phosphorylation of Parkin also reduces its E3 ubiquitin ligase activity, but how this directly contributes to neuronal loss remains to be explored.

regulate dopaminergic transmission and dopamine downstream signaling through phosphorylation of DARPP-32 (Chergui *et al.* 2004, Bibb *et al.* 1999). Furthermore, both dopamine and tyrosine hydroxylase have been identified as Cdk5 substrates (Zhen *et al.* 2004, Kansy *et al.* 2004). It will thus be important to further examine the effect of Cdk5 on dopaminergic transmission in PD models, and investigate the possibility that Cdk5 modulators may regulate dopamine levels to alleviate PD symptoms. Together with the apparent neuroprotective effect of Cdk5 against neuronal loss in PD through acting on multiple cellular events that are aberrant in PD, Cdk5 may emerge as an important target for future development of therapeutics against PD.

5. Acknowledgement

We apologize to the many researchers whose works were not cited due to space limitation. We would like to thank Ka-Chun Lok for his excellent help on preparing the figure. The studies by Z.H. Cheung and N.Y. Ip were supported in part by the Research Grants Council of Hong Kong (HKUST 661007, 660309, 661109, 660810 and 660210), the Area of Excellence Scheme of the University Grants Committee (AoE/B-15/01) and Hong Kong Jockey Club. N.Y. Ip and Z.H. Cheung are Croucher Foundation Senior Research Fellow and Croucher Foundation Fellow, respectively.

6. References

Andres-Mateos, E., Perier, C., Zhang, L., Blanchard-Fillion, B., Greco, T. M., Thomas, B., Ko, H. S., Sasaki, M., Ischiropoulos, H., Przedborski, S., Dawson, T. M. and Dawson, V. L. (2007) DJ-1 gene deletion reveals that DJ-1 is an atypical peroxiredoxin-like peroxidase. *Proc Natl Acad Sci U S A* 104, 14807-14812.

Arif, A., Jia, J., Moodt, R. A., DiCorleto, P. E. and Fox, P. L. (2011) Phosphorylation of glutamyl-prolyl tRNA synthetase by cyclin-dependent kinase 5 dictates transcript-selective translational control. *Proc Natl Acad Sci U S A* 108, 1415-1420.

Asada, A., Yamamoto, N., Gohda, M., Saito, T., Hayashi, N. and Hisanaga, S. (2008) Myristoylation of p39 and p35 is a determinant of cytoplasmic or nuclear localization of active cyclin-dependent kinase 5 complexes. *J Neurochem* 106, 1325-1336.

Avraham, E., Rott, R., Liani, E., Szargel, R. and Engelender, S. (2007) Phosphorylation of Parkin by the cyclin-dependent kinase 5 at the linker region modulates its ubiquitin-ligase activity and aggregation. *J Biol Chem* 282, 12842-12850.

Bibb, J. A., Snyder, G. L., Nishi, A., Yan, Z., Meijer, L., Fienberg, A. A., Tsai, L. H., Kwon, Y. T., Girault, J. A., Czernik, A. J., Huganir, R. L., Hemmings, H. C., Jr., Nairn, A. C. and Greengard, P. (1999) Phosphorylation of DARPP-32 by Cdk5 modulates dopamine signalling in neurons. *Nature* 402, 669-671.

Bredesen, D. E., Rao, R. V. and Mehlen, P. (2006) Cell death in the nervous system. *Nature* 443, 796-802.

Chae, T., Kwon, Y. T., Bronson, R., Dikkes, P., Li, E. and Tsai, L. H. (1997) Mice lacking p35, a neuronal specific activator of Cdk5, display cortical lamination defects, seizures, and adult lethality. *Neuron* 18, 29-42.

Chergui, K., Svenningsson, P. and Greengard, P. (2004) Cyclin-dependent kinase 5 regulates dopaminergic and glutamatergic transmission in the striatum. *Proc Natl Acad Sci U S A* 101, 2191-2196.

Cheung, Z. H., Chin, W. H., Chen, Y., Ng, Y. P. and Ip, N. Y. (2007) Cdk5 is involved in BDNF-stimulated dendritic growth in hippocampal neurons. *PLoS Biol* 5, e63.

Cheung, Z. H., Gong, K. and Ip, N. Y. (2008) Cyclin-dependent kinase 5 supports neuronal survival through phosphorylation of Bcl-2. *J Neurosci* 28, 4872-4877.

Cheung, Z. H. and Ip, N. Y. (2004) Cdk5: mediator of neuronal death and survival. *Neurosci Lett* 361, 47-51.

Cheung, Z. H. and Ip, N. Y. (2007) The roles of cyclin-dependent kinase 5 in dendrite and synapse development. *Biotechnol J*.

Cheung, Z. H. and Ip, N. Y. (2009) The emerging role of autophagy in Parkinson's disease. *Mol Brain* 2, 29.

Cho, D. H., Nakamura, T. and Lipton, S. A. (2010) Mitochondrial dynamics in cell death and neurodegeneration. *Cell Mol Life Sci* 67, 3435-3447.

Choi, J. H., Banks, A. S., Estall, J. L., Kajimura, S., Bostrom, P., Laznik, D., Ruas, J. L., Chalmers, M. J., Kamenecka, T. M., Bluher, M., Griffin, P. R. and Spiegelman, B. M. (2010) Anti-diabetic drugs inhibit obesity-linked phosphorylation of PPARgamma by Cdk5. *Nature* 466, 451-456.

Choubey, V., Safiulina, D., Vaarmann, A., Cagalinec, M., Wareski, P., Kuum, M., Zharkovsky, A. and Kaasik, A. (2011) Mutant A53T {alpha}-synuclein induces neuronal death by increasing mitochondrial autophagy. *J Biol Chem*.

Cruz, J. C. and Tsai, L. H. (2004) A Jekyll and Hyde kinase: roles for Cdk5 in brain development and disease. *Curr Opin Neurobiol* 14, 390-394.

Cuddeback, S. M., Yamaguchi, H., Komatsu, K., Miyashita, T., Yamada, M., Wu, C., Singh, S. and Wang, H. G. (2001) Molecular cloning and characterization of Bif-1. A novel Src homology 3 domain-containing protein that associates with Bax. *J Biol Chem* 276, 20559-20565.

Cuervo, A. M., Stefanis, L., Fredenburg, R., Lansbury, P. T. and Sulzer, D. (2004) Impaired degradation of mutant alpha-synuclein by chaperone-mediated autophagy. *Science* 305, 1292-1295.

Dauer, W. and Przedborski, S. (2003) Parkinson's disease: mechanisms and models. *Neuron* 39, 889-909.

de Rijk, M. C., Tzourio, C., Breteler, M. M., Dartigues, J. F., Amaducci, L., Lopez-Pousa, S., Manubens-Bertran, J. M., Alperovitch, A. and Rocca, W. A. (1997) Prevalence of parkinsonism and Parkinson's disease in Europe: the EUROPARKINSON Collaborative Study. European Community Concerted Action on the Epidemiology of Parkinson's disease. *J Neurol Neurosurg Psychiatry* 62, 10-15.

Dhavan, R. and Tsai, L. H. (2001) A decade of CDK5. *Nat Rev Mol Cell Biol* 2, 749-759.

Endo, R., Saito, T., Asada, A., Kawahara, H., Ohshima, T. and Hisanaga, S. (2009) Commitment of 1-methyl-4-phenylpyrinidinium ion-induced neuronal cell death by proteasome-mediated degradation of p35 cyclin-dependent kinase 5 activator. *J Biol Chem* 284, 26029-26039.

Fu, A. K., Cheung, J., Smith, F. D., Ip, F. C. and Ip, N. Y. (2001) Overexpression of muscle specific kinase increases the transcription and aggregation of acetylcholine receptors in Xenopus embryos. *Brain Res Mol Brain Res* 96, 21-29.

Fu, W. Y., Chen, Y., Sahin, M., Zhao, X. S., Shi, L., Bikoff, J. B., Lai, K. O., Yung, W. H., Fu, A. K., Greenberg, M. E. and Ip, N. Y. (2007) Cdk5 regulates EphA4-mediated dendritic spine retraction through an ephexin1-dependent mechanism. *Nat Neurosci* 10, 67-76.

Geisler, S., Holmstrom, K. M., Skujat, D., Fiesel, F. C., Rothfuss, O. C., Kahle, P. J. and Springer, W. (2010) PINK1/Parkin-mediated mitophagy is dependent on VDAC1 and p62/SQSTM1. *Nat Cell Biol* 12, 119-131.

Gong, X., Tang, X., Wiedmann, M., Wang, X., Peng, J., Zheng, D., Blair, L. A., Marshall, J. and Mao, Z. (2003) Cdk5-mediated inhibition of the protective effects of transcription factor MEF2 in neurotoxicity-induced apoptosis. *Neuron* 38, 33-46.

Hara, T., Nakamura, K., Matsui, M., Yamamoto, A., Nakahara, Y., Suzuki-Migishima, R., Yokoyama, M., Mishima, K., Saito, I., Okano, H. and Mizushima, N. (2006) Suppression of basal autophagy in neural cells causes neurodegenerative disease in mice. *Nature* 441, 885-889.

Hawasli, A. H. and Bibb, J. A. (2007) Alternative roles for Cdk5 in learning and synaptic plasticity. *Biotechnol J* 2, 941-948.

Herzog, K. H., Chong, M. J., Kapsetaki, M., Morgan, J. I. and McKinnon, P. J. (1998) Requirement for Atm in ionizing radiation-induced cell death in the developing central nervous system. *Science* 280, 1089-1091.

Huang, E., Qu, D., Zhang, Y., Venderova, K., Haque, M. E., Rousseaux, M. W., Slack, R. S., Woulfe, J. M. and Park, D. S. (2010) The role of Cdk5-mediated apurinic/apyrimidinic endonuclease 1 phosphorylation in neuronal death. *Nat Cell Biol* 12, 563-571.

Jin, S. M., Lazarou, M., Wang, C., Kane, L. A., Narendra, D. P. and Youle, R. J. (2010) Mitochondrial membrane potential regulates PINK1 import and proteolytic destabilization by PARL. *J Cell Biol* 191, 933-942.

Kansy, J. W., Daubner, S. C., Nishi, A., Sotogaku, N., Lloyd, M. D., Nguyen, C., Lu, L., Haycock, J. W., Hope, B. T., Fitzpatrick, P. F. and Bibb, J. A. (2004) Identification of tyrosine hydroxylase as a physiological substrate for Cdk5. *J Neurochem* 91, 374-384.

Karbowski, M., Jeong, S. Y. and Youle, R. J. (2004) Endophilin B1 is required for the maintenance of mitochondrial morphology. *J Cell Biol* 166, 1027-1039.

Kirik, D., Rosenblad, C., Burger, C., Lundberg, C., Johansen, T. E., Muzyczka, N., Mandel, R. J. and Bjorklund, A. (2002) Parkinson-like neurodegeneration induced by targeted overexpression of alpha-synuclein in the nigrostriatal system. *J Neurosci* 22, 2780-2791.

Kitada, T., Asakawa, S., Hattori, N., Matsumine, H., Yamamura, Y., Minoshima, S., Yokochi, M., Mizuno, Y. and Shimizu, N. (1998) Mutations in the parkin gene cause autosomal recessive juvenile parkinsonism. *Nature* 392, 605-608.

Knott, A. B., Perkins, G., Schwarzenbacher, R. and Bossy-Wetzel, E. (2008) Mitochondrial fragmentation in neurodegeneration. *Nat Rev Neurosci* 9, 505-518.

Ko, J., Humbert, S., Bronson, R. T., Takahashi, S., Kulkarni, A. B., Li, E. and Tsai, L. H. (2001) p35 and p39 are essential for cyclin-dependent kinase 5 function during neurodevelopment. *J Neurosci* 21, 6758-6771.

Kobayashi, S., Ishiguro, K., Omori, A., Takamatsu, M., Arioka, M., Imahori, K. and Uchida, T. (1993) A cdc2-related kinase PSSALRE/cdk5 is homologous with the 30 kDa subunit of tau protein kinase II, a proline-directed protein kinase associated with microtubule. *FEBS Lett* 335, 171-175.

Komatsu, M., Waguri, S., Chiba, T., Murata, S., Iwata, J., Tanida, I., Ueno, T., Koike, M., Uchiyama, Y., Kominami, E. and Tanaka, K. (2006) Loss of autophagy in the central nervous system causes neurodegeneration in mice. *Nature* 441, 880-884.

Kruman, II, Wersto, R. P., Cardozo-Pelaez, F., Smilenov, L., Chan, S. L., Chrest, F. J., Emokpae, R., Jr., Gorospe, M. and Mattson, M. P. (2004) Cell cycle activation linked to neuronal cell death initiated by DNA damage. *Neuron* 41, 549-561.

Lai, K. O. and Ip, N. Y. (2009) Recent advances in understanding the roles of Cdk5 in synaptic plasticity. *Biochim Biophys Acta* 1792, 741-745.

Lee, J. Y., Nagano, Y., Taylor, J. P., Lim, K. L. and Yao, T. P. (2010) Disease-causing mutations in parkin impair mitochondrial ubiquitination, aggregation, and HDAC6-dependent mitophagy. *J Cell Biol* 189, 671-679.

Lee, Y., Chong, M. J. and McKinnon, P. J. (2001) Ataxia telangiectasia mutated-dependent apoptosis after genotoxic stress in the developing nervous system is determined by cellular differentiation status. *J Neurosci* 21, 6687-6693.

Leroy, E., Boyer, R., Auburger, G., Leube, B., Ulm, G., Mezey, E., Harta, G., Brownstein, M. J., Jonnalagada, S., Chernova, T., Dehejia, A., Lavedan, C., Gasser, T., Steinbach, P. J., Wilkinson, K. D. and Polymeropoulos, M. H. (1998) The ubiquitin pathway in Parkinson's disease. *Nature* 395, 451-452.

Levy, O. A., Malagelada, C. and Greene, L. A. (2009) Cell death pathways in Parkinson's disease: proximal triggers, distal effectors, and final steps. *Apoptosis* 14, 478-500.

Lew, J., Beaudette, K., Litwin, C. M. and Wang, J. H. (1992) Purification and characterization of a novel proline-directed protein kinase from bovine brain. *J Biol Chem* 267, 13383-13390.

Li, B. S., Ma, W., Jaffe, H., Zheng, Y., Takahashi, S., Zhang, L., Kulkarni, A. B. and Pant, H. C. (2003a) Cyclin-dependent kinase-5 is involved in neuregulin-dependent activation of phosphatidylinositol 3-kinase and Akt activity mediating neuronal survival. *J Biol Chem* 278, 35702-35709.

Li, G., Faibushevich, A., Turunen, B. J., Yoon, S. O., Georg, G., Michaelis, M. L. and Dobrowsky, R. T. (2003b) Stabilization of the cyclin-dependent kinase 5 activator, p35, by paclitaxel decreases beta-amyloid toxicity in cortical neurons. *J Neurochem* 84, 347-362.

Lilja, L., Yang, S. N., Webb, D. L., Juntti-Berggren, L., Berggren, P. O. and Bark, C. (2001) Cyclin-dependent kinase 5 promotes insulin exocytosis. *J Biol Chem* 276, 34199-34205.

McNaught, K. S. and Jenner, P. (2001) Proteasomal function is impaired in substantia nigra in Parkinson's disease. *Neurosci Lett* 297, 191-194.

Meuer, K., Suppanz, I. E., Lingor, P., Planchamp, V., Goricke, B., Fichtner, L., Braus, G. H., Dietz, G. P., Jakobs, S., Bahr, M. and Weishaupt, J. H. (2007) Cyclin-dependent kinase 5 is an upstream regulator of mitochondrial fission during neuronal apoptosis. *Cell Death Differ* 14, 651-661.

Meyerson, M., Enders, G. H., Wu, C. L., Su, L. K., Gorka, C., Nelson, C., Harlow, E. and Tsai, L. H. (1992) A family of human cdc2-related protein kinases. *Embo J* 11, 2909-2917.

Mizushima, N. (2007) Autophagy: process and function. *Genes Dev* 21, 2861-2873.

Mizushima, N., Levine, B., Cuervo, A. M. and Klionsky, D. J. (2008) Autophagy fights disease through cellular self-digestion. *Nature* 451, 1069-1075.

Narendra, D., Tanaka, A., Suen, D. F. and Youle, R. J. (2008) Parkin is recruited selectively to impaired mitochondria and promotes their autophagy. *J Cell Biol* 183, 795-803.

Narendra, D. P., Jin, S. M., Tanaka, A., Suen, D. F., Gautier, C. A., Shen, J., Cookson, M. R. and Youle, R. J. (2010) PINK1 is selectively stabilized on impaired mitochondria to activate Parkin. *PLoS Biol* 8, e1000298.

Nguyen, M. D., Mushynski, W. E. and Julien, J. P. (2002) Cycling at the interface between neurodevelopment and neurodegeneration. *Cell Death Differ* 9, 1294-1306.

O'Hare, M. J., Kushwaha, N., Zhang, Y., Aleyasin, H., Callaghan, S. M., Slack, R. S., Albert, P. R., Vincent, I. and Park, D. S. (2005) Differential roles of nuclear and cytoplasmic cyclin-dependent kinase 5 in apoptotic and excitotoxic neuronal death. *J Neurosci* 25, 8954-8966.

Obeso, J. A., Rodriguez-Oroz, M. C., Goetz, C. G., Marin, C., Kordower, J. H., Rodriguez, M., Hirsch, E. C., Farrer, M., Schapira, A. H. and Halliday, G. (2010) Missing pieces in the Parkinson's disease puzzle. *Nat Med* 16, 653-661.

Ohshima, T., Ward, J. M., Huh, C. G., Longenecker, G., Veeranna, Pant, H. C., Brady, R. O., Martin, L. J. and Kulkarni, A. B. (1996) Targeted disruption of the cyclin-dependent kinase 5 gene results in abnormal corticogenesis, neuronal pathology and perinatal death. *Proc Natl Acad Sci U S A* 93, 11173-11178.

Patrick, G. N., Zhou, P., Kwon, Y. T., Howley, P. M. and Tsai, L. H. (1998) p35, the neuronal-specific activator of cyclin-dependent kinase 5 (Cdk5) is degraded by the ubiquitin-proteasome pathway. *J Biol Chem* 273, 24057-24064.

Patrick, G. N., Zukerberg, L., Nikolic, M., de la Monte, S., Dikkes, P. and Tsai, L. H. (1999) Conversion of p35 to p25 deregulates Cdk5 activity and promotes neurodegeneration. *Nature* 402, 615-622.

Patzke, H. and Tsai, L. H. (2002) Calpain-mediated cleavage of the cyclin-dependent kinase-5 activator p39 to p29. *J Biol Chem* 277, 8054-8060.

Peterson, D. W., Ando, D. M., Taketa, D. A., Zhou, H., Dahlquist, F. W. and Lew, J. (2010) No difference in kinetics of tau or histone phosphorylation by CDK5/p25 versus CDK5/p35 in vitro. *Proc Natl Acad Sci U S A* 107, 2884-2889.

Poewe, W., Antonini, A., Zijlmans, J. C., Burkhard, P. R. and Vingerhoets, F. (2010) Levodopa in the treatment of Parkinson's disease: an old drug still going strong. *Clin Interv Aging* 5, 229-238.

Qu, D., Rashidian, J., Mount, M. P., Aleyasin, H., Parsanejad, M., Lira, A., Haque, E., Zhang, Y., Callaghan, S., Daigle, M., Rousseaux, M. W., Slack, R. S., Albert, P. R., Vincent, I., Woulfe, J. M. and Park, D. S. (2007) Role of Cdk5-mediated phosphorylation of Prx2 in MPTP toxicity and Parkinson's disease. *Neuron* 55, 37-52.

Rashidian, J., Rousseaux, M. W., Venderova, K., Qu, D., Callaghan, S. M., Phillips, M., Bland, R. J., During, M. J., Mao, Z., Slack, R. S. and Park, D. S. (2009) Essential role of cytoplasmic cdk5 and Prx2 in multiple ischemic injury models, in vivo. *J Neurosci* 29, 12497-12505.

Ravikumar, B., Vacher, C., Berger, Z., Davies, J. E., Luo, S., Oroz, L. G., Scaravilli, F., Easton, D. F., Duden, R., O'Kane, C. J. and Rubinsztein, D. C. (2004) Inhibition of mTOR induces autophagy and reduces toxicity of polyglutamine expansions in fly and mouse models of Huntington disease. *Nat Genet* 36, 585-595.

Rubinsztein, D. C. (2006) The roles of intracellular protein-degradation pathways in neurodegeneration. *Nature* 443, 780-786.

Rubio de la Torre, E., Luzon-Toro, B., Forte-Lago, I., Minguez-Castellanos, A., Ferrer, I. and Hilfiker, S. (2009) Combined kinase inhibition modulates parkin inactivation. *Hum Mol Genet* 18, 809-823.

Sasaki, Y., Cheng, C., Uchida, Y., Nakajima, O., Ohshima, T., Yagi, T., Taniguchi, M., Nakayama, T., Kishida, R., Kudo, Y., Ohno, S., Nakamura, F. and Goshima, Y. (2002) Fyn and Cdk5 mediate semaphorin-3A signaling, which is involved in regulation of dendrite orientation in cerebral cortex. *Neuron* 35, 907-920.

Schulz, J. B. (2008) Update on the pathogenesis of Parkinson's disease. *J Neurol* 255 Suppl 5, 3-7.

Shimura, H., Hattori, N., Kubo, S., Mizuno, Y., Asakawa, S., Minoshima, S., Shimizu, N., Iwai, K., Chiba, T., Tanaka, K. and Suzuki, T. (2000) Familial Parkinson disease gene product, parkin, is a ubiquitin-protein ligase. *Nat Genet* 25, 302-305.

Smith, P. D., Crocker, S. J., Jackson-Lewis, V., Jordan-Sciutto, K. L., Hayley, S., Mount, M. P., O'Hare, M. J., Callaghan, S., Slack, R. S., Przedborski, S., Anisman, H. and Park, D. S. (2003) Cyclin-dependent kinase 5 is a mediator of dopaminergic neuron loss in a mouse model of Parkinson's disease. *Proc Natl Acad Sci U S A* 100, 13650-13655.

Smith, P. D., Mount, M. P., Shree, R., Callaghan, S., Slack, R. S., Anisman, H., Vincent, I., Wang, X., Mao, Z. and Park, D. S. (2006) Calpain-regulated p35/cdk5 plays a central role in dopaminergic neuron death through modulation of the transcription factor myocyte enhancer factor 2. *J Neurosci* 26, 440-447.

Stefanis, L., Larsen, K. E., Rideout, H. J., Sulzer, D. and Greene, L. A. (2001) Expression of A53T mutant but not wild-type alpha-synuclein in PC12 cells induces alterations of the ubiquitin-dependent degradation system, loss of dopamine release, and autophagic cell death. *J Neurosci* 21, 9549-9560.

Takahashi, M., Iseki, E. and Kosaka, K. (2000) Cyclin-dependent kinase 5 (Cdk5) associated with Lewy bodies in diffuse Lewy body disease. *Brain Res* 862, 253-256.

Takahashi, Y., Coppola, D., Matsushita, N., Cualing, H. D., Sun, M., Sato, Y., Liang, C., Jung, J. U., Cheng, J. Q., Mul, J. J., Pledger, W. J. and Wang, H. G. (2007) Bif-1 interacts with Beclin 1 through UVRAG and regulates autophagy and tumorigenesis. *Nat Cell Biol* 9, 1142-1151.

Takahashi, Y., Karbowski, M., Yamaguchi, H., Kazi, A., Wu, J., Sebti, S. M., Youle, R. J. and Wang, H. G. (2005) Loss of Bif-1 suppresses Bax/Bak conformational change and mitochondrial apoptosis. *Mol Cell Biol* 25, 9369-9382.

Tandon, A., Yu, H., Wang, L., Rogaeva, E., Sato, C., Chishti, M. A., Kawarai, T., Hasegawa, H., Chen, F., Davies, P., Fraser, P. E., Westaway, D. and St George-Hyslop, P. H. (2003) Brain levels of CDK5 activator p25 are not increased in Alzheimer's or other neurodegenerative diseases with neurofibrillary tangles. *J Neurochem* 86, 572-581.

Tang, X., Wang, X., Gong, X., Tong, M., Park, D., Xia, Z. and Mao, Z. (2005) Cyclin-dependent kinase 5 mediates neurotoxin-induced degradation of the transcription factor myocyte enhancer factor 2. *J Neurosci* 25, 4823-4834.

Tian, B., Yang, Q. and Mao, Z. (2009) Phosphorylation of ATM by Cdk5 mediates DNA damage signalling and regulates neuronal death. *Nat Cell Biol* 11, 211-218.

Tsai, L. H., Takahashi, T., Caviness, V. S., Jr. and Harlow, E. (1993) Activity and expression pattern of cyclin-dependent kinase 5 in the embryonic mouse nervous system. *Development* 119, 1029-1040.

Vogiatzi, T., Xilouri, M., Vekrellis, K. and Stefanis, L. (2008) Wild type alpha-synuclein is degraded by chaperone-mediated autophagy and macroautophagy in neuronal cells. *J Biol Chem* 283, 23542-23556.

Webb, J. L., Ravikumar, B., Atkins, J., Skepper, J. N. and Rubinsztein, D. C. (2003) Alpha-Synuclein is degraded by both autophagy and the proteasome. *J Biol Chem* 278, 25009-25013.

Wong, A. S., Lee, R. H., Cheung, A. Y., Yeung, P. K., Chung, S. K., Cheung, Z. H. and Ip, N. Y. (2011) Cdk5-mediated phosphorylation of endophilin B1 is required for induced autophagy in models of Parkinson's disease. *Nat Cell Biol.*

Xilouri, M., Vogiatzi, T., Vekrellis, K., Park, D. and Stefanis, L. (2009) Abberant alpha-synuclein confers toxicity to neurons in part through inhibition of chaperone-mediated autophagy. *PLoS One* 4, e5515.

Yang, Q., She, H., Gearing, M., Colla, E., Lee, M., Shacka, J. J. and Mao, Z. (2009) Regulation of neuronal survival factor MEF2D by chaperone-mediated autophagy. *Science* 323, 124-127.

Youle, R. J. and Narendra, D. P. (2011) Mechanisms of mitophagy. *Nat Rev Mol Cell Biol* 12, 9-14.

Zhang, J. and Herrup, K. (2008) Cdk5 and the non-catalytic arrest of the neuronal cell cycle. *Cell Cycle* 7, 3487-3490.

Zhang, J., Li, H. and Herrup, K. (2010a) Cdk5 nuclear localization is p27-dependent in nerve cells: implications for cell cycle suppression and caspase-3 activation. *J Biol Chem* 285, 14052-14061.

Zhang, P., Yu, P. C., Tsang, A. H., Chen, Y., Fu, A. K., Fu, W. Y., Chung, K. K. and Ip, N. Y. (2010b) S-nitrosylation of cyclin-dependent kinase 5 (cdk5) regulates its kinase activity and dendrite growth during neuronal development. *J Neurosci* 30, 14366-14370.

Zhen, X., Goswami, S., Abdali, S. A., Gil, M., Bakshi, K. and Friedman, E. (2004) Regulation of cyclin-dependent kinase 5 and calcium/calmodulin-dependent protein kinase II by phosphatidylinositol-linked dopamine receptor in rat brain. *Mol Pharmacol* 66, 1500-1507.

Ziviani, E., Tao, R. N. and Whitworth, A. J. (2010) Drosophila parkin requires PINK1 for mitochondrial translocation and ubiquitinates mitofusin. *Proc Natl Acad Sci U S A* 107, 5018-5023.

8

Role of FKBPs in Parkinson's Disease

Souvik Chattopadhaya, Amaravadhi Harikishore and Ho Sup Yoon
School of Biological Sciences, Nanyang Technological University
Singapore

1. Introduction

Parkinson's disease (PD) is the second most common neurodegenerative disease among the elderly. While sporadic PD constitutes 99% of the cases, the remaining 1% is of genetic origin. The neuropathological hallmarks of PD are progressive degeneration of dopaminergic (DA) neurons and presence of Lewy neurites and Lewy bodies (LBs) - intracytoplasmic proteinaceous inclusions that contain α-synuclein (SYN), synphilin-1, components of the ubiquitin proteasomal pathway and parkin (Dawson, 2006). The loss of DA neurons in substantia nigra pars compacta (SNpc) results in decreased signalling in the striatum thereby giving rise to motor defects like resting tremor, bradykinesia, rigidity and posture instability. Besides DA neuronal loss, microglial activation and increased astroglial and lymphocyte infiltration also occur in PD. A role for inflammation in PD has been inferred from the identification of human leukocyte antigen (HLA)-DR positive reactive microglia in the brains of PD patients (McGeer *et al.*, 1988). Additionally, levels of pro-inflammatory cytokines like IL-6, IL-1β, TNFα have been found to be elevated in the blood and cerebrospinal fluid (CSF) of PD patients (Nagatsu & Sawada, 2005; Dawson, 2006) Although these inflammatory components might serve as useful biomarkers, the aetiology of striatal DA degeneration still remains enigmatic.

In the last decade, identification of mutations in several distinct genes (*LRRK2, parkin, PINK1, DJ-1, α-synuclein, MAPT, UCHL1* etc) linked to different forms of familial Parkinsonism has imparted a new direction to understanding PD pathogenesis (Tong & Shen, 2009). The question as to how seemingly divergent genes cause PD still remains unanswered, as there is no common molecular pathway involving these gene products. While parkin, α-synuclein (SYN) and ubiquitin C-terminal hydrolase L1 (UCHL1) are functionally associated with the cellular ubiquitin proteasomal system (UPS), DJ-1 and PINK1 protect against oxidative stress and mitochondrial dysfunction. More recently, microarray analysis of SNpc from parkinsonian brain (Mandel *et al.*, 2005) has shown that 68 genes related to protein degradation, signal transduction, dopaminergic transmission, iron transport and glycolysis are downregulated. Prominent among these are the protein chaperone HSC-70, subunits of the UPS and SKP1A, a member of the E3 ubiquitin ligase complex. Therefore, it is most likely that impairment in energy metabolism and/or alterations in UPS are the underlying mechanisms for PD pathogenesis (Eriksen *et al.*, 2005; Mandel *et al.*, 2005).

Current PD treatment regimes can be divided into three categories: symptomatic, protective and restorative. Only symptomatic treatment via the administration of L-dopa and other drugs affecting neurological transmission have shown efficacy. However, side effects like dyskinesia, motor fluctuations and neurological complications limit their long-term use (Gold & Nutt, 2002). The neuroimmunophilins ligands (NILs) are a promising new class of drugs for treatment of PD as well as other neurodegenerative diseases. NILs are derived from the immunosuppressant, FK506 (tacrolimus) and exert their activity not via any cellular mechanism involving the immune system but by binding to a group of proteins termed FK506 binding proteins (FKBPs). When compared to the immune system, FKBP expression levels are highly enriched (10-50 fold greater) in both the central and peripheral nervous system. In this chapter, we review our current understanding of the role of FKBPs in the nervous system with an emphasis on the protein partners that interface with FKBPs inside cells. For brevity, we limit our discussions to FKBPs that are enriched in the nervous systems and may have important role in Parkinson's disease pathogenesis. We also highlight the mode of action of the NILs with the hope that knowledge of such interaction will enable rationale design of new drugs with improved efficacy for treatment of Parkinson's disease as well as other neurodegenerative disorders.

2. Role of FKBPs in the nervous system

FKBPs together with cyclophilins (CyPs) comprise a family of phylogenetically conserved immunophilins that have peptidyl prolyl isomerase activity (PPIase; EC 5.2.1.8), producing the *cis-trans* isomerization of X-Pro peptide bond, an essential but rate-limiting step in the protein folding process (Barik, 2006). Initial isolation and purification of immunophilins were based on their differential affinity towards the principal immunosuppressant drugs - rapamycin, FK506 and cyclosporin A (CsA). While CyPs bind to only CsA, FKBPs have affinities for both FK506 and rapamycin. Immunosuppressive activity mediated by these drugs is brought about by their binding to the cognate immunophilins. The FK506/FKBP or CsA/CyP binary complexes bind to the Ca^{2+}/calmodulin dependent protein serine/threonine phosphatase, calcineurin (CaN) and inhibit its phosphatase activity. The resulting FKBP-FK506-CaN ternary complex cannot dephosphorylate the key transcription factor, nuclear factor of activated T-cells (NF-AT). Inactive NF-AT remains in the cytoplasm thereby preventing interleukin-2 (IL-2) secretion (**Figure 1**). Consequently, both T-cell activation and proliferation is inhibited. On the other hand, FKBP-rapamycin complex exerts immunosuppression by inhibiting the serine/threonine kinase activity of mammalian target of rapamycin (mTOR) (Sharma et al., 1994).

The role of FKBPs in the nervous system was initiated by observations that the brain is abundantly enriched in CyPs and FKBPs (Maki et al., 1990; Steiner et al., 1992; Dawson et al., 1994). The importance of immunophilins in the nervous system was firmly established from studies showing that FK506 potently (as low as 0.1 nM) increases neurite outgrowth in both PC-12 (Lyons et al., 1994) and SH-SY5Y cell culture models as well as in primary cultures of chick dorsal root ganglion and hippocampal neurons (Hamilton and Steiner, 1998). Efforts to explain this neurotrophic effect focussed on the calcineurin-dependent pathway involving the CaN substrate, GAP-43 (growth-associated protein-43). GAP-43 selectively localizes to developing neurons and its phosphorylation is known to enhance its neurite extension activity (Meiri et al., 1991). Though initially tenable, the hypothesis was challenged when it was shown that both CsA (Gold, 1997) and non-immunosuppressive (hence non-calcineurin binding) derivatives of FK506 exhibit neurotrophic effect with similar potencies as that of FK506. Therefore, it is most likely that nerve growth proceeds via a calcineurin-independent pathway.

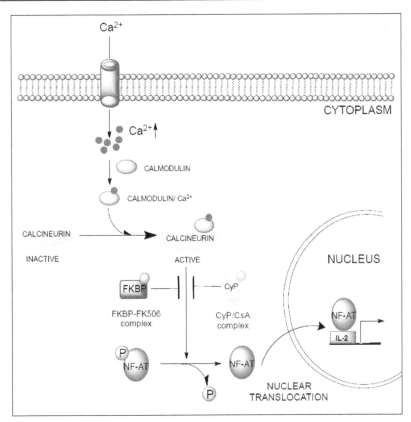

Fig. 1. Immunosuppressive effect of neuroimmunophilin ligands: T-cell receptor activation leads to a rapid increase in intracellular calcium levels with concomitant activation of the Ca^{2+}/calmodulin-dependent phosphatase, calcineurin (CaN). Active CaN dephosphorylates the transcription factor NF-AT, allowing its nuclear translocation and thereby upregulating IL-2 expression. Addition of FK506 or CsA results in formation of FKBP-FK506-CaN/CyP-CsA-CaN ternary complexes that inhibits CaN-dependent NF-AT dephosphorylation, as a result T-cell activation and IL-2 secretion does not occur.

When FK506-treated brain lysates were probed for proteins with increased phosphorylation levels, one of the identified targets was neuronal nitric oxide synthase (nNOS). In the brain, nNOS catalyzes the formation of nitric oxide (NO) from arginine and its catalytic activity is inhibited by phosphorylation. Following cerebral vascular occlusion, there is a massive increase in the excitatory neurotransmitter glutamate. Elevated glutamate levels, acting through the N-methyl-D-aspartate (NMDA) receptor, activates nNOS resulting in increased NO formation and neurotoxicity **(Figure 2)**. Toxicity may involve NO itself or its combination with superoxide free radical (O_2^-) to form peroxy-nitrite that decomposes to hydroxide (OH^-) and NO_2 (NO_2^-) free radicals with subsequent cellular damage by oxidation of nucleic acids, proteins and membrane lipids (Snyder, 1992). By enhancing phospho nNOS levels, FKBPs inhibit NO formation and thereby attenuate glutamate toxicity following vascular stroke (Snyder et al., 1998). Contrary to nerve regeneration, FKBP-mediated neuroprotection proceeds via calcineurin inhibition as anti-stroke effects were also seen with CsA.

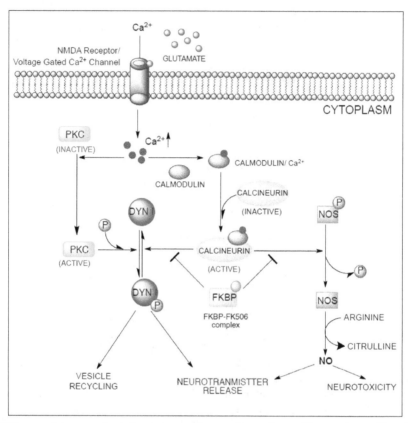

Fig. 2. NILs regulate neurotoxicity and neurotransmitter release: Glutamate-mediated influx of calcium through the NMDA receptor activates calcineurin (CaN) that in turn dephosphorylates nNOS and increases its catalytic activity. nNOS activation leads to increased NO formation and subsequent neurotoxicity and neurotransmitter release. FK506/CsA can counteract this neuronal toxicity by inhibiting CaN-dependent nNOS activation. Influx of Ca2+ also activates PKC and CaN that have opposing effect on phosphorylation state of the GTPase, dynamin I. While PKC-mediated phosphorylation of dynamin I increases its GTPase activity and leads to increased neurotransmitter release, CaN dephosphorylates and inactivates dynamin I. By inhibiting CaN, FK506 and CsA enhances phospho-dynamin I levels and subsequent depolarization-evoked neurotransmitter release.

FK506 has contradictory roles in neurotransmitter release - it inhibits NMDA induced neurotransmitter release while augmenting depolarization-induced release. Since neurotransmitter release proceeds via calcineurin-dependent pathway, this discrepancy in FK506 response can be attributed to the involvement of distinct calcineurin substrates, nNOS and dynamin I **(Figure 2)**. FK506 reduces glutamate release from NMDA-stimulated striatal synaptosomes as well as acetylcholine and dopamine release from PC12 cells that have been differentiated by NGF (Steiner *et al.*, 1996). Similar reductions seen with the nNOS inhibitor, nitro-L-arginine, indicates that NO regulates neurotransmitter release in PC12 and synaptosomes. In presence of FK506 and CsA, inhibition of calcineurin and subsequent reduction of nNOS activity results in decreased NO levels and therefore reduced neurotransmitter release.

In contrast, FK506 fails to inhibit potassium depolarization-evoked neurotransmitter release. Both CsA and L-683590 (FK506 analog that inhibits calcineurin), augment glutamate release from synaptosomes that have been treated with the K^+-channel blocker, 4-aminopyridine. In this case, the *bona fide* calcineurin substrate, dynamin I and not nNOS is involved (Nichols *et al.*, 1994). Dynamin I, a GTPase that regulates vesicular recycling, is active in its phosphorylated form; enhanced GTPase activity results in greater synaptic vesicular trafficking and increased rate of neurotransmitter release. CsA and FK506 mediated inhibition of calcineurin enhances dynamin I phosphorylation and hence its activity.

FK506 and its derivatives have also shown neuroprotective activity in neuropathy models mimicking stroke and dementia. For example, FK506-mediated calcineurin inhibition protects against ischemic brain injury (Sharkey & Butcher, 1994), desensitizes NMDA receptors (Tong *et al.*, 1995), prevents long-term depression (LTD) in rat hippocampus (Hodgkiss & Kelly, 1995) and modulates long-term potentiation (LTP) in rat visual cortex (Funauchi *et al.*, 1994). Stabilization of mitochondrial function was suggested to account for the anti-ischemic activities of FK506. FK506 does not target the mitochondrial potential transition pore (MTP) but prevents deterioration in mitochondrial respiration while maintaining cellular ATP levels and Ca^{2+} homeostasis. Furthermore, the role of FKBPs in the central nervous system has been extensively probed using 1-methyl-4-phenyl-1,2,3,6-tetrahydropyridine (MPTP) or 6-hydroxydopamine (6-OHDA) induced lesions of dopaminergic neurons. Both agents cause massive degeneration of nigrostriatal DA neurons thereby making MPTP and 6-OHDA treatment experimental paradigms for Parkinson's disease (Gerlach *et al.*, 1991). Treatment with GPI-1046, a FK506 analog was able to substantially recover the MPTP-damaged DA neurons as evidenced by increased tyrosine hydroxylase staining while rats lesioned with 6-OHDA showed morphological and functional recovery with increased striatal catecholamine levels and reduced amphetamine-induced rotations (Steiner *et al.*, 1997).

How might immunophilin ligands exert their neurotrophic and neuroprotective actions? The data suggests that PPIase activity of FKBPs maybe involved but no conclusive evidence has been provided so far. Several studies have tried to identify the FKBP(s) involved and elucidate the mechanism-of-action. This has proved particularly difficult as (1) most of the FKBP family members bind FK506 or its derivatives, albeit with varying degrees of affinity; (2) activities of both FKBPs and the protein phosphatase, calcineurin are inhibited by FK506 and its analogues and (3) FKBPs perform multifarious roles in protein folding, translocation and regulation as well as have a wide range of tissue/organellar distribution. Initial studies implicated a role for FKBP12 as elevated mRNA and proteins levels were observed in 6-OHDA model of PD (Nilsson *et al.*, 2007). Moreover, higher levels of FKBP12 have also been reported in brains of PD patients (Avramut & Achim, 2002). Therefore, a possible link between FKBPs and PD might stem from the increase in expression or redistribution of chaperone proteins in stress conditions. In addition to FKBP12, the human brain is enriched in FKBP38, FKBP51, FKBP52 and FKBP65 (Charters *et al.*, 1994; Coss *et al.*, 1998; Chambraud *et al.*, 2010; Jinwal *et al.*, 2010). Collectively, these immunophilins enriched in the nervous system are termed neuroimmunophilins. In the following sections, we will discuss the role of only those neuroimmunophilins that may be important for PD pathogenesis.

3. Molecular interacting partners of neuroimmunophilins

The neuroprotective and neurotrophic functions observed with NILs together with studies showing that chaperone proteins like HSP70 can suppresses α-synuclein (α-SYN) mediated loss of dopaminergic neurons in Drosophila model of PD (Auluck *et al.*, 2002; Muchowski, 2002), posits that FKBPs may have important role(s) in preventing PD-associated neurodegeneration. FKBPs, together with other chaperones may convert the toxic conformations of misfolded proteins to non-toxic form that is tolerated by cells. Alternatively, they may prevent the formation of toxic pre-fibrillar intermediates, or accelerate their conversion to nontoxic, amorphous aggregates that can be degraded by the cellular proteolytic machinery.

3.1 FKBPs interact with α-synuclein both *in vitro* and *in vivo*

α-SYN is a small (140 amino acid) intrinsically disordered protein predominantly localized to the presynaptic terminals. α-SYN regulates the functions of several other proteins - synphilin-1, parkin, tyrosine hydroxylase, dopamine transporter and phospholipase D, via stoichiometric protein-protein and protein-lipid interactions (Goedert, 2001; Ischiropoulos, 2003). In PD, α-SYN aggregates into characteristic fibrillar β-pleated structures in Lewy bodies. Besides LBs, α-SYN also forms intermediate-state oligomers that when released from the neurons activate microglia leading to an increased production of ROS and proinflammatory cytokines (Glass *et al.*, 2010). Activated microglia further amplifies this inflammatory response in a positive feedback loop. In α-SYN, the ability of the central hydrophobic NAC (non Aβ-component of amyloid plaques in Alzheimer's disease) domain to aggregate is normally counteracted by the highly charged hydrophilic C-terminal domain. Interestingly, all 5 proline residues (Pro^{108}, Pro^{117}, Pro^{120}, Pro^{128}, Pro^{138}) of α-SYN are located at the C-terminal of the protein. Changes to the C-terminal domain through deletion, point mutations or via posttranslational modifications such as phosphorylation (Kragh *et al.*, 2009) expose the NAC domain leading to hydrophobic interaction driven aggregation. For example, the E3-ubiquitin ligase, parkin can protect against α-SYN-induced toxicity by altering the phosphorylation levels of α-SYN (**Figure 3**). By simultaneously reducing PLK2 levels and activating PP2A, parkin decreases Ser^{87} and Ser^{129} phosphorylation thereby decreasing aggregation of phosphorylated α-SYN in LBs (Khandelwal *et al.*, 2010). The role of FKBPs in synucleinopathy has been probed both *in vitro* (Gerard *et al.*, 2006) and *in vivo* (Gerard *et al.*, 2010). *In vitro*, fluorescence correlation spectroscopy (FCS) measurements showed that addition of FKBP12 accelerates α-SYN aggregation into fibrillar structures that mimic aggregates formed in LBs. FKBP12 significantly alters the rate for both the nucleation and fibril formation stages (Gerard *et al.*, 2008). Since FKBPs catalyze the cis-trans isomerization of X-Pro peptide bond, the importance of C-terminal proline residues of α-SYN was also investigated. Changing one or more proline residues to alanine increased the aggregation kinetics of mutant α-SYN (Meuvis *et al.*, 2010). Additionally, FKBP12 did not interact with a proline deficient α-SYN mutant and this mutant was also found to be more structured.

Using a neuronal model of synucleinopathy in which α-SYN aggregation and cell death was induced by oxidative stress, Gerard and coworkers have shown that both FK506 and knockdown of FKBP12/FKBP52 can counter the effects of oxidative stress. Likewise, it was shown that overexpression of FKBP12 and -52 enhances α-SYN aggregation. FKBP52 was less potent than FKBP12 in inducing fibrillar aggregation. *In vivo*, FKBP12 was shown to colocalize with α-SYN in the brain of A30P-α-SYN transgenic mice model. Furthermore, FK506 administration reduced both the α-SYN aggregation in cells as well as increased survival of α-SYN overexpressing neurons in the striatum. Collectively, these studies validate FKBPs as a novel target for PD.

Besides α-SYN, other interacting partners of FKBP12 identified from 6-OHDA treated rat model of PD include 1-*cys* peroxyredoxin, HSP70, 14-3-3 zeta, M2-type pyruvate kinase (PKM2), annexin A2 and α-enolase (ENO1) (Nilsson *et al.*, 2007). It has been known that levels of PKM2, 14-3-3 zeta and ENO1 are altered during neurodegenerative diseases like PD and Alzheimer's (Poon *et al.*, 2006).

Given that FKBPs are chaperone proteins having important roles in protein folding, it is counterintuitive to note that the interaction between FKBP(s) and α-SYN results in α-SYN aggregation. Its is likely that α-SYN inclusions may not result simply from precipitated misfolded protein but rather from an active process meant to sequester soluble misfolded proteins from the cellular milieu (Kopito, 2000). Accordingly, inclusion body formation might serve as a cellular defense mechanism aimed at removing toxic insoluble proteins.

3.2 FKBP52 interacts with RET51 in a phosphorylation-dependent manner

RET51, a tyrosine kinase (TK) receptor, has important roles in the development and maintenance of the nervous system. Recently, FKBP52 was found to be novel interacting partner for RET51 in a split ubiquitin two-hybrid screen (Fusco *et al.*, 2010). Neurotrophins like NGF and glial-cell line derived neurotrophic factor (GDNF) promote the phosphorylation driven formation of RET51/FKBP52 complex; phosphorylation occurs on Tyr^{905} within the TK domain of RET51 and is a pre-requisite for complex formation. Association of RET51 with FKBP52 does not depend on HSP90 or other chaperones. The involvement of RET51 in PD comes from the genetic analysis of an early onset-PD patient heterozygous for mutations on both *RET51* and *FKBP52* genes (Fusco *et al.*, 2010). Mutations on both proteins disrupt formation of RET51/FKBP52 complex and its downstream signaling pathway. The detail of this signaling mechanism remains to be elucidated.

3.3 FKBP38 promotes trafficking of membrane channels

FKBP38 is distributed to both the mitochondria (Shirane & Nakayama, 2003) and endoplasmic reticulum (Wang *et al.*, 2005). Only the C-terminal tail is membrane anchored while the bulk of the protein is exposed to the cytosol. The unique topology of FKBP38 allows it to juxtapose between cytosolic and ER chaperone proteins. FKBP38 functions as a co-chaperone to HSC70/HSP90 complex to mediate proper folding and trafficking of membrane proteins like the multidomain cAMP-regulated chloride channel, CFTR (Wang *et al.*, 2006) and the voltage-dependent K^+ channel, HERG (Walker *et al.*, 2007). The immature form of HERG localizes to the endoplasmic reticulum whereas the fully glycosylated mature protein is present in the Golgi or the cell surface. While siRNA mediated knockdown of FKBP38 reduced HERG maturation, overexpression of FKBP38 was able to rescue the HERG F805C trafficking mutant. FKBP38 is involved in the late stages of HERG folding and ER export, as majority of FKBP38 has been found to associate with immature HERG. It is likely that natively folded HERG is released from its final chaperone complex while still attached with FKBP38. The bound FKBP38 could further mediate the attachment of HERG with the motor protein kinesin for transport to the plasma membrane. HERG mutations have been associated with the Long QT syndrome, a cardiac disorder characterized by long QT intervals. PD patients have an increased susceptibility to cardiac arrest as is evident from a prolongation of the QT interval (Hurst *et al.*, 2003). Therefore, it is likely that FKBP38-mediated HERG trafficking plays an important role in PD pathogenesis.

3.4 FKBP mediated regulation of Tau function and its effect on microtubule dynamics

Tau, a member of the microtubule-associated protein family (MAP), binds and stabilizes microtubules (MTs) and is therefore intrinsically linked with MT dynamics. Six isoforms of tau are present in humans, the longest one having four MT-binding repeat motifs. Normal biological functions of tau are dependent on its phosphorylation state. Involvement of tau in PD pathogenesis comes from the observations that (1) it accumulates in LBs together with α-SYN (Ishizawa *et al.*, 2003); (2) analysis of synapse-enriched fractions from PD brains show an increased phosphorylation for both tau and α-SYN (Muntane *et al.*, 2008) and (3) tau and synuclein synergistically promote *in vitro* fibrillization of each other (Giasson *et al.*, 2003). α-SYN mediates tau phosphorylation at $Ser^{262/356}$ by activating protein kinase A (PKA)(Jensen *et al.*, 1999) while in MPTP models of PD, α-SYN recruits $GSK\beta3$ kinase to phosphorylate tau at $Ser^{396/404}$ (Duka *et al.*, 2009). Hyperphosphorylation of tau results in MT destabilization by interfering with its binding.

Recent studies have shown that both FKBP51 (Jinwal *et al.*, 2010) and FKBP52 (*Chambraud et al.*, 2007; Chambraud *et al.*, 2010) can interact with tau. FKBP52 preferentially binds to hyperphosphorylated tau and colocalizes with tau at the growth cones in both cortical neurons and PC12 cells. Interestingly, FKBP52 could inhibit tau-mediated tubulin polymerization *in vitro*. This is consistent with the observation that overexpression of FKBP52 impairs neurite outgrowth in cultured neurons (Chambraud *et al.*, 2010). Interaction of FKBP52 with tau was mapped to the C-terminal TPR domain of FKBP52 (Chambraud *et al.*, 2007). Currently it is not known if the neuroprotection mediated by "anti-tau" activity of FKBP52 is linked to proteasomal degradation of hyperphosphorylated tau via enhanced trafficking or by increased aggregation of toxic tau into fibrillary tangles.

FKBP51, a member of the HSP90 chaperone complex, directly associates with tau and its overexpression significantly increases the levels of phospho- and total tau in cells. Contrary to FKBP52, FKBP51 enhances the tau-mediated MT polymerization and the PPIase activity of FKBP51 is crucial for its function in tau processing. The data by Dickey and coworkers suggest a model whereby binding of FKBP51-HSP90 complex to phosphorylated tau triggers its dephosphorylation and recycling to the microtubules thereby facilitating MT polymerization and stabilization (Jinwal *et al.*, 2010). HSP90-FKBP51 binding also shields tau from CHIP (carboxy terminus of the HSC70-interacting protein) mediated ubiquitination and subsequent proteasomal degradation (**Figure 3**).

3.5 FKBP38 anchors Bcl-2 to the mitochondria and regulates apoptosis

The C-terminal tail of the noncanonical FKBP, FKBP38, localizes the protein to the ER and mitochondrial membrane where it interacts with the anti-apoptotic proteins, Bcl-2 and Bcl-x$_L$ and regulates their functions. FKB38 is critical for the mitochondrial localization of Bcl-2 and Bcl-x$_L$; expression of mitochondrial targeting defective FKBP38 mutants and RNAi mediated

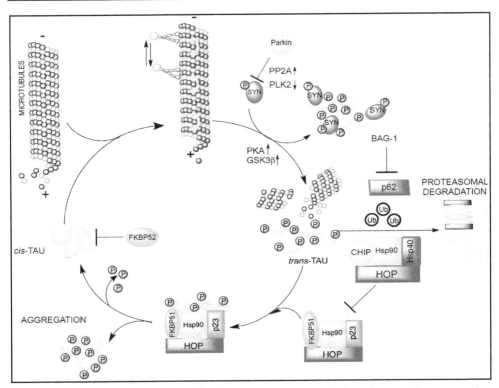

Fig. 3. FKBPs regulate microtubule stability by interacting with the microtubule-associated protein, tau. FKBP51 and FKBP52 have opposing effects on microtubule (MT) stability. FKBP52 exhibits "anti-tau" activity; by sequestering tau, it prevents its association with MT thereby destabilizing MTs. Together with the HSP90 complex, FKBP51 binds phosphorylated tau in its *trans*-conformation, isomerizes it to the *cis*-form and recycles it back to the MTs. Alternatively FKBP51 can accelerate aggregation of phospho-tau species. Phospho-tau can also be degraded by the cellular proteasomal system following CHIP-mediated polyubiquitination. Binding of FKBP51 and CHIP to phosphorylated tau is mutually exclusive. By recruiting PKA/GSK3β, α-SYN promotes tau-phosphorylation within the MT-binding domain and its subsequent removal from MTs. Activity of α-SYN is in turn regulated by the E3 ubiquitin ligase, Parkin. By inhibiting PLK2 kinase and enhancing PP2A phosphatase activity, Parkin decreases α-SYN phosphorylation and interferes with its activity.

knockdown of FKBP38 causes the cellular redistribution of these proteins. Furthermore FKBP38-mediated mitochondrial targeting is responsible for the anti-apoptotic activity of FKBP38 (Shirane & Nakayama, 2003; Kang *et al.*, 2005). Nishimura and colleagues have shown FKBP38 is a *bona fide* substrate for the aspartyl protease, presenilin 1 and 2 (PS1/2) (Wang *et al.*, 2005). Under physiological conditions PS1/2 forms macromolecular heteromeric complexes with FKBP38 and Bcl-2 and sequesters them in the ER/Golgi via a γ-secretase independent mechanism. Thus by inhibiting the FKBP38 mediated mitochondrial targeting of Bcl-2, PS1/2 antagonizes the anti-apoptotic effect of FKBP38.

In neuroblastoma cells, FKBP38 exhibits Ca2+/CaM stimulated PPIase activity and the FKBP38/Ca2+/CaM ternary complex binds Bcl-2. This binding is interrupted by GPI-1046, indicating that the active site of FKBP38 is involved in Bcl-2 interaction. HSP90 in the HSP90/Bcl-2/Ca^{2+}/CaM ternary complex has also been shown to inhibit the Bcl-2-FKBP38 interaction by blocking access to the enzyme active site (Edlich et al., 2007). GPI-1046 and RNAi-mediated depletion of FKBP38 activity was able to promote neuronal cell survival thus indicating that, in neuronal cells, FKBP38 has proapoptotic function. This observation contradicts earlier reports wherein it was shown that FKBP38 has anti-apoptotic effect (Shirane & Nakayama, 2003; Kang et al., 2005). One plausible explanation for this discrepancy could be explained on the basis of the different cell lines, neuronal versus non-neuronal, used in these studies. The potent neuroprotective and neuroregenerative effects of low molecular weight FKBP38 inhibitors in neuroblastoma cells concur well with the proapoptotic role of FKBP38. Furthermore, the ability of the FKBP38 inhibitor - N-(N',N'-dimethylcarboxamidomethyl)-cycloheximide to elicit neural stem proliferation and neuronal differentiation in a rat model of transient cerebral ischemia underscores the importance of FKBP38 in neuronal apoptosis (Edlich et al., 2006).

4. Neuroimmunophilin ligands as therapeutics for PD

Currently available drugs aimed at PD treatment do not have the capacity to inhibit PD progression but can only alleviate symptoms and/or delay neuronal atrophy by altering neurotransmitter metabolism. Neuroimmunophilin ligands are non-immunosuppressive and mediate the beneficial effects by multiple mechanisms that include inhibition of apoptosis, increased neurotrophic signaling and/or reducing oxidative stress by interfering with mitochondrial dysfunction (Tanaka & Ogawa, 2004). Several groups have reported that NILs like FK506, GPI-1046 and V-10367 (**Figure 4A**) promote striatal dopaminergic innervations in MPTP- or 6-OHDA models of PD (Kitamura et al., 1994; Steiner et al., 1997; Costantini et al., 1998; Guo et al., 2001). Studies have also shown that GPI-1046 protects against the p-chloroamphetamine-induced destruction of central serotoninergic neurons and

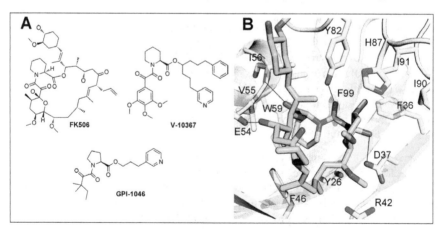

Fig. 4. (A) Structure of the neuroimmunophilin ligand FK506 and its non-immunosuppressive derivatives, GPI-1046 and V-10367. (B) Binding of FK506 (green) into the active site pocket of FKBP12 "(represented by cartoon model).

senescence-related atrophy of medial septal cholinergic neurons (Sauer *et al.*, 1999). Furthermore, rotational behavior and loss of corticostriatal long-term potentiation (LTP) in 6-OHDA treated rats was alleviated by GPI-1046. However, as similar efficacy was obtained with an analog that does not bind FKBP12 (V-13670), the importance of FKBP12 in mediating neurotrophic effects is debatable. Besides FK506 derivatives, CsA has been shown to protect against dopaminergic degeneration, promote regeneration of DA neurons and even suppress microglial cytotoxicity, as activated microglia has been known to generate free radicals (Banati *et al.*, 1993).

The binding mode of FK506 and its non-immunosuppressive counterpart, GPI-1046 has been elucidated (Van Duyne *et al.*, 1993; Sich *et al.*, 2000). Minimal binding motif comprises of the central pipecolic acid ring, the α-dicarbonyl amide linkage and pyranose ring. In the FK506-FKBP12 crystal structure (Van Duyne *et al.*, 1993), the pipecoline ring sits in the cavity defined by Trp^{59} and Tyr^{26}, Phe^{46}, Val^{55}, Ile^{56}, Phe^{99} side chains, whereas the α-dicarbonyl amide is hydrogen-bonded to –COOH and –OH group of Asp^{37} and Tyr^{82}, respectively (**Figure 4B**). The hydrophobic pocket formed by Phe^{36}, Asp^{37}, Tyr^{82}, His^{87}, Ile^{90} and Ile^{91} buries the pyranose ring while the cyclohexyl ester chain is engaged in hydrophobic interactions within a shallow surface groove. SAR studies have shown that the α-dicarbonyl amide functionality is indispensible for enzyme inhibition as replacement of either one or both carbonyl groups reduces potency. Similarly, pipecolic ring opening drastically increases the inhibition constant of the derivatives. GPI-1046 binds in a manner analogous to that of FK506 with the amide bond in *trans* configuration; the only exception being the replacement of pipecolyl moiety of FK506 by the prolyl ring of GPI-1046. Even though GPI-1046 has fewer favorable protein-ligand interactions, its effect on protein dynamics is essentially same as FK506, that is, stabilize the conformation of solvent exposed residues that are important in protein-protein and protein-ligand interactions.

The therapeutic utility of NILs has been questioned by work from other groups (Harper *et al.*, 1999; Parker *et al.*, 2000; Bocquet *et al.*, 2001) as many of the initial observations could not be replicated in identical systems. For instance, Harper and colleagues observed that GPI-1046 causes only a marginal increase in neurite outgrowth of chick dorsal root ganglia in culture under conditions where a very robust effect of nerve growth factor was seen. GPI-1046 did not restore tyrosine hydroxylase-positive fibers after 6-OHDA administration neither did it protect cultured dopaminergic neurons against MPTP induced toxicity. One possibility for the observed differences could be the levels of dopaminergic dysfunction. GPI-1046 provided neuroprotection in cases when the degradation was mild to moderate; it has no effect in severe cases when DA neuron levels deplete to 20% of that in normal controls. Other parameters like variability in culture conditions, differences in days *in vitro* prior to experimentation, can potentially account for the contrasting observations (Pong and Zaleska, 2003). Furthermore, neuroprotective effects of GPI-1046 could not be replicated in monkey model of MPTP toxicity (Emborg *et al.*, 2001) suggesting species-specific differences with respect to GPI-1046 activity.

5. Conclusion

FKBPs have emerged as novel cellular target for treatment of Parkinson's disease and other neurological disorders. The extraordinary unmet need for therapeutic intervention in PD continues to drive the search for potential drug candidates. Non-immunosuppressive NILs with their small size, target specificity, bioavailability and stability provide excellent scaffolds for the development of new drugs. Although our present knowledge of the mode of action of NILs is still fragmentary, there is increasing evidence that the neurotrophic, neuroprotective and restorative potential of these compounds is mediated by signaling pathways that can have antagonistic or additive effect. For example, multiple pathways may crosstalk via common integral components such as c-Jun (Gold *et al.*, 1999; Winter *et al.*, 2000). So far, the nervous system has been found to be enriched in only five FKBPs – FKBP-12, -38, -51, -52 and -65. Much work needs to be done so as to identify unique neuroimmunophilins and their interacting partners, assess their cellular function as well as their response to injury. Furthermore, issues such as reproducibility of pre-clinical data, structure-activity relationship studies, drug evaluation in appropriate animal models, and implementation of proper clinical designs and endpoints needs immediate attention as such information will aid in the development of novel NILs with improved efficacies, target selectivity and potency. FKBPs and NILs seem to be a promising area for therapeutic intervention of PD and other neurodegenerative disorders.

6. Acknowledgment

The authors would like to acknowledge the support from Ministry of Health-National Medical Research Council, Singapore for funding (NMRC/1177/2008).

7. References

Auluck, P.K., Chan, H.Y., Trojanowski, J.Q., Lee, V.M. & Bonini, N.M. (2002). Chaperone suppression of alpha-synuclein toxicity in a Drosophila model for Parkinson's disease. *Science*, Vol 295, pp 865-868.

Avramut, M. & Achim, C.L. (2002). Immunophilins and their ligands: insights into survival and growth of human neurons. *Physiol Behav*, Vol 77, pp 463-468.

Banati, R.B., Gehrmann, J., Schubert, P. & Kreutzberg, G.W. (1993). Cytotoxicity of microglia. *Glia*, Vol 7, pp 111-118.

Barik, S. (2006). Immunophilins: for the love of proteins. *Cell Mol. Life Sci.*, Vol 63, pp 2889-2900.

Bocquet, A., Lorent, G., Fuks, B., Grimee, R., Talaga, P., Daliers, J. & Klitgaard, H. (2001). Failure of GPI compounds to display neurotrophic activity in vitro and in vivo. *Eur. J Pharmacol.*, Vol 415, pp 173-180.

Chambraud, B., Belabes, H., Fontaine-Lenoir, V., Fellous, A. & Baulieu, E.E. (2007). The immunophilin FKBP52 specifically binds to tubulin and prevents microtubule formation. *FASEB J.*, Vol 21, pp 2787-2797.

Chambraud, B., Sardin, E., Giustiniani, J., Dounane, O., Schumacher, M., Goedert, M. & Baulieu, E.E. (2010). A role for FKBP52 in Tau protein function. *Proc. Natl. Acad. Sci. USA*, Vol 107, pp 2658-2663.

Charters, A.R., Kobayashi, M. & Butcher, S.P. (1994). Immunochemical analysis of FK506 binding proteins in neuronal cell lines and rat brain. *Biochem. Soc. Trans.*, Vol 22, pp 411S.

Coss, M.C., Stephens, R.M., Morrison, D.K., Winterstein, D., Smith, L.M. & Simek, S.L. (1998). The immunophilin FKBP65 forms an association with the serine/threonine kinase c-Raf-1. *Cell Growth Differ.*, Vol 9, pp 41-48.

Costantini, L.C., Chaturvedi, P., Armistead, D.M., McCaffrey, P.G., Deacon, T.W. & Isacson, O. (1998). A novel immunophilin ligand: distinct branching effects on dopaminergic neurons in culture and neurotrophic actions after oral administration in an animal model of Parkinson's disease. *Neurobiol. Dis* Vol 5, pp 97-106.

Dawson, T.M., Steiner, J.P., Lyons, W.E., Fotuhi, M., Blue, M. & Snyder, S.H. (1994). The immunophilins, FK506 binding protein and cyclophilin, are discretely localized in the brain: relationship to calcineurin. *Neuroscience*, Vol 62, pp 569-580.

Dawson, T.M. (2006). Parkin and defective ubiquitination in Parkinson's disease. *J. Neural Transm. Suppl,* Vol 209-213.

Duka, T., Duka, V., Joyce, J.N. & Sidhu, A. (2009). Alpha-Synuclein contributes to GSK-3beta-catalyzed Tau phosphorylation in Parkinson's disease models. *FASEB J,* Vol 23, pp 2820-2830.

Edlich, F., Weiwad, M., Erdmann, F., Fanghanel, J., Jarczowski, F., Rahfeld, J.U. & Fischer, G. (2005). Bcl-2 regulator FKBP38 is activated by Ca2+/calmodulin. *EMBO J,* Vol 24, pp 2688-2699.

Edlich, F., Weiwad, M., Wildemann, D., Jarczowski, F., Kilka, S., Moutty, M.C., Jahreis, G., Lucke, C., Schmidt, W., Striggow, F. & Fischer, G. (2006). The specific FKBP38 inhibitor   N-(N',N'-dimethylcarboxamidomethyl)cycloheximide   has   potent neuroprotective and neurotrophic properties in brain ischemia. *J Biol. Chem.* Vol 281, pp 14961-14970.

Edlich, F., Erdmann, F., Jarczowski, F., Moutty, M.C., Weiwad, M. & Fischer, G. (2007). The Bcl-2 regulator FKBP38-calmodulin-Ca2+ is inhibited by Hsp90. *J Biol. Chem.,* Vol 282, pp 15341-15348.

Emborg, M.E., Shin, P., Roitberg, B., Sramek, J.G., Chu, Y., Stebbins, G.T., Hamilton, J.S., Suzdak, P.D., Steiner, J.P. & Kordower, J.H. (2001). Systemic administration of the immunophilin ligand GPI 1046 in MPTP-treated monkeys. *Exp. Neurol.,* Vol 168, pp 171-182.

Eriksen, J.L., Wszolek, Z. & Petrucelli, L. (2005). Molecular pathogenesis of Parkinson disease. *Arch. Neurol.* Vol 62, pp 353-357.

Funauchi, M., Haruta, H. & Tsumoto, T. (1994). Effects of an inhibitor for calcium/calmodulin-dependent protein phosphatase, calcineurin, on induction of long-term potentiation in rat visual cortex. *Neurosci. Res.,* Vol 19, pp 269-278.

Fusco, D., Vargiolu, M., Vidone, M., Mariani, E., Pennisi, L.F., Bonora, E., Capellari, S., Dirnberger, D., Baumeister, R., Martinelli, P. & Romeo, G. (2010). The RET51/FKBP52 complex and its involvement in Parkinson disease. *Hum. Mol. Genet.,* Vol 19, pp 2804-2816.

Gerard, M., Debyser, Z., Desender, L., Kahle, P.J., Baert, J., Baekelandt, V. & Engelborghs, Y. (2006). The aggregation of alpha-synuclein is stimulated by FK506 binding proteins as shown by fluorescence correlation spectroscopy. *FASEB J.,* Vol 20, pp 524-526.

Gerard, M., Debyser, Z., Desender, L., Baert, J., Brandt, I., Baekelandt, V. & Engelborghs, Y. (2008). FK506 binding protein 12 differentially accelerates fibril formation of wild type alpha-synuclein and its clinical mutants A30P or A53T. *J Neurochem.,* Vol 106, pp 121-133.

Gerard, M., Deleersnijder, A., Daniels, V., Schreurs, S., Munck, S., Reumers, V., Pottel, H., Engelborghs, Y., Van den Haute, C., Taymans, J.M., Debyser, Z. & Baekelandt, V. (2010). Inhibition of FK506 binding proteins reduces alpha-synuclein aggregation and Parkinson's disease-like pathology. *J Neurosci.,* Vol 30, pp 2454-2463.

Gerlach, M., Riederer, P., Przuntek, H. & Youdim, M.B. (1991). MPTP mechanisms of neurotoxicity and their implications for Parkinson's disease. *Eur. J Pharmacol.,* Vol 208, pp 273-286.

Giasson, B.I., Forman, M.S., Higuchi, M., Golbe, L.I., Graves, C.L., Kotzbauer, P.T., Trojanowski, J.Q. & Lee, V.M. (2003). Initiation and synergistic fibrillization of tau and alpha-synuclein. *Science,* Vol 300, pp 636-640.

Glass, C.K., Saijo, K., Winner, B., Marchetto, M.C. & Gage, F.H. (2010). Mechanisms underlying inflammation in neurodegeneration. *Cell,* Vol 140, pp 918-934.

Goedert, M. (2001). Alpha-synuclein and neurodegenerative diseases. *Nat. Rev. Neurosci.*, Vol 2, pp 492-501.

Gold, B.G. (1997). FK506 and the role of immunophilins in nerve regeneration. *Mol. Neurobiol.*, Vol 15, pp 285-306.

Gold, B.G. & Nutt, J.G. (2002). Neuroimmunophilin ligands in the treatment of Parkinson's disease. *Curr. Opin. Pharmacol.*, Vol 2, pp 82-86.

Gold, B.G., Densmore, V., Shou, W., Matzuk, M.M. & Gordon, H.S. (1999). Immunophilin FK506-binding protein 52 (not FK506-binding protein 12) mediates the neurotrophic action of FK506. *J Pharmacol. Exp. Ther.*, Vol 289, pp 1202-1210.

Guo, X., Dawson, V.L. & Dawson, T.M. (2001). Neuroimmunophilin ligands exert neuroregeneration and neuroprotection in midbrain dopaminergic neurons. *Eur. J Neurosci.*, Vol 13, pp 1683-1693.

Hamilton, G.S. & Steiner, J.P. (1998). Immunophilins: beyond immunosuppression. *J Med. Chem.*, Vol 41, pp 5119-5143.

Harper, S., Bilsland, J., Young, L., Bristow, L., Boyce, S., Mason, G., Rigby, M., Hewson, L., Smith, D., O'Donnell, R., O'Connor, D., Hill, R.G., Evans, D., Swain, C., Williams, B. & Hefti, F. (1999). Analysis of the neurotrophic effects of GPI-1046 on neuron survival and regeneration in culture and in vivo. *Neuroscience*, Vol 88, pp 257-267.

Hodgkiss, J.P. & Kelly, J.S. (1995). Only 'de novo' long-term depression (LTD) in the rat hippocampus in vitro is blocked by the same low concentration of FK506 that blocks LTD in the visual cortex. *Brain Res.*, Vol 705, pp 241-246.

Hurst, R.S., Higdon, N.R., Lawson, J.A., Clark, M.A., Rutherford-Root, K.L., McDonald, W.G., Haas, J.V., McGrath, J.P. & Meglasson, M.D. (2003). Dopamine receptor agonists differ in their actions on cardiac ion channels. *Eur. J Pharmacol.*, Vol 482, pp 31-37.

Ischiropoulos, H. (2003). Oxidative modifications of alpha-synuclein. *Ann. N. Y. Acad. Sci.*, Vol 991, pp 93-100.

Ishizawa, T., Mattila, P., Davies, P., Wang, D. & Dickson, D.W. (2003). Colocalization of tau and alpha-synuclein epitopes in Lewy bodies. *J Neuropathol. Exp. Neurol.*, Vol 62, pp 389-397.

Jensen, P.H., Hager, H., Nielsen, M.S., Hojrup, P., Gliemann, J. & Jakes, R. (1999). Alpha-synuclein binds to Tau and stimulates the protein kinase A-catalyzed tau phosphorylation of serine residues 262 and 356. *J Biol. Chem.*, Vol 274, pp 25481-25489.

Jinwal, U.K., Koren, J., Borysov, S.I., Schmid, A.B., Abisambra, J.F., Blair, L.J., Johnson, A.G., Jones, J.R., Shults, C.L., O'Leary, J.C., Jin, Y., Buchner, J., Cox, M.B. & Dickey, C.A. (2010). The Hsp90 cochaperone, FKBP51, increases Tau stability and polymerizes microtubules. *J Neurosci.*, Vol 30, pp 591-599.

Kang, C.B., Feng, L., Chia, J. & Yoon, H.S. (2005). Molecular characterization of FK-506 binding protein 38 and its potential regulatory role on the anti-apoptotic protein Bcl-2. *Biochem. Biophys. Res. Commun.*, Vol 337, pp 30-38.

Khandelwal, P.J., Dumanis, S.B., Feng, L.R., Maguire-Zeiss, K., Rebeck, G., Lashuel, H.A. & Moussa, C.E. (2010). Parkinson-related parkin reduces alpha-Synuclein phosphorylation in a gene transfer model. *Mol. Neurodegener.* Vol 5, pp 47.

Kitamura, Y., Itano, Y., Kubo, T. & Nomura, Y. (1994). Suppressive effect of FK-506, a novel immunosuppressant, against MPTP-induced dopamine depletion in the striatum of young C57BL/6 mice. *J Neuroimmunol.*, Vol 50, pp 221-224.

Kopito, R.R. (2000). Aggresomes, inclusion bodies and protein aggregation. *Trends Cell Biol.*, Vol 10, pp 524-530.

Kragh, C.L., Lund, L.B., Febbraro, F., Hansen, H.D., Gai, W.P., El-Agnaf, O., Richter-Landsberg, C. & Jensen, P.H. (2009). {alpha}-Synuclein Aggregation and Ser-129 Phosphorylation-dependent Cell Death in Oligodendroglial Cells. *J Biol. Chem.*, Vol 284, pp 10211-10222.

Lyons, W.E., George, E.B., Dawson, T.M., Steiner, J.P. & Snyder, S.H. (1994). Immunosuppressant FK506 promotes neurite outgrowth in cultures of PC12 cells and sensory ganglia. *Proc. Natl. Acad. Sci. USA,* Vol 91, pp 3191-3195.

Maki, N., Sekiguchi, F., Nishimaki, J., Miwa, K., Hayano, T., Takahashi, N. & Suzuki, M. (1990). Complementary DNA encoding the human T-cell FK506-binding protein, a peptidylprolyl cis-trans isomerase distinct from cyclophilin. *Proc. Natl. Acad. Sci. USA,* Vol 87, pp 5440-5443.

Mandel, S., Grunblatt, E., Riederer, P., Amariglio, N., Jacob-Hirsch, J., Rechavi, G. & Youdim, M.B. (2005). Gene expression profiling of sporadic Parkinson's disease substantia nigra pars compacta reveals impairment of ubiquitin-proteasome subunits, SKP1A, aldehyde dehydrogenase, and chaperone HSC-70. *Ann. N. Y. Acad. Sci.,* Vol 1053, pp 356-375.

McGeer, P.L., Itagaki, S., Boyes, B.E. & McGeer, E.G. (1988). Reactive microglia are positive for HLA-DR in the substantia nigra of Parkinson's and Alzheimer's disease brains. *Neurology,* Vol 38, pp 1285-1291.

Meiri, K.F., Bickerstaff, L.E. & Schwob, J.E. (1991). Monoclonal antibodies show that kinase C phosphorylation of GAP-43 during axonogenesis is both spatially and temporally restricted in vivo. *J Cell Biol.,* Vol 112, pp 991-1005.

Meuvis, J., Gerard, M., Desender, L., Baekelandt, V. & Engelborghs, Y. (2010). The conformation and the aggregation kinetics of alpha-synuclein depend on the proline residues in its C-terminal region. *Biochemistry,* Vol 49, pp 9345-9352.

Muchowski, P.J. (2002). Protein misfolding, amyloid formation, and neurodegeneration: a critical role for molecular chaperones? *Neuron,* Vol 35, pp 9-12.

Muntane, G., Dalfo, E., Martinez, A. & Ferrer, I. (2008). Phosphorylation of tau and alpha-synuclein in synaptic-enriched fractions of the frontal cortex in Alzheimer's disease and in Parkinson's disease and related alpha-synucleinopathies. *Neuroscience,* Vol 152, pp 913-923.

Nagatsu, T. & Sawada, M. (2005) Inflammatory process in Parkinson's disease: role for cytokines. *Curr. Pharm. Des.,* Vol 11, pp 999-1016.

Nichols, R.A., Suplick, G.R. & Brown, J.M. (1994). Calcineurin-mediated protein dephosphorylation in brain nerve terminals regulates the release of glutamate. *J Biol. Chem.,* Vol 269, pp 23817-23823.

Nilsson, A., Skold, K., Sjogren, B., Svensson, M., Pierson, J., Zhang, X., Caprioli, R.M., Buijs, J., Persson, B., Svenningsson, P & Andren, P.E. (2007). Increased striatal mRNA and protein levels of the immunophilin FKBP-12 in experimental Parkinson's disease and identification of FKBP-12-binding proteins. *J Proteome Res.,* Vol 6, pp 3952-3961.

Parker, E.M., Monopoli, A., Ongini, E., Lozza, G. & Babij. C.M. (2000). Rapamycin, but not FK506 and GPI-1046, increases neurite outgrowth in PC12 cells by inhibiting cell cycle progression. *Neuropharmacology,* Vol 39, pp 1913-1919.

Pong, K. & Zaleska, M.M. (2003). Therapeutic implications for immunophilin ligands in the treatment of neurodegenerative diseases. *Curr. Drug Targets CNS Neurol. Disord .,* Vol 2, pp 349-356.

Poon, H.F., Shepherd, H.M., Reed, T.T., Calabrese, V., Stella, A.M., Pennisi, G., Cai, J., Pierce, W.M., Klein, J.B. & Butterfield, D.A. (2006). Proteomics analysis provides insight into caloric restriction mediated oxidation and expression of brain proteins associated with age-related impaired cellular processes: Mitochondrial dysfunction, glutamate dysregulation and impaired protein synthesis. *Neurobiol. Aging.,*Vol 27, pp 1020-1034.

Sauer, H., Francis, J.M., Jiang, H., Hamilton, G.S. & Steiner, J.P. (1999). Systemic treatment with GPI 1046 improves spatial memory and reverses cholinergic neuron atrophy in the medial septal nucleus of aged mice. *Brain Res.*, Vol 842, pp 109-118.

Sharkey, J. & Butcher, S.P. (1994). Immunophilins mediate the neuroprotective effects of FK506 in focal cerebral ischaemia. *Nature*, Vol 371, pp 336-339.

Sharma, V.K., Li, B., Khanna, A., Sehajpal, P.K. & Suthanthiran, M. (1994). Which way for drug-mediated immunosuppression? *Curr. Opin. Immunol.*, Vol 6, pp 784-790.

Shirane, M. & Nakayama, K.I. (2003). Inherent calcineurin inhibitor FKBP38 targets Bcl-2 to mitochondria and inhibits apoptosis. *Nat. Cell Biol.*, Vol 5, pp 28-37.

Sich, C., Improta, S., Cowley, D.J., Guenet, C., Merly, J.P., Teufel, M & Saudek, V. (2000). Solution structure of a neurotrophic ligand bound to FKBP12 and its effects on protein dynamics. *Eur. J Biochem.*, Vol 267, pp 5342-5355.

Snyder, S.H. (1992). Nitric Oxide: first in a new class of neurotransmitters. *Science*, Vol 257, pp 494-496.

Snyder, S.H., Lai, M.M. & Burnett, P.E. (1998). Immunophilins in the nervous system. *Neuron*, Vol 21, pp 283-294.

Steiner, J.P., Dawson, T.M., Fotuhi, M., Glatt, C.E., Snowman, A.M., Cohen, N & Snyder, S.H. (1992). High brain densities of the immunophilin FKBP colocalized with calcineurin. *Nature*, Vol 358, pp 584-587.

Steiner, J.P., Dawson, T.M., Fotuhi, M & Snyder, S.H. (1996). Immunophilin regulation of neurotransmitter release. *Mol. Med.*, Vol 2, pp 325-333.

Steiner, J.P., Hamilton, G.S., Ross, D.T., Valentine, H.L., Guo, H., Connolly, M.A., Liang, S., Ramsey, C., Li, J.H., Huang, W., Howorth, P., Soni, R., Fuller, M., Sauer, H., Nowotnik, A.C. & Suzdak, P.D. (1997). Neurotrophic immunophilin ligands stimulate structural and functional recovery in neurodegenerative animal models. *Proc. Natl. Acad. Sci. USA*, Vol 94, pp 2019-2024.

Tanaka, K. & Ogawa, N. (2004). Possibility of non-immunosuppressive immunophilin ligands as potential therapeutic agents for Parkinson's disease. *Curr. Pharm. Des.*, Vol 10, pp 669-677.

Tong, G., Shepherd, D. & Jahr, C.E. (1995). Synaptic desensitization of NMDA receptors by calcineurin. *Science*, Vol 267, pp 1510-1512.

Tong, Y. & Shen, J. (2009). Alpha-synuclein and LRRK2: partners in crime. *Neuron*, Vol 64, pp 771-773.

Van Duyne, G.D., Standaert, R.F., Karplus, P.A., Schreiber, S.L. & Clardy, J. (1993). Atomic structures of the human immunophilin FKBP-12 complexes with FK506 and rapamycin. *J Mol. Biol.*, Vol 229, pp 105-124.

Walker, V.E., Atanasiu, R., Lam, H. & Shrier, A. (2007). Co-chaperone FKBP38 promotes HERG trafficking. *J Biol. Chem.*, Vol 282, pp 23509-23516.

Wang, H.Q., Nakaya, Y., Du, Z., Yamane, T., Shirane, M., Kudo, T., Takeda, M., Takebayashi, K., Noda, Y., Nakayama, K.I. & Nishimura, M. (2005). Interaction of presenilins with FKBP38 promotes apoptosis by reducing mitochondrial Bcl-2. *Hum. Mol. Genet.*, Vol 14, pp 1889-1902.

Wang, X., Venable, J., LaPointe, P., Hutt, D.M., Koulov, A.V., Coppinger, J., Gurkan, C., Kellner, W., Matteson, J., Plutner, H., Riordan, J.R., Kelly, J.W., Yates, JR. & Balch, W.E. (2006). Hsp90 cochaperone Aha1 downregulation rescues misfolding of CFTR in cystic fibrosis. *Cell*, Vol 127, pp 803-815.

Winter, C., Schenkel, J., Burger, E., Eickmeier, C., Zimmermann, M & Herdegen, T. (2000). The immunophilin ligand FK506, but not GPI-1046, protects against neuronal death and inhibits c-Jun expression in the substantia nigra pars compacta following transection of the rat medial forebrain bundle. *Neuroscience*, Vol 95, pp 753-762.

9

Regulation of α-Synuclein Membrane Binding and Its Implications

Robert H.C. Chen[1], Sabine Wislet-Gendebien[1,2],
Howard T.J. Mount[1] and Anurag Tandon[1]
[1]Tanz Centre for Research in Neurodegenerative Diseases, University of Toronto,
[2]GIGA Neurosciences, University of Liège,
[1]Canada
[2]Belgium

1. Introduction

1.1 Parkinson's disease and Lewy bodies

Parkinson's disease (PD) is the most prevalent neurodegenerative disease that affects motor control, although dementia, depression, and other psychiatric symptoms are occasionally present (reviewed in Jankovic, 2008). The motor symptoms include resting tremors, bradykinesia/akinesia, rigidity, and postural instability, and are associated with the death of dopaminergic neurons in the substantia nigra pars compacta (SNpc) (Lloyd and Hornykiewicz, 1970; reviewed in Saper, 1999) and noradrenergic neurons in the locus coeruleus (Mann and Yates, 1983; Gaspar et al., 1991). Degeneration of these neurons disrupts basal ganglia circuitry of the brain and interferes with the initiation of voluntary movement (Levy et al., 1997).

Another pathological characteristic of the disease is the presence of the intracellular protein aggregates known as Lewy bodies and Lewy neurites (Hughes et al., 1992), described initially by Frederick Lewy in 1912, that were associated with dying dopaminergic neurons in the SNpc by Tretiakoff (reviewed in Holdorff, 2006). Lewy bodies are also present in other brain regions outside the SNpc, and may appear first in the glossopharyngeal, vagal, and olfactory centres (Braak et al., 2003). The disruption of these regions is now linked to a preclinical phase of PD that includes perturbations of smell, gastrointestinal motility, and sleep patterns prior to the development of motor impairments coincident with neurodegeneration and inclusions in the midbrain. These intraneuronal aggregates are composed of lipids and various proteins including α-synuclein, ubiquitin, and neurofilaments (Spillantini et al., 1998; reviewed in Cookson, 2005). Whether Lewy bodies directly cause cytotoxicity or are formed as compensatory activation of survival pathways remains under debate. Nevertheless, the presence of Lewy bodies is an essential component of post-mortem diagnoses of PD (Christine and Aminoff, 2004; reviewed in Jankovic, 2008).

1.2 α-Synuclein in Parkinson's disease

α-Synuclein is important to understanding the etiology of PD both because it is the main pathological component of Lewy bodies and because mutations and changes in its expression are linked to familial PD. Three missense mutations causing single amino acid substitutions in α-synuclein are linked to autosomal dominant forms of familial PD: A53T, A30P, and E46K (Polymeropoulos et al., 1997; Kruger et al., 1998; Zarranz et al., 2004). Interestingly, in many mammalian species, including mice and new world primates, threonine is the normal residue at position 53, which suggest some kind of corrective mechanism elsewhere in the coding sequence to reduce the toxicity of the A53T mutation (Hamilton, 2004). Elevated expression of normal α-synuclein is also pathogenic as gene triplication or duplication is linked to early- or late-onset PD, respectively (Singleton et al., 2003; Chartier-Harlin et al., 2004).

Despite the efforts of many research laboratories since its initial discovery as an abundant presynaptic protein in cholinergic nerve terminals innervating the *Torpedo* electric organic (Maroteax et al, 1988), α-synuclein's function still remains somewhat of a mystery. Mice deficient in α-synuclein are unremarkable, but exhibit increased release of dopamine under paired-pulse stimuli and reduced striatal tissue content of dopamine (Abeliovich et al., 2000). Over-expression of α-synuclein in yeast leads to aggregation of vesicles, disruption in vesicular transport, and death (Gitler et al., 2008; Soper et al., 2008). Similarly, moderate α-synuclein over-expression in mammalian neurons reduces transmitter release and the number of synaptic vesicles arrayed at presynaptic active zones (Nemani et al., 2010). These reports clearly implicate α-synuclein in synaptic vesicle mobilization or fusion, but offer little information about its pathogenic role.

In vitro studies revealed that A30P and A53T mutant α-synuclein form oligomers at a faster rate than wild-type α-synuclein (Conway et al., 2000). Post-translational modifications may also affect α-synuclein aggregation, as phosphorylation of serine at position 129 is highly upregulated in Lewy bodies (Fujiwara et al., 2002). Phosphomimic residue changes, such as serine 129 to aspartate, which simulates the charge distribution of phosphorylation, cause neuronal loss in fruit flies and substitution of serine 129 with alanine, which prevents phosphorylation, rescues this cell loss (Chen and Feany, 2005). However, experimental evidence for the toxicity of serine 129 phosphorylation is somewhat equivocal in rodents, because expression of α-synuclein with alanine 129 is as toxic as aspartate 129 (Gorbatyuk et al, 2008; McFarland et al., 2009).

Although α-synuclein is decreased in the cerebrospinal fluid of PD patients (Mollenhauer et al, 2011), there is an increase in α-synuclein oligomers suggesting that α-synuclein aggregation and its leakage from neurons is accelerated in PD (Tokuda et al., 2010). However, the mechanistic contribution of α-synuclein to neuronal death in PD still remains unclear. Low nanomolar concentrations of α-synuclein are neuroprotective against the oxidative insults of hydrogen peroxide and 6-hydroxydopamine, whereas higher micromolar concentrations are toxic (Batelli et al., 2008). This suggests that α-synuclein may be neuroprotective and toxic at low and high levels, respectively, and is in accord with the pathogenic effects of SNCA duplication or triplication. α-Synuclein has also been shown to cause oxidative stress through direct damage to mitochondria. For example, mitochondrial import of α-synuclein mediated by a cryptic targeting signal can disrupt complex 1 activity (Devi et al., 2008), and α-synuclein over-expression in nematodes and mammalian cells induced fragmentation of mitochondria (Kamp et al., 2010; Nakamura et al., 2011). Co-expression of PINK1, parkin, and DJ-1 protect against mitochondrial fragmentation, consistent with the notion that these three proteins function in a common mitochondrial pathway leading to PD pathology. The convergence of α-synuclein to a mitochondrial role when expressed at sufficient levels could therefore be viewed as a pathogenic pathway that diverges from its normal physiological role in vesicle trafficking.

1.3 α-Synuclein outside of disease

A role in synaptic function is implicated from the observation that α-synuclein is highly concentrated in pre-synaptic terminals (Jakes et al., 1994; George et al., 1995) and that α-synuclein disperses reversibly from these presynaptic terminals in response to brief neural activity (Fortin et al., 2005). The dispersion is attenuated by tetanus toxin, which inactivates vesicle fusion but not the preceding ion fluxes, suggesting that α-synuclein solubility is directly linked to exocytosis. While these results do not suggest a presynaptic function for α-synuclein, other studies with α-synuclein knockout mice reveal increased nigrostriatal dopamine release induced by paired-pulse stimuli (Abeliovich et al., 2000), implicating α-synuclein as a negative regulator of a readily-releasable vesicle pool of dopamine. In contrast, another line of α-synuclein null mice showed normal response to single or paired stimuli, but deficits in response to trains of stimuli which rely on reserve vesicle recruitment and a reduction in the number distal vesicles (Cabin et al., 2002). To explore whether β-synuclein compensates for loss of α-synuclein, removal of both α- and β-synuclein decreased total brain dopamine by 20% as well as complexins and 14-3-3 proteins (Chandra et al., 2004). Complexins are a regulatory component of the SNARE (soluble N-ethylmaleimide-sensitive attachment protein receptor) complexes involved in synaptic vesicle fusion (Hu et al., 2002). However, the other previously described aberrations such as synaptic vesicle reduction, electrophysiological changes, and dopamine re-uptake were not observed in these α-synuclein knockout mice. Despite the differences, α-synuclein knockout mice display subtle alterations in vesicle storage and dynamics.

The converse experimental paradigm using over-expression of α-synuclein also suggests that it inhibits synaptic transmission in primary neurons and intact *ex vivo* brain (Nemani et al., 2010). Morphological and electrophysiological analyses indicate that the reduction was due to decreased readily-releasable synaptic vesicles, but not the overall number of synaptic vesicles, consistent with the notion that α-synuclein is a negative regulator of the synaptic vesicle mobilization.

Recent studies using biochemical approaches have reported that α-synuclein disrupts arachidonic acid-mediated stabilization of soluble N-ethylmaleimide sensitive fusion protein receptor (SNARE) complex (comprised of syntaxin-1, SNAP25, and synaptobrevin-2) that is essential for synaptic vesicle fusion (Darios et al., 2010). Although this study did not co-immunoprecipitate α-synuclein with members of the SNARE complex, thus suggesting an indirect interaction, others have reported α-synuclein binding with synaptobrevin-2 and proposed that this binding stabilizes the SNARE complex (Burre et al., 2010). Interestingly, loss of assembled SNARE complexes in mice deficient for cysteine-string protein alpha (CSPα) can be rescued by α-synuclein over-expression and worsened by its knockdown. The loss of all three synucleins (α-, β-, and γ-) causes premature death due to neurological symptoms, suggesting that β- and/or γ-synuclein perform redundant functions and compensate for α-synuclein deficiency in the single knockout animals. Thus, α-synuclein exerts a regulatory effect on SNARE complex formation, but its mechanism remains poorly defined.

Some studies have suggested that α-synuclein may regulate vesicle trafficking more broadly that just in synaptic transmission. Expression of α-synuclein in yeast and mammalian cells causes delays in ER-to-Golgi vesicle trafficking, an effect that was more striking with the A53T mutant (Cooper et al., 2006; Thayanidhi et al., 2010). These changes in ER-to-Golgi trafficking by α-synuclein may be caused by immobilizing vesicles in the cytoplasm (Soper et al., 2008). The mechanism appears to involve rab proteins, small GTPases that regulate vesicle trafficking, as the impairment is rescued by overexpressing certain rab proteins (Gitler et al., 2008). Furthermore, as yeast do not express α-synuclein endogenously, these studies suggest that α-synuclein can interact with both constitutive and Ca²⁺-dependent vesicle trafficking machineries that is conserved between yeast and higher organisms.

2. α-Synuclein and membrane-binding

2.1 The structure of α-synuclein and how it contributes to membrane-binding

The structure of α-synuclein can be divided into three domains: an amino-terminal domain with seven imperfect KTKEGV repeats, a central domain essential for aggregation called the non-amyloidβ component (NAC), and a hydrophilic carboxyl-terminal tail (Clayton and George, 1998) (**Fig. 1.1A**). The amino-terminal repeats, which are similar to sequences found in apolipoproteins, form amphipathic helices with polar and non-polar residues aligned in opposing direction and allow α-synuclein to immerse partially into lipid membranes (**Fig. 1.1B**). The capacity of α-synuclein to bind freely to membranes has been demonstrated (Jo et al., 2000; Conway et al., 2000). The helical structure of α-synuclein upon binding to sodium dodecyl sulfate (SDS)-soluble micelles has been established using nuclear magnetic

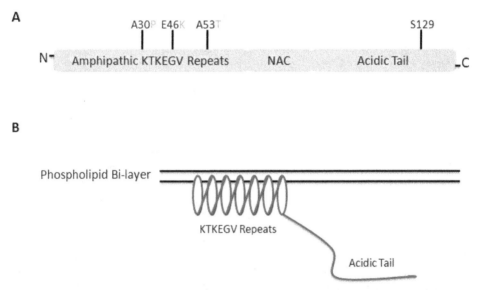

Fig. 1. The primary structure of human α-synuclein. (A) The structure itself can be divided into three unequal regions: the imperfect KTKEGV repeats believed to form a helical structure on phospholipid membranes, the non-Aβ component (NAC) seen in Alzheimer disease-associated plaques, and a non-membrane-associated acidic c-terminal tail. (B) Upon binding to membranes, α-synuclein assumes a helical conformation due to the amphipathic nature of the KTKEGV repeats. All three amino acid substitution sites associated with familial forms of PD (A30P, E46K, and A53T) can be found in the amphipathic repeat region. The serine 129 site commonly found to be phosphorylated in Lewy bodies can be found in the acidic tail. Note that the residue in position 53 is naturally a threonine instead of an alanine in many mammalian species, including rodents.

resonance and electron spin resonance studies (Jao et al., 2004; Ulmer et al., 2005; Borbat et al., 2006). The helical conformation is energetically favourable when compared to the unstructured conformation of cytosolic α-synuclein.

2.2 Implications of α-synuclein membrane-binding

Binding to and dissociation from the synaptic membrane may be linked to regulating the still-undefined function of α-synuclein. Using fluorescent imaging to visualize GFP-tagged α-synuclein, depolarization reversibly induced the redistribution of α-synuclein from synaptic boutons to the perisynaptic region (Fortin et al., 2005), consistent with the dissociation of α-synuclein from synaptic vesicles prior to exocytosis. This link between α-synuclein, its membrane binding, and exocytosis is consistent with other reports that α-synuclein regulates SNARE complex assembly (Darios et al., 2010; Burre et al, 2010).

The membrane-binding properties of α-synuclein may also have implications in PD pathogenesis. The addition of lipid vesicles causes a greater proportion of α-synuclein to assume an α-helical conformation and decreases the fibrillization of α-synuclein (Zhu et al., 2003); Jo et al., 2004), suggesting that increased membrane binding may be protective against Lewy body pathology. However, other studies adding phospholipids to α-synuclein induced fibril formation (Narayanan and Scarlata, 2001; Cole et al., 2002). Mutant A30P α-synuclein exhibits a lower propensity to bind to phospholipid membranes as determined in vitro (Jo et al., 2002), but forms oligomers faster than wild-type or A53T α-synuclein (Conway et al., 2000). Nevertheless, the A53T mutant α-synuclein forms fibrils (the likely precursor to Lewy bodies) at a higher rate. Furthermore, a rotenone model of PD revealed that lipids co-stained with α-synuclein aggregates (Lee et al., 2002), suggesting that lipids may enable Lewy body formation. Taken together, the evidence is conflicting on whether the membrane-bound or cytosolic α-synuclein is the precursor for aggregated α-synuclein and Lewy body pathology, although it remains possible that oligomerization and fibrillization could occur in distinct cellular compartments (Auluck et al., 2010).

2.3 Regulation of α-synuclein membrane-binding

While there remains some uncertainty as to whether the membrane-bound or cytosolic α-synuclein is more pathologically relevant, it is also important to understand the mechanisms regulating the exchange between these two pools. We have previously suggested that brain cytosolic factors are critical in facilitating α-synuclein dissociation and association from synaptic membranes (Wislet-Gendebien et al., 2006; 2008). The remainder of this chapter will be devoted to describing some of these cytosolic factors that were characterized using our cell-free assays.

3. Key techniques for examining the regulation of membrane-binding

3.1 Fractionation into membrane-bound and cytosolic proteins

Much of our current understanding of α-synuclein conformation and membrane interactions are based on studies with recombinant α-synuclein purified from bacteria and bound to artificial membranes. This approach has yielded a wealth of information on the biophysical characteristics of normal and mutant α-synuclein and their affinity for specific lipids. However, recombinant α-synuclein and artificial membranes provide no basis for the understanding α-synuclein behaviour *in vivo*, in particular its ability to exchange between membrane and cytosol within neurons, where the compartmentalization of α-synuclein is modulated by intracellular components and neuronal activity.

To understand endogenous intracellular regulation of α-synuclein dynamics, reconstitution of its membrane binding and dissociation can be studied using semi-intact or cell-free assays. For example, the use of hypotonic lysis to disrupt neuronal plasma membrane releases freely-diffusible cytoplasmic components and permits measurement of subtle shifts in α-synuclein membrane-binding (Fig. 2). Experiments of this type are best done with endogenously expressed α-synuclein, although where exogenous expression is required, consideration should be given to the extent of α-synuclein overexpression so as not to saturate the membrane compartment and cause artifactually low membrane-bound to cytosolic ratio of α-synuclein, as excess α-synuclein will accumulate in cytosol. Measurement of α-synuclein dynamics in intact cells may be limited by an inability to assess whether changes in membrane-bound and cytosolic α-synuclein are caused by perturbations in α-synuclein dissociation or binding kinetics. This can be overcome by using cell-free assays (such as those described below) that monitor the unidirectional movement of α-synuclein from a "donor" fraction expressing α-synuclein to an "acceptor" fraction derived from an α-synuclein-deficient mouse or cells.

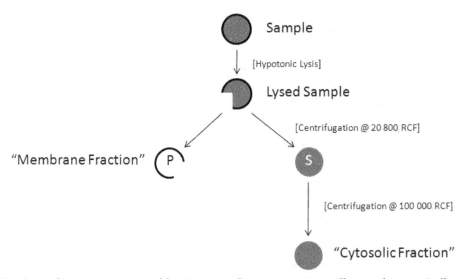

Fig. 2. A schematic overview of fractionation. Synaptosomes or cells were hypotonically lysed in either distilled water or a hypotonic buffer. The lysates were centrifuged and the supernatant (S) and pellet (P) fractions were processed separately. S fractions were centrifuged again to remove residual synaptic vesicles and supernatants were kept as cytosolic fractions. The P fractions were resuspended in buffer containing 1% CHAPS or 1% Triton X-100. Lysates were centrifuged and the supernatants were kept as membrane fraction.

3.2 α-Synuclein dissociation and binding assays

While analyzing the ratio of membrane-bound to cytosolic α-synuclein can yield useful data in an *in-vivo* or *ex-vivo* setting, it does not provide information on whether effects are taking place in the membrane-dissociation or membrane-binding step of α-synuclein dynamics. This question can be answered by employing cell-free assays we have previously published

(Wislet-Gendebien et al., 2006). To measure α-synuclein dissociation, synaptosomal membranes from either non-transgenic or α-synuclein transgenic mice are incubated with brain cytosol isolated from α-synuclein deficient mice. By measuring the amount of α-synuclein dissociated from the membrane and into the cytosol under different conditions, it is possible to determine whether specific cellular factors affect α-synuclein membrane-dissociation.

A converse protocol was developed to assess α-synuclein binding to synaptic membrane (Wislet-Gendebien et al., 2008). In this assay, α-synuclein can be prepared from 2 different origins: either 1) purified *E.coli*-expressed α-synuclein mixed with cytosol from α-synuclein deficient mouse brains, or 2) cytosol prepared from transgenic mice overexpressing the human form of wild-type or mutant α-synuclein. Either of the two sources of α-synuclein is then combined with synaptic membrane prepared from α-synuclein deficient mouse synaptosomes. Membrane-bound α-synuclein can then be analyzed as a measure of α-synuclein membrane-binding in response to various controlled factors such as pharmacological agents or lipids. This assay can provide information on whether a certain condition or factor is affecting α-synuclein membrane-binding.

The key benefit of these dissociation and binding assays is the ability to probe the intracellular milieu with specific reagents, such as antibodies, recombinant mutants, or peptide domains, which are membrane impermeant. However, because these assays depends on mixing separately-derived membrane and cytosolic fractions, one of which must be α-synuclein-deficient, there is an inherent limitation to assess the dissociation or binding of other synaptic proteins due to their presence in both the membrane and the cytosol of both assays. However, these assays can be adapted to analyze the dissociation and binding of other synaptic proteins provided that transgenic animals deficient in the protein of interest are available.

4. Factors involved in regulating α-synuclein membrane-binding

4.1 Brain cytosol

The α-synuclein dissociation assay revealed that stably membrane-bound α-synuclein can be recruited into the cytosol in the presence of brain cytosolic proteins (Wislet-Gendebien et al., 2006). Pre-digestion with trypsin or preheating at 95 °C of the cytosol eliminated its ability to induce α-synuclein dissociation, directly implicating a role for specific cytosolic proteins in controlling α-synuclein solubility. Moreover, the permissive factors required to mediate α-synuclein dissociation from the membrane appeared to be enriched in brain cytosol, as a 6-fold greater concentration of liver cytosol was required to achieve equivalent α-synuclein dissociation using brain cytosol. The proteins triggering α-synuclein dissociation were in limited quantity in cytosol and were not regenerated under our assay conditions. A single exposure to synaptosomal membranes was sufficient to deplete the capacity of the cytosol to extract membrane α-synuclein so that subsequent incubations with fresh membranes yielded no additional dissociated α-synuclein. In contrast, presynaptic membranes retained ample extractable α-synuclein, which could be dissociated with subsequent applications of fresh cytosol. We also showed that the cytosolic activity that mediated α-synuclein dissociation clearly distinguished between wild-type α-synuclein and PD-associated mutants. The cytosol-dependent off-rate for both A30P and A53T α-synuclein mutant was double that of the wild-type, but had no effect on cytosol-independent dissociation.

4.2 Cytosolic lipids

Using our α-synuclein binding assay, we observed that cytosol-mediated α-synuclein membrane-binding was heat stable and protease insensitive. Further characterization revealed that ATP and lipids are two of the main cytosolic components that modulate α-synuclein binding to synaptic membranes (Wislet-Gendebien et al., 2008). We proposed that endogenous cytosolic lipids transferred to membranes prior to α-synuclein recruitment or bound directly to cytosolic α-synuclein may aid α-synuclein folding at the lipid-cytoplasm interface so that it is more amenable to binding directly to synaptic membranes. To provide further insight into this novel protein-lipid-protein interaction, we profiled glycerophosphocholines bound to proteins in α-synuclein-deficient cytosol by nanoflow LC-ESI-MS and precursor ion scan. Our analysis identified 24 species that can potentially affect α-synuclein membrane interactions, including platelet activating factor, which was able to reconstitute the activity of delipidated cytosol.

4.3 Rab3a

Interestingly, our binding experiments also revealed that the association of α-synuclein to synaptic membranes could be stabilized by brief formaldehyde-induced cross-linking, which generates very short intermolecular covalent bonds. This suggested that α-synuclein binding is partly dependent on one or more synaptic vesicle proteins for recruitment. There are several candidate vesicular proteins that have been proposed to interact with α-synuclein, including cysteine string protein, rab3a, and synaptobrevin-2 (Chandra et al., 2005; Gitler et al., 2008; Burre et al., 2010). As a potential test to identify the α-synuclein receptive component on synaptic vesicles, when we screened the ability of antibodies against synaptic vesicle proteins to inhibit α-synuclein membrane binding, rab3a antibodies effectively reduced α-synuclein membrane binding. Moreover, exposure of membranes to rab3a antibody prior to incubation with α-synuclein was sufficient, whereas treatment of α-synuclein-containing cytosol with the antibody has no effect, suggesting that α-synuclein binding is facilitated by vesicle bound rab3a (Chen and Tandon, unpublished).

Similarities in localization and membrane-binding have previously suggested an interaction between rab3a and α-synuclein, at least under pathological conditions. Immunoprecipitation studies revealed α-synuclein interaction with rabphilin in brains from individuals with diffuse Lewy body disease and multiple system atrophy (Dalfo et al., 2004a; 2005). In addition, A30P α-synuclein in transgenic mouse brain was found to co-elute with rab3a, rab5, and rab8, suggesting that α-synuclein may interact with a broad range of rab proteins (Dalfo et al., 2004b). From a functional perspective, α-synuclein appears to antagonize rab3a function. For example, over-expression of α-synuclein in yeast interfered with ER-to-Golgi vesicle trafficking that was corrected by the simultaneous over-expression of the yeast homologue of rab1 (Cooper et al., 2006; Soper et al., 2008). Similarly, elevated toxicity in nematodes and rat primary neurons engineered to express wild-type or A53T α-synuclein was rescued by the addition of rab8 or rab3a (Gitler et al., 2008). In all these studies, α-synuclein toxicity was corrected by over-expressing rab proteins, suggesting that the over-expression of α-synuclein disrupted rab-mediated vesicle targeting and docking.

Rab3a is a small GTPase that regulates synaptic vesicle targeting, docking, and fusion, and like other members of the rab family, it's cycling between vesicles and cytosol is regulated by the phosphorylation state of its guanine nucleotide (GTP/GDP). Dissociation of rab3a from synaptic vesicles is coupled to the calcium-influx that initiates exocytosis (Fischer von

Mollard et al., 1991). The molecular machinery that mediates rab3a cycling has been extensively characterized. After GTP cleavage, rab3a is retrieved off vesicles by guanine-nucleotide dissociation inhibitor (GDI) complex that includes Hsp90, such that the Hsp90 inhibitors radicicol and geldanamycin prevent rab3a dissociation from synaptic membranes (Sakisaka et al., 2002). Using our α-synuclein dissociation assay, we found that the Hsp90 inhibitors also caused an accumulation of α-synuclein on synaptic membranes, providing support for argument that α-synuclein membrane association is closely linked to that of rab3a and is regulated by the GDI/Hsp90 chaperone complex (Chen and Tandon, unpublished). In accordance with this, expression of a constitutively GTP-bound, dominant-negative rab3a mutant also induced an increase in membrane-bound α-synuclein suggesting that GTP/GDP conversion by rab3a is a precondition for the liberation of vesicular α-synuclein. Together, our results suggest that rab3a and its recycling machinery regulate α-synuclein membrane-binding and dissociation (Fig. 3).

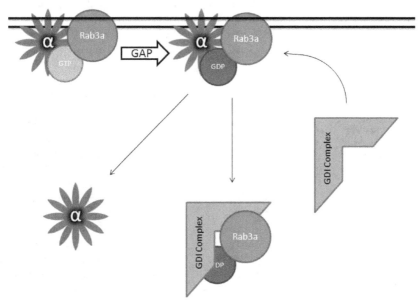

Fig. 3. A model whereby rab3a regulates dissociation of α-synuclein from synaptic membranes. GTP-bound rab3a binds to α-synuclein on the membrane. After GTP-hydrolysis mediated by a GTPase activating protein (GAP), rab3a is chaperoned off of the membrane by the GDP-dissociation inhibitor complex (GDI complex) and α-synuclein also dissociates from the membrane. Whether α-synuclein dissociation is transiently mediated by the GDI complex or is because of the loss of membrane-bound rab3a is yet to be determined.

Whether these results have any implications on the etiology of synucleinopathies is unclear and there are no rab3a mutations linked to PD. However, the interaction with rab3a reinforces α-synuclein's close relationship with the machinery controlling synaptic vesicle trafficking. Further research is needed on how α-synuclein fits into the broader picture of the exocytic pathway and how subtle changes to α-synuclein disposition may disturb vesicle dynamics and lead to pathology.

5. Conclusion

There is now ample evidence that α-synuclein is involved in the regulation of synaptic vesicle trafficking and, more recently, in mitochondrial fission/fusion machinery. Whether its role in maintaining these different organelles occurs concurrently in healthy neurons is not known, though it may be instructive to consider the levels of expression required for apparent modulation of vesicle mobilization or mitochondrial dynamics. The effects of α-synuclein on mitochondrial morphology have been noted in only two studies thus far, both requiring transient overexpression and not in models of normal or stable α-synuclein expression (Kamp et al., 2010; Nakamura et al., 2011). If this observation holds in future analyses, it may represent a segregation of α-synuclein activity based on its expression level, whereby lower levels of α-synuclein impart direct effects on synaptic vesicle behaviour and high α-synuclein concentration disrupts normal mitochondrial division and turnover. This dual activity may also explain the biphasic nature of α-synuclein toxicity, being beneficial at lower expression levels and increasing in toxicity at higher concentration, particularly in combination with oxidative stress. Moreover, a gain-of-function pathogenic link between α-synuclein and mitochondria fits well into a biological cascade that is opposed by expression of PINK1, parkin, or DJ-1, which are now recognized as controlling mitochondrial fission/fusion and mitophagy.

It is clear that direct interaction of α-synuclein with lipid membranes is necessary to propagate its biological function. Regardless of the organelle interaction, it is reasonable to assume that the binding α-synuclein to various organelle membranes is likely to involve a common mechanism whereby the amino-terminal half of α-synuclein folds into an amphipathic α-helix for partial immersion into the lipid bilayer. However, additional selective molecular requirements for stable α-synuclein binding and retrieval may vary between different organelles, such as vesicles or mitochondria, each regulated by organelle-specific factors present on the membrane or in the cytosol. One potential means to characterize α-synuclein compartmentalization on discrete organelles is by further refining the cell-free binding and dissociation assays, as described above using hypotonically permeabilized mouse brain synaptosomes, to specific organelles that are first isolated by differential density and centrifugation protocols. Alternatively, detection of organelle-specific interactors could be done by using inhibitory antibodies to screen for candidates known to exist only on defined organelles, as we have done to identify rab3a as an α-synuclein binding partner on synaptic vesicles. Finally, these cell-free assays also offer an approach to validate the functional effects of α-synuclein interactions identified by various genetic or biochemical methodologies by characterizing their consequences on α-synuclein membrane distribution.

6. Acknowledgements

This work was supported by operating grants to AT from the Canadian Institutes for Health Research and from the Parkinson Society of Canada.

7. References

Abeliovich, A., Schmitz, Y., Farinas, I., Choi-Lundberg, D., Ho, W. H., Castillo, P. E., Shinsky, N., Verdugo, J. M., Armanini, M., Ryan, A., Hynes, M., Phillips, H., Sulzer,

D., and Rosenthal, A. (2000). Mice lacking alpha-synuclein display functional deficits in the nigrostriatal dopamine system. *Neuron* 25(1), 239-52.

Auluck, P. K., Caraveo, G., and Lindquist, S. (2010). alpha-Synuclein: membrane interactions and toxicity in Parkinson's disease. *Annu Rev Cell Dev Biol* 26, 211-33.

Batelli, S., Albani, D., Rametta, R., Polito, L., Prato, F., Pesaresi, M., Negro, A., and Forloni, G. (2008). DJ-1 modulates alpha-synuclein aggregation state in a cellular model of oxidative stress: relevance for Parkinson's disease and involvement of HSP70. *PLoS ONE* 3(4), e1884.

Borbat, P., Ramlall, T. F., Freed, J. H., and Eliezer, D. (2006). Inter-helix distances in lysophospholipid micelle-bound alpha-synuclein from pulsed ESR measurements. *J Am Chem Soc* 128(31), 10004-5.

Braak, H., Del Tredici, K., Rub, U., de Vos, R. A., Jansen Steur, E. N., and Braak, E. (2003). Staging of brain pathology related to sporadic Parkinson's disease. *Neurobiol Aging* 24(2), 197-211.

Burre, J., Sharma, M., Tsetsenis, T., Buchman, V., Etherton, M., and Sudhof, T. C. (2010). {alpha}-Synuclein Promotes SNARE-Complex Assembly in Vivo and in Vitro. *Science*.

Cabin, D. E., Shimazu, K., Murphy, D., Cole, N. B., Gottschalk, W., McIlwain, K. L., Orrison, B., Chen, A., Ellis, C. E., Paylor, R., Lu, B., and Nussbaum, R. L. (2002). Synaptic vesicle depletion correlates with attenuated synaptic responses to prolonged repetitive stimulation in mice lacking alpha-synuclein. *J Neurosci* 22(20), 8797-807.

Chandra, S., Chen, X., Rizo, J., Jahn, R., and Sudhof, T. C. (2003). A broken alpha -helix in folded alpha -Synuclein. *J Biol Chem* 278(17), 15313-8.

Chandra, S., Fornai, F., Kwon, H. B., Yazdani, U., Atasoy, D., Liu, X., Hammer, R. E., Battaglia, G., German, D. C., Castillo, P. E., and Sudhof, T. C. (2004). Double-knockout mice for alpha- and beta-synucleins: effect on synaptic functions. *Proc Natl Acad Sci U S A* 101(41), 14966-71.

Chandra S, Gallardo G, Fernandez-Chacon R, Schluter OM, Sudhof TC (2005) Alpha-synuclein cooperates with CSP alpha in preventing neurodegeneration. Cell, 123:383-396.

Chartier-Harlin, M. C., Kachergus, J., Roumier, C., Mouroux, V., Douay, X., Lincoln, S., Levecque, C., Larvor, L., Andrieux, J., Hulihan, M., Waucquier, N., Defebvre, L., Amouyel, P., Farrer, M., and Destee, A. (2004). Alpha-synuclein locus duplication as a cause of familial Parkinson's disease. *Lancet* 364(9440), 1167-9.

Chen, C. Y., and Balch, W. E. (2006). The Hsp90 chaperone complex regulates GDI-dependent Rab recycling. *Mol Biol Cell* 17(8), 3494-507.

Chen, C. Y., Sakisaka, T., and Balch, W. E. (2005). Use of Hsp90 inhibitors to disrupt GDI-dependent Rab recycling. *Methods Enzymol* 403, 339-47.

Chen, L., and Feany, M. B. (2005). Alpha-synuclein phosphorylation controls neurotoxicity and inclusion formation in a Drosophila model of Parkinson disease. *Nat Neurosci* 8(5), 657-63.

Christine, C. W., and Aminoff, M. J. (2004). Clinical differentiation of parkinsonian syndromes: prognostic and therapeutic relevance. *Am J Med* 117(6), 412-9.

Clayton, D. F., and George, J. M. (1998). The synucleins: a family of proteins involved in synaptic function, plasticity, neurodegeneration and disease. *Trends Neurosci* 21(6), 249-54.

Cole, N. B., Murphy, D. D., Grider, T., Rueter, S., Brasaemle, D., and Nussbaum, R. L. (2002). Lipid droplet binding and oligomerization properties of the Parkinson's disease protein alpha-synuclein. *J Biol Chem* 277(8), 6344-52.

Conway, K. A., Lee, S. J., Rochet, J. C., Ding, T. T., Williamson, R. E., and Lansbury, P. T., Jr. (2000). Acceleration of oligomerization, not fibrillization, is a shared property of both alpha-synuclein mutations linked to early-onset Parkinson's disease: implications for pathogenesis and therapy. *Proc Natl Acad Sci U S A* 97(2), 571-6.

Cookson, M. R. (2005). The biochemistry of Parkinson's disease. *Annu Rev Biochem* 74, 29-52.

Cooper, A. A., Gitler, A. D., Cashikar, A., Haynes, C. M., Hill, K. J., Bhullar, B., Liu, K., Xu, K., Strathearn, K. E., Liu, F., Cao, S., Caldwell, K. A., Caldwell, G. A., Marsischky, G., Kolodner, R. D., Labaer, J., Rochet, J. C., Bonini, N. M., and Lindquist, S. (2006). Alpha-synuclein blocks ER-Golgi traffic and Rab1 rescues neuron loss in Parkinson's models. *Science* 313(5785), 324-8.

Dalfo, E., Barrachina, M., Rosa, J. L., Ambrosio, S., and Ferrer, I. (2004a). Abnormal alpha-synuclein interactions with rab3a and rabphilin in diffuse Lewy body disease. *Neurobiol Dis* 16(1), 92-7.

Dalfo, E., and Ferrer, I. (2005). Alpha-synuclein binding to rab3a in multiple system atrophy. *Neurosci Lett* 380(1-2), 170-5.

Dalfo, E., Gomez-Isla, T., Rosa, J. L., Nieto Bodelon, M., Cuadrado Tejedor, M., Barrachina, M., Ambrosio, S., and Ferrer, I. (2004b). Abnormal alpha-synuclein interactions with Rab proteins in alpha-synuclein A30P transgenic mice. *J Neuropathol Exp Neurol* 63(4), 302-13.

Darios, F., Ruiperez, V., Lopez, I., Villanueva, J., Gutierrez, L. M., and Davletov, B. (2010). Alpha-synuclein sequesters arachidonic acid to modulate SNARE-mediated exocytosis. *EMBO Rep* 11(7), 528-33.

Davidson, W. S., Jonas, A., Clayton, D. F., and George, J. M. (1998). Stabilization of alpha-synuclein secondary structure upon binding to synthetic membranes. *J Biol Chem* 273(16), 9443-9.

Devi, L., Raghavendran, V., Prabhu, B. M., Avadhani, N. G., and Anandatheerthavarada, H. K. (2008). Mitochondrial import and accumulation of alpha-synuclein impair complex I in human dopaminergic neuronal cultures and Parkinson disease brain. *J Biol Chem* 283(14), 9089-100.

Fischer von Mollard, G., Sudhof, T. C., and Jahn, R. (1991). A small GTP-binding protein dissociates from synaptic vesicles during exocytosis. *Nature* 349(6304), 79-81.

Fortin, D. L., Nemani, V. M., Voglmaier, S. M., Anthony, M. D., Ryan, T. A., and Edwards, R. H. (2005). Neural activity controls the synaptic accumulation of alpha-synuclein. *J Neurosci* 25(47), 10913-21.

Fujiwara, H., Hasegawa, M., Dohmae, N., Kawashima, A., Masliah, E., Goldberg, M. S., Shen, J., Takio, K., and Iwatsubo, T. (2002). alpha-Synuclein is phosphorylated in synucleinopathy lesions. *Nat Cell Biol* 4(2), 160-4.

George, J. M., Jin, H., Woods, W. S., and Clayton, D. F. (1995). Characterization of a novel protein regulated during the critical period for song learning in the zebra finch. *Neuron* 15(2), 361-72.

Georgieva, E. R., Ramlall, T. F., Borbat, P. P., Freed, J. H., and Eliezer, D. (2010). The lipid-binding domain of wild type and mutant alpha-synuclein: compactness and interconversion between the broken and extended helix forms. *J Biol Chem* 285(36), 28261-74.

Geppert, M., Bolshakov, V. Y., Siegelbaum, S. A., Takei, K., De Camilli, P., Hammer, R. E., and Sudhof, T. C. (1994). The role of Rab3A in neurotransmitter release. *Nature* 369(6480), 493-7.

Geppert, M., Goda, Y., Stevens, C. F., and Sudhof, T. C. (1997). The small GTP-binding protein Rab3A regulates a late step in synaptic vesicle fusion. *Nature* 387(6635), 810-4.

Gitler, A. D., Bevis, B. J., Shorter, J., Strathearn, K. E., Hamamichi, S., Su, L. J., Caldwell, K. A., Caldwell, G. A., Rochet, J. C., McCaffery, J. M., Barlowe, C., and Lindquist, S. (2008). The Parkinson's disease protein alpha-synuclein disrupts cellular Rab homeostasis. *Proc Natl Acad Sci U S A* 105(1), 145-50.

Gorbatyuk, O. S., Li, S., Sullivan, L. F., Chen, W., Kondrikova, G., Manfredsson, F. P., Mandel, R. J., and Muzyczka, N. (2008). The phosphorylation state of Ser-129 in human alpha-synuclein determines neurodegeneration in a rat model of Parkinson disease. *Proc Natl Acad Sci U S A* 105(2), 763-8.

Hamilton, B. A. (2004). alpha-Synuclein A53T substitution associated with Parkinson disease also marks the divergence of Old World and New World primates. *Genomics* 83(4), 739-42.

Hashimoto, M., Hsu, L. J., Rockenstein, E., Takenouchi, T., Mallory, M., and Masliah, E. (2002). alpha-Synuclein protects against oxidative stress via inactivation of the c-Jun N-terminal kinase stress-signaling pathway in neuronal cells. *J Biol Chem* 277(13), 11465-72.

Holdorff, B. (2006). Fritz Heinrich Lewy (1885-1950). *J Neurol* 253(5), 677-8.

Hu, K., Carroll, J., Rickman, C., and Davletov, B. (2002). Action of complexin on SNARE complex. *J Biol Chem* 277(44), 41652-6.

Jakes, R., Spillantini, M. G., and Goedert, M. (1994). Identification of two distinct synucleins from human brain. *FEBS Lett* 345(1), 27-32.

Jao, C. C., Der-Sarkissian, A., Chen, J., and Langen, R. (2004). Structure of membrane-bound alpha-synuclein studied by site-directed spin labeling. *Proc Natl Acad Sci U S A* 101(22), 8331-6.

Jankovic, J. (2008). Parkinson's disease: clinical features and diagnosis. *J Neurol Neurosurg Psychiatry* 79(4), 368-76.

Jo, E., McLaurin, J., Yip, C. M., St George-Hyslop, P., and Fraser, P. E. (2000). alpha-Synuclein membrane interactions and lipid specificity. *J Biol Chem* 275(44), 34328-34.

Jo, E., Fuller, N., Rand, R. P., St George-Hyslop, P., and Fraser, P. E. (2002). Defective membrane interactions of familial Parkinson's disease mutant A30P alpha-synuclein. *J Mol Biol* 315(4), 799-807.

Jo, E., Darabie, A. A., Han, K., Tandon, A., Fraser, P. E., and McLaurin, J. (2004). alpha-Synuclein-synaptosomal membrane interactions: implications for fibrillogenesis. *Eur J Biochem* 271(15), 3180-9.

Johannes, L., Doussau, F., Clabecq, A., Henry, J. P., Darchen, F., and Poulain, B. (1996). Evidence for a functional link between Rab3 and the SNARE complex. *J Cell Sci* 109 (Pt 12), 2875-84.

Johannes, L., Lledo, P. M., Roa, M., Vincent, J. D., Henry, J. P., and Darchen, F. (1994). The GTPase Rab3a negatively controls calcium-dependent exocytosis in neuroendocrine cells. *Embo J* 13(9), 2029-37.

Kamp, F., Exner, N., Lutz, A. K., Wender, N., Hegermann, J., Brunner, B., Nuscher, B., Bartels, T., Giese, A., Beyer, K., Eimer, S., Winklhofer, K. F., and Haass, C. (2010). Inhibition of mitochondrial fusion by alpha-synuclein is rescued by PINK1, Parkin and DJ-1. *Embo J* 29(20), 3571-89.

Kanda, S., Bishop, J. F., Eglitis, M. A., Yang, Y., and Mouradian, M. M. (2000). Enhanced vulnerability to oxidative stress by alpha-synuclein mutations and C-terminal truncation. *Neuroscience* 97(2), 279-84.

Kruger, R., Kuhn, W., Muller, T., Woitalla, D., Graeber, M., Kosel, S., Przuntek, H., Epplen, J. T., Schols, L., and Riess, O. (1998). Ala30Pro mutation in the gene encoding alpha-synuclein in Parkinson's disease. *Nat Genet* 18(2), 106-8.

Lee, H. J., Choi, C., and Lee, S. J. (2002). Membrane-bound alpha-synuclein has a high aggregation propensity and the ability to seed the aggregation of the cytosolic form. *J Biol Chem* 277(1), 671-8.

Leenders, A. G., Lopes da Silva, F. H., Ghijsen, W. E., and Verhage, M. (2001). Rab3a is involved in transport of synaptic vesicles to the active zone in mouse brain nerve terminals. *Mol Biol Cell* 12(10), 3095-102.

Maroteaux L, Campanelli JT, Scheller RH (1988). Synuclein: a neuron-specific protein localized to the nucleus and presynaptic nerve terminal. *J Neurosci* 8, 2804-2815.

McFarland, N. R., Fan, Z., Xu, K., Schwarzschild, M. A., Feany, M. B., Hyman, B. T., and McLean, P. J. (2009). Alpha-synuclein S129 phosphorylation mutants do not alter nigrostriatal toxicity in a rat model of Parkinson disease. *J Neuropathol Exp Neurol* 68(5), 515-24.

Mollenhauer, B., Locascio, J. J., Schulz-Schaeffer, W., Sixel-Doring, F., Trenkwalder, C., and Schlossmacher, M. G. (2011). alpha-Synuclein and tau concentrations in cerebrospinal fluid of patients presenting with parkinsonism: a cohort study. *Lancet Neurol* 10(3), 230-40.

Nakamura, K., Nemani, V. M., Azarbal, F., Skibinski, G., Levy, J. M., Egami, K., Munishkina, L., Zhang, J., Gardner, B., Wakabayashi, J., Sesaki, H., Cheng, Y., Finkbeiner, S., Nussbaum, R. L., Masliah, E., and Edwards, R. H. (2011). Direct membrane association drives mitochondrial fission by the Parkinson Disease-associated protein {alpha}-synuclein. *J Biol Chem* (Epub ahead of print).

Narayanan, V., and Scarlata, S. (2001). Membrane binding and self-association of alpha-synucleins. *Biochemistry* 40(33), 9927-34.

Nemani, V. M., Lu, W., Berge, V., Nakamura, K., Onoa, B., Lee, M. K., Chaudhry, F. A., Nicoll, R. A., and Edwards, R. H. (2010). Increased expression of alpha-synuclein reduces neurotransmitter release by inhibiting synaptic vesicle reclustering after endocytosis. *Neuron* 65(1), 66-79.

Polymeropoulos, M. H., Lavedan, C., Leroy, E., Ide, S. E., Dehejia, A., Dutra, A., Pike, B., Root, H., Rubenstein, J., Boyer, R., Stenroos, E. S., Chandrasekharappa, S., Athanassiadou, A., Papapetropoulos, T., Johnson, W. G., Lazzarini, A. M., Duvoisin, R. C., Di Iorio, G., Golbe, L. I., and Nussbaum, R. L. (1997). Mutation in the alpha-synuclein gene identified in families with Parkinson's disease. *Science* 276(5321), 2045-7.

Sakisaka, T., Meerlo, T., Matteson, J., Plutner, H., and Balch, W. E. (2002). Rab-alphaGDI activity is regulated by a Hsp90 chaperone complex. *Embo J* 21(22), 6125-35.

Saper, C. B. (1999). 'Like a thief in the night': the selectivity of degeneration in Parkinson's disease. *Brain* 122 (Pt 8), 1401-2.

Singleton, A. B., Farrer, M., Johnson, J., Singleton, A., Hague, S., Kachergus, J., Hulihan, M., Peuralinna, T., Dutra, A., Nussbaum, R., Lincoln, S., Crawley, A., Hanson, M., Maraganore, D., Adler, C., Cookson, M. R., Muenter, M., Baptista, M., Miller, D., Blancato, J., Hardy, J., and Gwinn-Hardy, K. (2003). alpha-Synuclein locus triplication causes Parkinson's disease. *Science* 302(5646), 841.

Soper, J. H., Roy, S., Stieber, A., Lee, E., Wilson, R. B., Trojanowski, J. Q., Burd, C. G., and Lee, V. M. (2008). Alpha-synuclein-induced aggregation of cytoplasmic vesicles in Saccharomyces cerevisiae. *Mol Biol Cell* 19(3), 1093-103.

Spillantini, M. G., Crowther, R. A., Jakes, R., Hasegawa, M., and Goedert, M. (1998). alpha-Synuclein in filamentous inclusions of Lewy bodies from Parkinson's disease and dementia with lewy bodies. *Proc Natl Acad Sci U S A* 95(11), 6469-73.

Thayanidhi, N., Helm, J. R., Nycz, D. C., Bentley, M., Liang, Y., and Hay, J. C. (2010). Alpha-synuclein delays endoplasmic reticulum (ER)-to-Golgi transport in mammalian cells by antagonizing ER/Golgi SNAREs. *Mol Biol Cell* 21(11), 1850-63.

Ulmer, T. S., Bax, A., Cole, N. B., and Nussbaum, R. L. (2005). Structure and dynamics of micelle-bound human alpha-synuclein. *J Biol Chem* 280(10), 9595-603.

Wislet-Gendebien, S., D'Souza, C., Kawarai, T., St George-Hyslop, P., Westaway, D., Fraser, P., and Tandon, A. (2006). Cytosolic proteins regulate alpha-synuclein dissociation from presynaptic membranes. *J Biol Chem* 281(43), 32148-55.

Wislet-Gendebien, S., Visanji, N. P., Whitehead, S. N., Marsilio, D., Hou, W., Figeys, D., Fraser, P. E., Bennett, S. A., and Tandon, A. (2008). Differential regulation of wild-type and mutant alpha-synuclein binding to synaptic membranes by cytosolic factors. *BMC Neurosci* 9, 92.

Zarranz, J. J., Alegre, J., Gomez-Esteban, J. C., Lezcano, E., Ros, R., Ampuero, I., Vidal, L., Hoenicka, J., Rodriguez, O., Atares, B., Llorens, V., Gomez Tortosa, E., del Ser, T., Munoz, D. G., and de Yebenes, J. G. (2004). The new mutation, E46K, of alpha-synuclein causes Parkinson and Lewy body dementia. *Ann Neurol* 55(2), 164-73.

Zhu, M., and Fink, A. L. (2003). Lipid binding inhibits alpha-synuclein fibril formation. *J Biol Chem* 278(19), 16873-7.

Permissions

The contributors of this book come from diverse backgrounds, making this book a truly international effort. This book will bring forth new frontiers with its revolutionizing research information and detailed analysis of the nascent developments around the world.

We would like to thank Dr. Juliana Dushanova, for lending her expertise to make the book truly unique. She has played a crucial role in the development of this book. Without her invaluable contribution this book wouldn't have been possible. She has made vital efforts to compile up to date information on the varied aspects of this subject to make this book a valuable addition to the collection of many professionals and students.

This book was conceptualized with the vision of imparting up-to-date information and advanced data in this field. To ensure the same, a matchless editorial board was set up. Every individual on the board went through rigorous rounds of assessment to prove their worth. After which they invested a large part of their time researching and compiling the most relevant data for our readers. Conferences and sessions were held from time to time between the editorial board and the contributing authors to present the data in the most comprehensible form. The editorial team has worked tirelessly to provide valuable and valid information to help people across the globe.

Every chapter published in this book has been scrutinized by our experts. Their significance has been extensively debated. The topics covered herein carry significant findings which will fuel the growth of the discipline. They may even be implemented as practical applications or may be referred to as a beginning point for another development. Chapters in this book were first published by InTech; hereby published with permission under the Creative Commons Attribution License or equivalent.

The editorial board has been involved in producing this book since its inception. They have spent rigorous hours researching and exploring the diverse topics which have resulted in the successful publishing of this book. They have passed on their knowledge of decades through this book. To expedite this challenging task, the publisher supported the team at every step. A small team of assistant editors was also appointed to further simplify the editing procedure and attain best results for the readers.

Our editorial team has been hand-picked from every corner of the world. Their multi-ethnicity adds dynamic inputs to the discussions which result in innovative outcomes. These outcomes are then further discussed with the researchers and contributors who give their valuable feedback and opinion regarding the same. The feedback is then collaborated with the researches and they are edited in a comprehensive manner to aid the understanding of the subject.

Apart from the editorial board, the designing team has also invested a significant amount of their time in understanding the subject and creating the most relevant covers. They scrutinized every image to scout for the most suitable representation of the subject and create an appropriate cover for the book.

The publishing team has been involved in this book since its early stages. They were actively engaged in every process, be it collecting the data, connecting with the contributors or procuring relevant information. The team has been an ardent support to the editorial, designing and production team. Their endless efforts to recruit the best for this project, has resulted in the accomplishment of this book. They are a veteran in the field of academics and their pool of knowledge is as vast as their experience in printing. Their expertise and guidance has proved useful at every step. Their uncompromising quality standards have made this book an exceptional effort. Their encouragement from time to time has been an inspiration for everyone.

The publisher and the editorial board hope that this book will prove to be a valuable piece of knowledge for researchers, students, practitioners and scholars across the globe.

List of Contributors

Fátima Carrillo and Pablo Mir
Unidad de Trastornos del Movimiento. Servicio de Neurología. Instituto de Biomedicina de Sevilla (IBiS). Hospital Universitario Virgen del Rocío/CSIC/Universidad de Sevilla, Spain

Roberta J. Ward and R.R. Crichton
Universite Catholique de Louvain, Louvain-la-Neuve, Belgium

D.T. Dexter
Centre for Neuroscience, Division of Experimental Medicine, Hammersmith Campus, Imperial College London, London, UK

Quincy J. Almeida
Sun Life Financial Movement Disorders Research & Rehabilitation Centre, Wilfrid Laurier University, Canada

Marisa G. Repetto, Raúl O. Domínguez, Enrique R. Marschoff and Jorge A. Serra
School of Pharmacy and Biochemistry, University of Buenos Aires (UBA) / PRALIB – CONICET, Argentina

Shunro Kohbata
Gifu University, Japan

Ryoichi Hayashi
Shinshu University, Japan

Tomokazu Tamura
Fuji National Hospital, Japan

Chitoshi Kadoya
Kamisone Hospital, Japan

Marco T. Núñez, Pamela Urrutia, Natalia Mena and Pabla Aguirre
University of Chile, Chile

Zelda H. Cheung and Nancy Y. Ip
Division of Life Science, State Key Laboratory of Molecular Neuroscience and Molecular, Neuroscience Center, Hong Kong University of Science and Technology, Clear Water Bay, Kowloon, Hong Kong, China

Souvik Chattopadhaya, Amaravadhi Harikishore and Ho Sup Yoon
School of Biological Sciences, Nanyang Technological University, Singapore

Robert H.C. Chen, Howard T.J. Mount and Anurag Tandon
Tanz Centre for Research in Neurodegenerative Diseases, University of Toronto, Canada

Sabine Wislet-Gendebien
GIGA Neurosciences, University of Liège, Belgium

Printed in the USA
CPSIA information can be obtained
at www.ICGtesting.com
JSHW011358221024
72173JS00003B/333